A Clinical Guide to Ophthalmology

A Clinical Guide to Ophthalmology

Editor: Ray George

AMERICAN
MEDICAL PUBLISHERS
www.americanmedicalpublishers.com

AMERICAN
MEDICAL PUBLISHERS
www.americanmedicalpublishers.com

Cataloging-in-publication Data

A clinical guide to ophthalmology / edited by Ray George.
p. cm.
Includes bibliographical references and index.
ISBN 978-1-63927-838-1
1. Eye--Diseases. 2. Ophthalmology. 3. Eye--Diseases--Treatment.
4. Eye--Diseases--Diagnosis. I. George, Ray.
RE46 .C55 2023
617.7--dc23

American Medical Publishers,
41 Flatbush Avenue,
1st Floor, New York,
NY 11217, USA

ISBN 978-1-63927-838-1 (Hardback)

Contents

Preface

This book has been a concerted effort by a group of academicians, researchers and scientists, who have contributed their research works for the realization of the book. This book has materialized in the wake of emerging advancements and innovations in this field. Therefore, the need of the hour was to compile all the required researches and disseminate the knowledge to a broad spectrum of people comprising of students, researchers and specialists of the field.

Ophthalmology is a medical specialty that deals with the diagnosis and treatment of eye disorders. It is also involved in the study of the anatomy and physiology of the eye. Cataracts, diabetic retinopathy, glaucoma, and age-related macular degeneration are the four most prevalent eye disorders that can cause vision loss or blindness. Ophthalmology encompasses the usage of both surgical procedures and pharmaceutical interventions. It also makes use of artificial intelligence. Approved AI-based devices can be used to detect disorders by analyzing images of the eye taken with a retinal camera and utilizing a system to analyze whether the patient has any abnormalities and whether therapy is required. This book unfolds some of the vital pieces of work being conducted worldwide on various topics related to ophthalmology. Such selected concepts that redefine the research in this field have been presented herein. As this field is emerging at a rapid pace, the contents of this book will help the readers understand the developments taking place in ophthalmology.

At the end of the preface, I would like to thank the authors for their brilliant chapters and the publisher for guiding us all-through the making of the book till its final stage. Also, I would like to thank my family for providing the support and encouragement throughout my academic career and research projects.

Editor

1

Imaging in Ophthalmology

Umit Yolcu, Omer Faruk Sahin and
Fatih C. Gundogan

1. Introduction

The imaging systems have a unique role in the ophthalmologic routine practice. While imaging has an auxiliary role in other branches of medicine, it is the most essential part of the ophthalmic examination. In other words, it can be said that ophthalmic examination is almost impossible without imaging. In this chapter, a basic review of the essentials of imaging techniques in ophthalmology will be presented.

2. Anterior segment imaging systems

2.1. Slit-lamp biomicroscopy

The slit lamp biomicroscopy is an important tool in ophthalmic practice. It is basically designed for examination of anterior segment but with the appropriate attachments, all ocular structures can be viewed. Most important advantage of biomicroscopy in examining the eye structures is stereopsis, in other words ophthalmologist can examine eye structures in three dimensions. It is a routine examination tool of most practitioners. In order to use all benefits of this tool, clinician should understand the basic imaging principle of the instrument.

Modern slit-lamp biomicroscopes have two major parts; observation and illumination systems. The illumination system of slit lamp projects bright slit light onto the focus plane. Illumination part delivers very sharp, thin and undistorted slit light in order to view true representation of the ocular structures. Blue and green filters are available in most slit-lamps to visualize fluorescein stain, micro-aneurysms and nerve fiber layer. In recent years LED illuminated slit lamps are also available. LED illuminated systems provides sharpest, brightest and most homogeneous slit beam. The other advantages LED systems on halogen lamps are last 100 times longer, have special light spectrum and they consume less energy.

Observation part comprises many optical lenses in order to deliver magnified view of ocular structures. Its magnification range differs between 5x to 40x depending on the manufacturer (Figure 1 A-F). It can enable magnification by flip-type, Galilean rotating barrel and continuous zoom methods [1]. High magnified view may be desirable for many clinicians however image quality compromises with high magnification. Therefore least required magnification should be used for the examination to achieve the best possible resolution. Resolution of a slit-lamp is depends on the wavelength of light used, the refractive index between the eye and objective, the working distance, and the diameter of the objective lens. Most biomicroscope oculars have 10 to 15 degree convergence angle to minimize convergence need of the examiner during the examination.

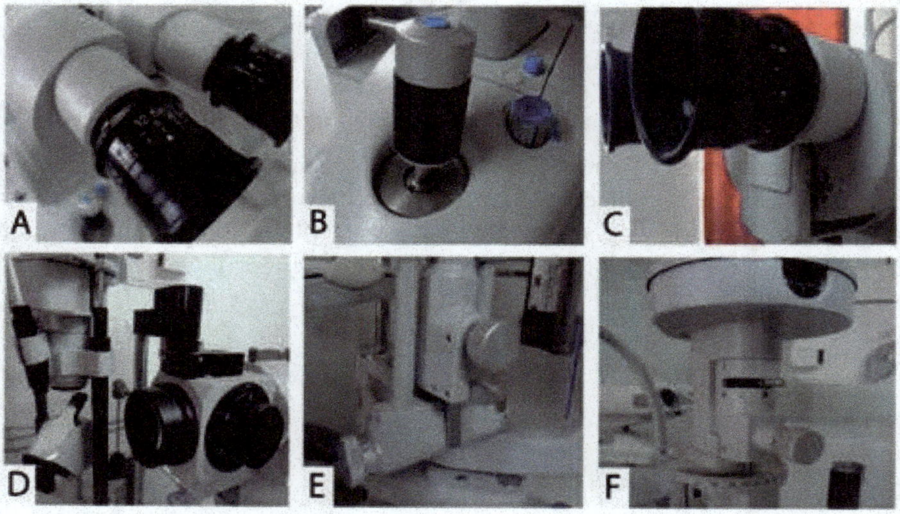

Figure 1. A. Binocular eyepieces provide stereoscopic vision and can be adjusted for examiners refraction. B. Joystick allows focusing with movement to forward, backward, laterally and diagonally. It can be rotated to lower or elevate the light beam. C. Eyepieces can be adjusted for Interpupillar distance of examiner D. Magnification can be changed with between 6x to 40 x. E. Releasing the knob allows separation of illumination and observation point. F. Slit height, color and angle can be adjusted with knurled knob.

In normal usage illumination system and observation system are coupled on a common focal plane and point. Both moves around a common focus point. It can horizontally uncoupled by releasing a knob. It is recommended that before using the slit lamp, distance between eyepieces should be adjusted for inter pupillary distance of the practitioner and focused by the help of a rod for his or her refraction. This procedure helps comfortable binocular viewing. Examination also should be conducted in semi-dark light conditions.

2.1.1. Examination techniques

2.1.1.1. Diffuse illumination

Diffuse illumination is a simple illumination method for examining the eye and surrounding structures. Slit width should be set to maximum, magnification to low and light at approximately 45-degree (Figure 2). Details cannot be viewed by this method; it just gives overview of eye and adnexia. High magnification should not be used with this method. Corneal scars, foreign bodies, pigmentary changes should be noted by this gross inspection method [2]. Findings obtained by the diffuse illumination should be investigated by other illumination techniques.

Cobalt blue filter and red free (green) filter can be used with this method. After instillation of fluorescein stain corneal epithelial defects, tear break up time and contact lens positioning can be viewed under cobalt blue light. With the green filter, bulbar conjunctival vessels and small hemorrhages and aneurysms can be viewed.

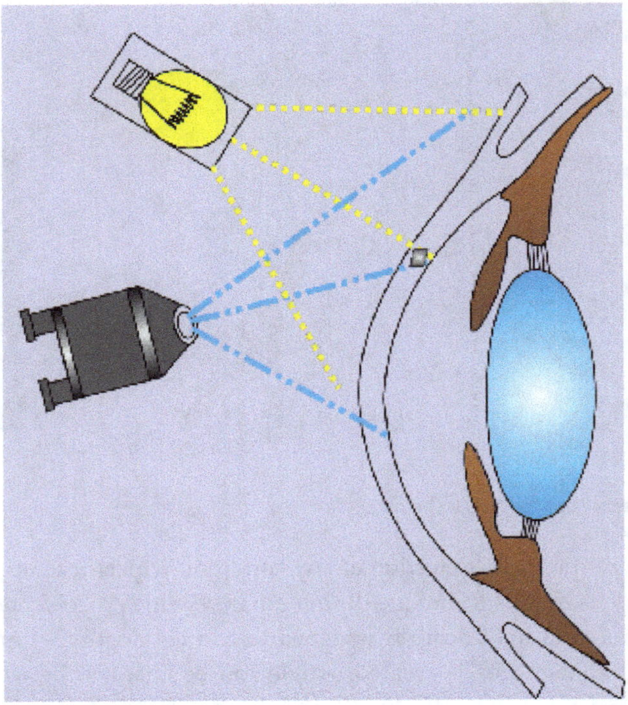

Figure 2. Diffuse illumination

a. Direct Illumination

Direct focal illumination is the most commonly used method. Observer focuses on the area directly illuminated by the slit light. Magnification can be increased to maximum if needed. Direct illumination can be used with different type of light beams.

Optic section of the cornea, anterior chamber and lens can be examined with optic section technique. Depth of any foreign body, stromal thinning, epithelial edema, layers of cornea, anterior chamber depth and different layers of lens can be determined. In this technique, illumination system is placed on the side of cornea or lens (i.e. temporal) and is set at angle between 30-60 degrees. Light beam is narrowed to minimum, light intensity is adjusted to maximum. Then examiner should focus on the middle point of horizontal corneal or lens section. Middle or maximum magnification can be used (Figure 3) [2].

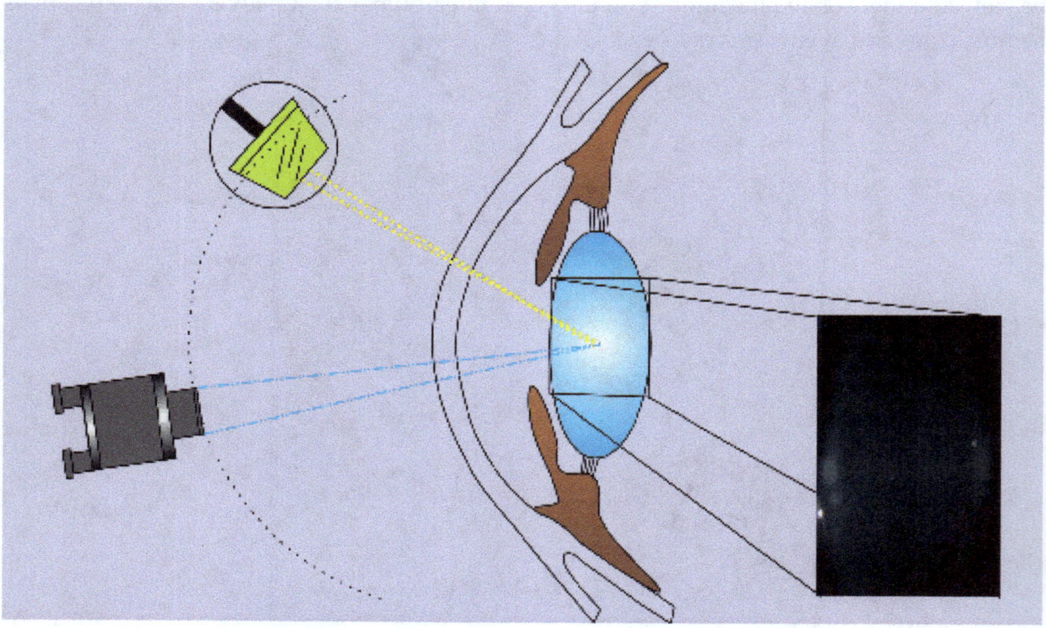

Figure 3. Direct illumination, optic section technique.

Parallelepiped technique provides detection of any condition which obscures corneal transparency or crystalline lens. In this technique illumination system is placed on the side of cornea or lens (i.e. temporal) and light beam is widened to corneal depth (3-4 mm). By this way a parallelepiped illuminated area is created. Angle can be changed between 30-60 degrees. Magnification may vary between 10x-40x (Figure 4). By focusing on the anterior side of the parallelepiped light, corneal epithelial alterations and protein deposits and debris in a contact lens wearer can be viewed. Endetolial pigment changes, keratic precipitates, other deposits and striations on the endotelium can be viewed by using parallelepiped technique [2].

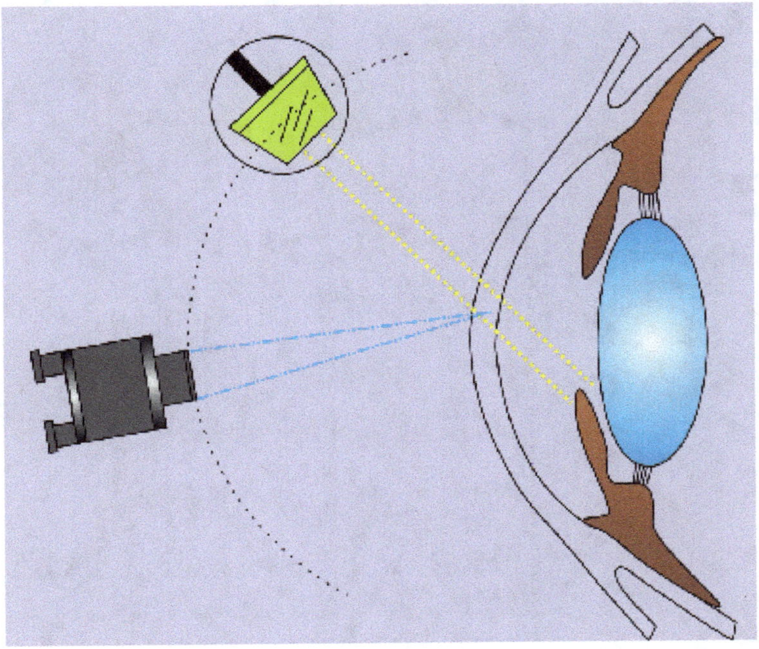

Figure 4. Direct illumination, parallelepiped technique

Crystalline lens transparency and opacities can be evaluated by using with a 0.5 to 2 mm wide beam. Different from the corneal examination illumination, system should be set to a smaller angle, 10 to 45 degree. Detailed examination can be performed by directing the light towards the pupil area and focusing different layers of the lens [2].

Wide beam illumination is useful for the inspection of contact lens surface. By this method, protein deposits, mucus secretion, corneal nerve fibers, infiltrative keratitis, corneal opacities, iris and lens surface can be viewed. Setup of the method is similar to parallelepiped method except slit width is wider then corneal depth. Light intensity should get reduced and angle of the illumination adjusted depending on the surface of under inspection, generally more than 45 degrees [2].

Conical beam illumination is useful in viewing the inflammatory cells and proteins in the anterior chamber. In this method width and height of the slit light beam is reduced until obtaining a point light. Height is reduced to 1-2 mm. Light intensity is set to maximum. Examination should be done in dark conditions (Figure 5) [2]. The number of cells in the anterior chamber is assessed from side to side of the anterior chamber in medium magnification and high-angle illumination.

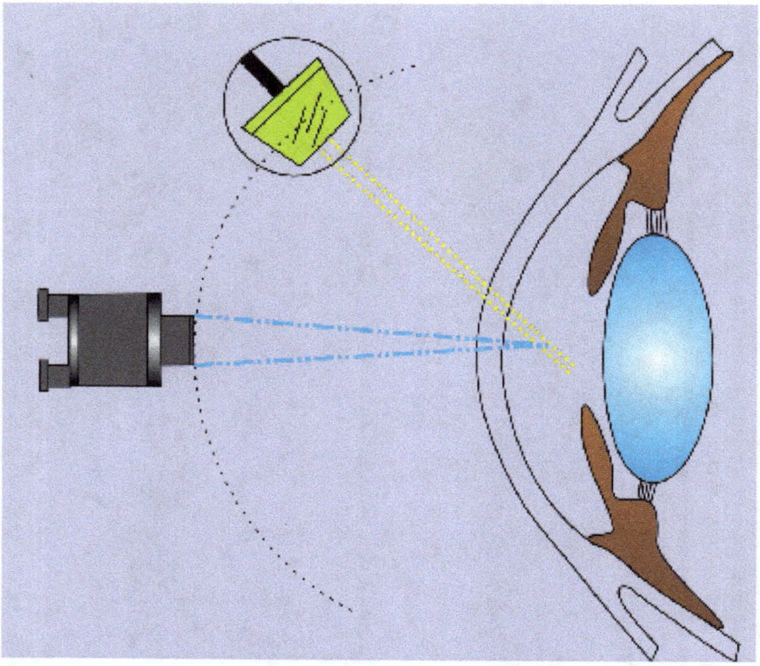

Figure 5. Conical beam illumination

b. Indirect illumination

In this technique light beam is projected to a different area other than the focal point of the observation system. Illumination system is get moved off from its click position by releasing a knob (Figure 6). Therefore two systems do not coincide at same point. Procedure is similar to parallelepiped illumination technique exceptionally, in this method, observed area is not directly the illuminated area but just beside the anterior border of parallelepiped area. With this method, transparency loss or loose contrast differences in transparent structures can be viewed such as subtle corneal opacities, bulbar conjunctival vessels and lens opacities [2].

Scleral scatter is used for especially small changes in large transparent areas. Central corneal clouding, bullous keratopathy, corneal scars, contact lens edges can be examined with this method. In this method, parallelepiped beam focused on central cornea then after releasing the knob illumination system moved out its click position and beam can be projected to nasal or temporal limbus (Figure 7). With correct positioning of the illumination system, a halo of scatter light around the cornea can be viewed [2]. Any condition which alters corneal transparency obstructs the internal reflecting light and becomes visible as a whitish color over pupil background.

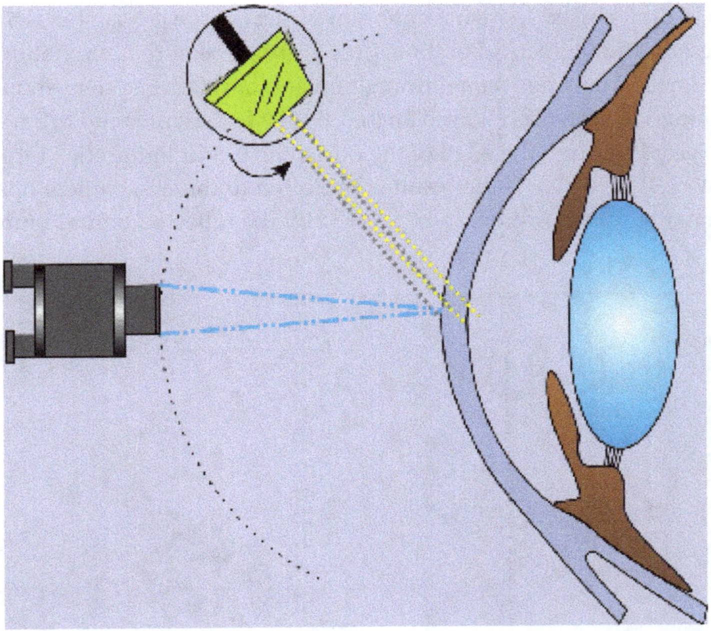

Figure 6. Indirect illumination

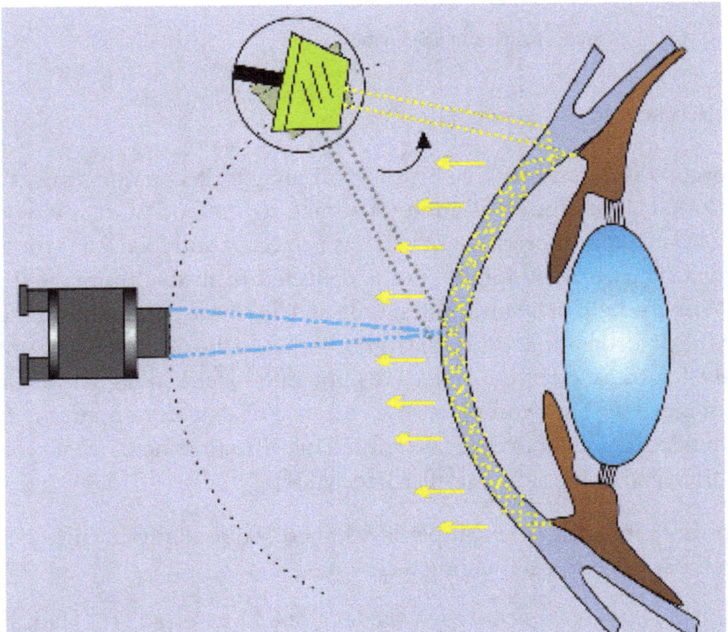

Figure 7. Indirect illumination, scleral scatter technique

Retro illumination can be used in visualization of central corneal opacities, lens and vitreous opacities, iris defects and pigment liberation. Procedure of the retro illumination is started with releasing of the knob. Angle between illumination and observing system should be set about zero. Then illumination system is focused on the object which is intended to be observed. When the beam is projected through the edge of the pupil, the bright light reflex returning from the retina can be seen (Figure 8A). If the beam is projected to the iris, corneal opacities and any vascularisation in the cornea or iris can be viewed by the reflected light (Figure 8 B) [2].

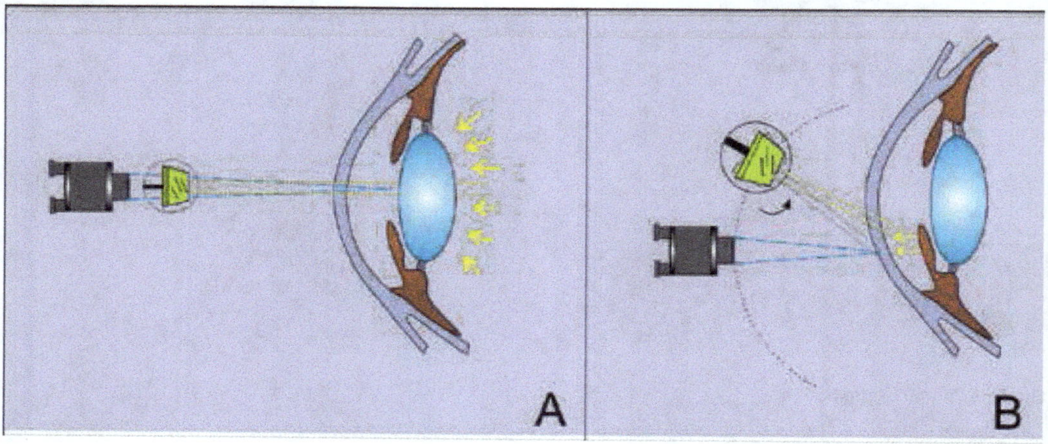

Figure 8. A. Fundus retro illumination. B. Iris retro illumination

2.2. Confocal microscopy

Confocal microscopy is a non-invasive histological imaging technique. It uses reflected light from the living tissue. Therefore, it is an in vivo imaging method of the living cornea. It uses focused light or laser beam. A bright light beam is projected and focused through an objective lens to the cornea. Then reflected light spot is collected from the illuminated tissue area by objective lens. With the help of beam splitter, reflected light is separated from the light mixture and directed to the detection unit. Reflected light reaches to the detection apparatus by passing a pin-hole. Detector transcodes the reflected light into electrical signal and records to the storage media (Figure 9). The pin-hole at the entrance of detector apparatus filters the light coming from outside the intended focal point. This filtration helps grabbing sharper and clearer images than conventional light microscopy [3].

For two-dimensional imaging, the sample is scanned sequentially in different focal planes. There are three types of confocal imaging techniques.

a. *Tandemn scanning confocal microscopy* was developed by Petran and Hadravsky [4]. Basic part of the system is the real time point illumination and point detection. It was developed by Nipkow in 1884 [5]. System provides real-time images at true color and marginal image quality based on the low intensity of reflected light [6]. Future development in tandemn

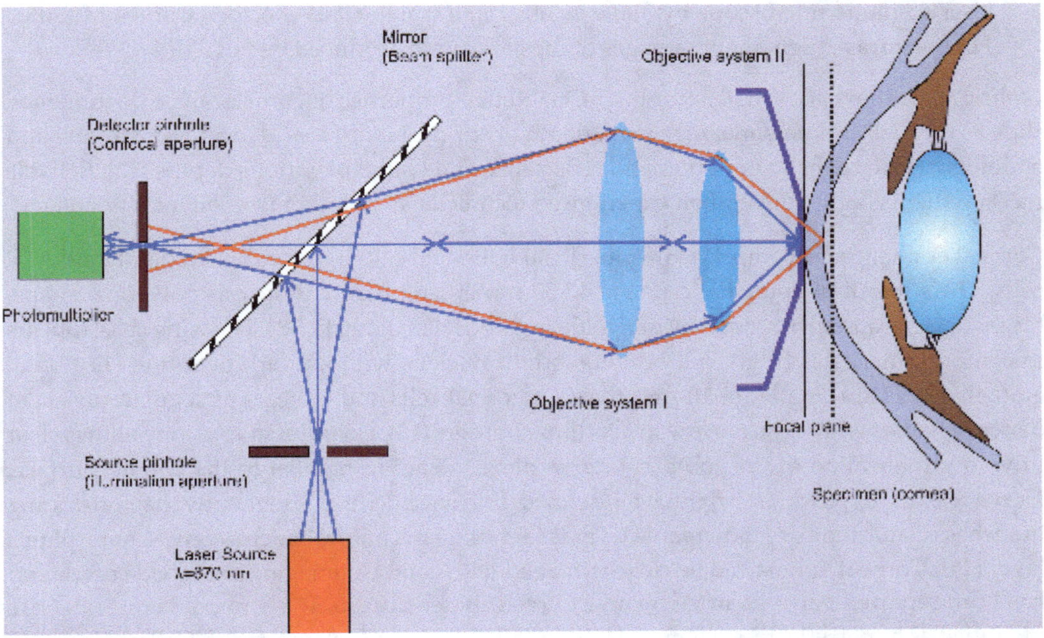

Figure 9. Working principle of confocal microscopy.

scanning was done by Xiao et al [7]. They used set of pin-holes on the same side of Nipkow disk for illumination and detection. The pinholes need to be as small as possible to eliminate the scattered light [4]. Design was simple but it has disadvantage of low intensity of illumination for image formation. Clinical version was produced but no longer in production [3].

b. *Scanning slit confocal microscopy* is an alternative scanning method to point scanning which uses a slit illumination. It scans over the back focal plane of the microscope. Advantage of slit scanning is that many points on the axis of the slit are scanned at the same time and therefore scanning time is markedly decreased. Scanning slit systems also have superior light brightness compared to point scanning. In comparison to pin-hole systems, slit scanning systems have lower axial and transverse resolution. Slit height, width and amount of light can be adjusted in slit scanning systems. By this way, visualization quality and optic section area can be modified based on the specimen i.e. transparent or opaque specimens.

c. *Laser scanning confocal microscopy* was developed by Webb in 1987 [8-10]. A coherent laser beam is used as a light source and specimen scanned by laser beam with the help of galvanometer scanning mirrors which provides fast scanning. Reflected light is refocused and projected to the photomultiplier through the pin-hole aperture. Heidelberg Retinal Tomograph is an example of in vivo confocal imaging systems. It uses 670 nm diode laser as a light source to acquire and analyze the optic nerve for glaucomatous damage. With the help of detachable optical attachment, HRT II was modified to high resolution confocal laser scanning microscope by Stave et. al. [11]. It is named as 'Rostock Cornea Module'. High-contrast, high quality images of the cornea are produced by HRT III.

Clinical applications of confocal microscopy: Qualitative properties of cornea can be documented such as corneal thickness measurement, depth of surgical interfaces, densities of stromal and endothelial cells, density or nerves and reflectance and scatter at various depths [12]. Reliable measurements highly depend on experienced technician and grabbing good quality images.

Corneal epithelium is comprised of superficial epithelial cells, wing cells and basal epithelial cells. The superficial epithelial cells are 40-50 μm in length and appear as polygonal shape, bright nucleus and surrounded by dark halo in confocal imaging [5, 13]. The wing cells appears in confocal images as bright cell borders, bright nucleus without dark oval ring [14]. Basal epithelial cells are smaller (8-10 μm) than superficial cells and appears as regular mosaic of dark cell bodies with light, narrow intercellular borders [13]. Confocal microscopy allows clear in vivo visualization of the sub-basal nerve plexus running parallel to the corneal surface. Nerve plexus appears as bright well-defined linear structures, frequently demonstrating branches or anastomoses. Bowman's layer is identified in confocal microscopy as amorphous layer [15]. Corneal stroma can be clearly imaged with confocal imaging and good correlation has been reported between in vivo and ex vivo cell density [16, 17]. Stromal keratocytes are identified as hyperreflective cell nuclei with poorly visualized cell processes. Cell process may become more visible in corneal edema or trauma [15, 18]. Descement membrane appears as an acellular layer between posterior stroma and endothelium [15]. Confocal microscopy provides clear images of the corneal endothelium despite of moderate corneal edema [19]. Endothelial cells appear in confocal imaging as hexagonal shape cells with a honeycomb order [15].

The introduction of confocal microscopy into the research and clinical practice, represented a revolutionary approach to the inherited corneal diseases. It allowed the clinician in vivo microscopic analysis of affected corneas and screening of unaffected family members [20]. Besides the inherited corneal diseases, confocal microscopy can be used in determining the acanthamoeba keratitis, fungal keratitis, bacterial and viral keratitis [3, 21, 22]. Wound healing response can be analyzed after refractive surgery with confocal microscopy [3].

2.3. Scheimpflug imaging

The Scheimpflug principle, first described by Theodor Scheimpflug, a cartographer of the Austrian navy [23]. According to him, obliquely tilted object can be documented with maximal possible depth of focus and minimal image distortion. In a normal imaging camera, all planes are parallel to each other. But in a Scheimpflug imaging principle, all planes cuts each other in an intersection point (Figure 10). Scheimpflug principle was first introduced in ophthalmology by Drews, Niesel, Brown, Dragomirescu and Hockwin [24-27]. Scheimpflug imaging technique provides high resolution and wide depth-of-focused sharp images from anterior corneal surface to the posterior crystalline lens capsule. In this technique camera rotates along with a monochromatic slit light source around the optical axis of the eye to obtain slit images. This system scans the cornea from zero to 180° and each one of the photographs belongs to the specific angle of corneal section (Figure 11). During the scanning process, a center placed static camera detects pupil contours and controls fixation.

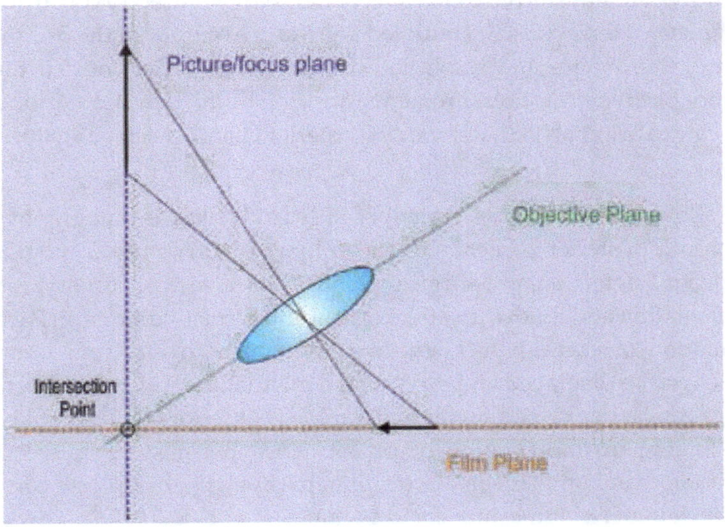

Figure 10. Scheimpflug principle imaging

Reconstruction of anterior and posterior corneal surface topography is done by analyzing of multiple photographs taken from specific angle. Corneal pachymetry, wavefront aberrations, densitometry of crystalline lens and anterior chamber calculations and measurements are provided by bundled software. Pentacam is a Scheimpflug imaging device available in market. There are three different model Pentacam versions available in the markets which are basic, classic and HR (high resolution). Differences between models are mostly in software but resolution upgrade is available in HR model [28].

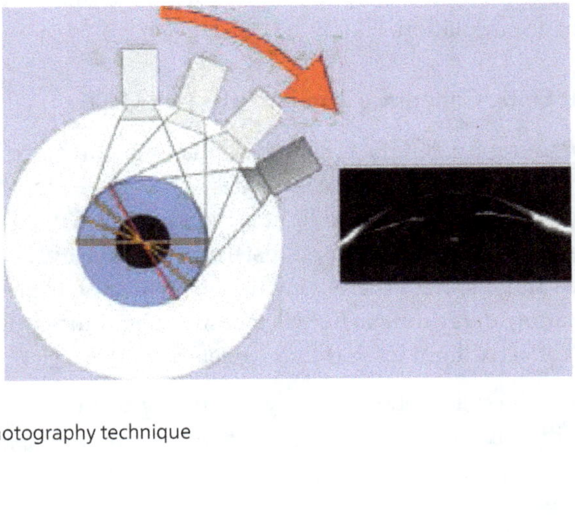

Figure 11. Scheimpflug photography technique

The other one is Galilei dual Scheimpflug analyzer which integrates a placido disc with a dual rotating Scheimpflug system [29]. Both systems acquire images simultaneously to obtain information on the curvature and elevation of the cornea. After scanning the anterior chamber, Scheimpflug images are transferred to PC to get analyzed and used to construct 3-D model of the anterior segment of the eye by the bundled software. Accuracy of the 3-D model increases with the count of the images and resolution of the camera. After constructing 3-D model, topographic and pachymetric measurements are done and entire anterior and posterior surfaces of the cornea are analyzed. Remodeled anterior chamber can be analyzed and viewed in any direction.

Basic software allows qualitative assessment of the cornea such as topography and elevation data of anterior and posterior corneal surface and pachymetry map. Topography maps are used for keratoconus detection, pre-surgical planning of refractive surgery, intra ocular lens (IOL) power calculation and follow-up after corneal and refractive surgery. Pachymetry maps allow representation of corneal thickness in color which covers from limbus to limbus. Measured values can be displayed and represented manually at any point. Corneal wavefront Zernike analysis can be performed by the software. 3-D anterior chamber analysis is used for pre-surgical planning of implantation of phakic IOLs, pre-post operative comparison of changes in anterior chamber, glaucoma screening, pachymetry-based IOP correction, assessment of anterior chamber volume, angle and volume.

Optional software modules such as Holladay Report, Holladay EKR Detail Report, Belin/Ambrosio Enhanced Ectasia Display, Contact Lens Fitting, 3D Posterior chamber IOL Simulation Software and 3D cataract analysis can be installed. The Holladay Report was developed by Jack T. Holladay, M.D [30]. It calculates the real relationship of the posterior corneal surface to the anterior corneal surface and provides data for calculating the optimal IOL refractive power for patients who have undergone refractive corneal surgeries. The Belin/Ambrosio display is the first keratoconus screening tool. It provides height data of the anterior and posterior corneal surface in combination with a progression analysis of the corneal thickness. It was developed by Michael W. Belin, M.D. and Renato Ambrosio Jr., M.D [31]. This module is used to early detection of keratoconus. Contact Lens Fitting module allows automatic display of all necessary measurement data for fitting contact lenses, automatic suggestions for contact lenses and realistic image simulation.

2.4. Anterior Segment Optic Coherence Tomography (AS-OCT)

Optical coherence tomography (OCT) is a non-contact imaging method which provides detailed cross-sectional images of biological tissues. It works with similar principle with ultrasound imaging. Delay time of reflected light is measured and used to visualize the target tissue in depth. A beam of infrared light is used instead of sound wave. Light travels extremely faster than sound wave and therefore measuring the delay time of infrared light is impossible. To overcome this limitation, delay time of light is measured by comparing the sample reflected light with a reference reflected light in an interferometer.

Resolution of OCT depends on the coherence length of the light and ranges from 2 μm to 20μm. High resolution capability and transparent structure of the anterior segment makes OCT an ideal imaging technology. High frequency ultrasound of anterior segment and confocal microscopy also can reach similar resolution but OCT is more practical, non-contact, and faster.

OCT was invented by David Huang and colleagues in 1991 [32]. Joseph Izatt described anterior segment OCT in 1994 [32, 33]. First anterior segment OCT was based on time domain technique and used 1310 nm wavelength infrared light. Time domain technique requires mechanical movement of a mirror to estimate the latency of every axial scan (A scan) in the projecting light. Wavelength of light that is used in this technique limits the resolution to 18 μm and the mechanical part limits the speed of A-scans performed by the device to 2000 scan/sec [34].

With the invention of spectral domain OCT (SD-OCT), axial resolution is increased to 5μm and the A-scan speed to about 26000 – 40000 (depends upon manufacturer) per second with the 840 nm light and without a movable mechanical part. In SD-OCT, reference mirror is fixed and A-scan is produced by Fourier transformation of spectral interference patterns between the sample and reference reflections. SD-OCT can visualize bowman layer as a parallel line, thickness profile of epithelial and stromal layer separately. However, time-domain OCT cannot easily visualize epithelial layer and stromal layer separately. Time-domain OCT still has advantage of visualizing deep tissue structures and anterior chamber biometry [34].

Newest technology for AS-OCT is Swept-Source OCT (SS-OCT). It uses 1310 nm infrared light source and categorized as fourier-domain OCT. SS-OCT makes possible to reconstruct the three dimensional images of the anterior segment of the eye more accurately [35]. SS-OCT has 10μm vertical resolution and capable to make 300.000 A-scan in one second for 16 mm section. Scan width of SS-OCT is higher than SD-OCT (16mm versus us 6 mm) [34]. It is quite simple and less expensive than SD-OCT. SS-OCT based OCT device has been announced in the market recently.

AS-OCT enables objective evaluation of anterior chamber. It provides comparable data of anterior chamber depth and irido-corneal angle dimensions with ultra sound biomicroscopy (UBM) [36]. Specific dimensions of the iris and chamber angle provided by AS-OCT can be used in predicting the development of angle-closure glaucoma [37]. AS-OCT is also useful in evaluating anterior chamber anatomy and positioning filtering devices after glaucoma surgery [37]. Anterior chamber measurements provided by AS-OCT are also useful in pre-operative evaluation of keratorefractive surgery. Measurement of chamber depth is useful in sizing and predicting the postoperative position of phakic intraocular lenses to the corneal endothelium [38, 39]. AS-OCT produced pachymetry map helps preoperative prediction of keratoconus and postoperative evaluation of ectasia and corneal thinning [40]. It is also useful in analysis of corneal wound structure after refractive surgery. AS-OCT is also useful in placement of intracorneal ring segments. It can identify incision depth and intrastromal position of the ring segments precisely. Assessment of segment position may help physician to avoid depth related complications [41].

AS-OCT can provide useful information before and after corneal surgery including corneal transplants. In preoperative setting, it is useful for evaluation of graft donor tissue for thickness and structural preservation [42]. After descement stripping endothelial keratoplasty, it detects posterior lamellar dislocation, primary graft failure and anterior chamber crowding with consequent chamber angle encroachment, possible descement membrane detachment and pupillary block [43]. It can successfully detect descement membrane detachment in case of corneal edema after corneal transplant or cataract extraction [44].

Beyond the surgeries, AS-OCT is a valuable tool in determining the hereditary or infective corneal pathologies. AS-OCT can visualize the full-thickness intrastromal deposits, and confirm the pattern and the depth of these intrastromal infiltrates in granular corneal dystrophy Type 2 [45]. It is ideal for evaluating the depth of injury due to a foreign body, laceration or ocular burn [46]. In microbial keratitis, AS-OCT can illustrate corneal infiltrates as hyper-reflective areas [47].

2.5. Ultrasound biomicroscopy (UBM)

Ultrasound biomicroscopy allows in vivo detailed assessment of anterior segment structures even if an optical opacity is presented. UBM was developed by Pavlin, Sherar and Foster [48]. It is based on 50-100 MHz transducers which are incorporated into a B mode clinical scanner [48-50]. Similar with other imaging techniques, penetration decreases but, resolution increases with the increasing frequency. It requires supine positioning of the patient and ocular contact with a coupling gel or fluid bath. One percent methyl cellulose is used for fluid bath but saline can also be used. During the examination, transducer moves continuously. Careful attention must be paid not to contact the transducer with the eye during the examination, otherwise corneal abrasion may occur. Most of the commercially available devices provide 25μm axial resolution and 50μm lateral resolution. Tissue penetrations of these devices are approximately 4-5 mm [51]. Scanning procedure can be viewed in real time and recorded on media. Qualitative measurements can be done with using electronic calipers of bundled software. UBM device can record the B-mode images to the media and software can reconstruct 3D anatomy model of the scanned area. The images can be viewed in any direction after examination. UBM also can be used for ocular biometry to calculate IOL power but popularity has reduced due to be a invasive technique and commercialization of partial coherent interferometry technique which is non-invasive.

UBM systems are also suitable for imaging other parts of the eye. With the eye movement, conjunctiva, underlying sclera and even peripheral retina can be examined. It can provide diagnostic images for corneal diseases, glaucoma, cysts, tumors and lens implants. Anterior chamber depth can easily be measured with UBM. Corneal layers can be identified in cross section. The first highly reflective layer is corneal epithelium. Under the epithelium, bowman layer also can be differentiated as a highly reflective layer. Corneal stroma reveals low reflectivity under the bowman layer. Endothelium cannot be differentiated from descement membrane by UBM, but both can be seen as a highly reflective layer at the posterior corneal margin [52]. Corneoscleral junction and scleral spur can be distinguished. Trabecular meshwork cannot be visualized with UBM but identification of scleral spur locates its posterior extent. Iris epithelium forms as highly reflective layer on the posterior iris surface. This layer is useful in determining the interaction of intra-irideal lesions from lesions behind the iris [52].

UBM provides valuable information about anterior segment related diseases. It allows classification of angle closure glaucoma based on their anatomic differences [53]. It can help to understand the mechanisms of angle closure glaucoma, pigmentary glaucoma, malignant glaucoma and other glaucoma types [53-55]. It can also help defining the mechanisms and results of various types of glaucoma surgery [56]. UBM appearance of filtration bleb is characterized by a fluid tract from the anterior chamber through the internal ostium, beneath the scleral flap and into the subconjunctival space. Low internal reflectivity is a sign of better IOP control. Location of accurate obstruction site of fluid flow can be determined by UBM imaging [51].

UBM can visualize patients with opaque corneas before making decision for corneal transplantation [57]. Depth of anterior chamber, state of the angle presence of synechiae and position of intraocular lens can be determined before surgery [52]. UBM is also useful in scleral diseases. It can differentiate extra-scleral and intra-scleral diseases and degree of scleral thinning [58].

In case of traumatic hypotony, UBM can detect cyclodialysis cleft even in the presence of anterior chamber swallowing [59]. After trauma, other causes of hypotony such as occult wound leakage, ciliary body membranes can also be detected. UBM can show the anterior chamber traumatic opacities and can detect small foreign bodies [60, 61]. UBM can provide valuable information in the management of anterior segment tumors [62].

3. Posterior segment and orbital imaging system

3.1. Fundus camera

Fundus camera is a specially designed low power microscope. It can take photo from surface to the posterior pole of the eye with an attached camera. It is used for imaging the eye, monitoring progression of a disease and screening purposes. With the retinal angiograph attachment, it can be used for diagnostic purposes. Most of the commercially available fundus cameras have 30-50 degrees view angle with magnification of 2.5x. Most of them have some modifications which allow visualizing 5x magnified view of 15 degree central retinal area. With the wide angle lenses, 140 degree retinal area can be visualized which minifies the image by half.

Fundus camera uses flash bulb as a light source. The light follows different paths in both observation and illumination systems. Observation light is focused via a series of lenses through a doughnut shaped aperture. When passing distance between the camera objective and corneal surface, it forms an annulus through central aperture. Reflected light coming back from the retina passes through the unilluminated hole in the doughnut formation [63]. Independent light travelling system minimizes the reflections of light source in the captured image. Retinal image projected through a low powered telescopic eye-piece allows selecting and focusing the retinal image. When the capture button is pressed, a mirror interrupts the illumination system and allows flash bulb light. Simultaneously, another mirror falls in front of the observation system which redirects the retinal image to the CCD camera. New devices use infrared light instead of a visible light to observe the retina to improve patient comfort, minimize reflections and to take undilated fundus images. Once the images have been captured, they are transferred to a connected PC for observation and analysis.

Bundled software's are capable of creating panoramic images of retina with processing multiple images taken from different areas of retina. Most of the fundus cameras have internal fixation point or external fixation point for taking images from different regions of retina and patient cooperation.

Digital SLR (single-lens-reflex) cameras provide superior image quality. They also require less illumination to capture photographs. This means less flash light requirement and better patient comfort. Recent devices combine digital SLR devices with fundus cameras to take digitally editable, high quality images. Capability of fundus camera instruments varies by model and manufacturer. They can perform color fundus photography, stereo fundus photography, red-free imaging, autoflourescence imaging and angiography of retina. Stereo fundus photography permits clinician to view the patient's fundus pathology in three dimensional from the print-out or computer screen.

In Recent years, usage of scanning laser technology in imaging of the posterior segment also allowed fast and wide field retinal image capturing. For example P200 (Optos PLC, Dunferline, Scotland) ultra-wide field non-contact retinal imaging camera uses red and green laser to scan the retina. It can produce up to 200 degree of high resolution retinal images in a single capture. It can also capture autofluorescence and fluorescein angiography images with additional modules [64].

Fundus photographs are visual records of the current opthalmoscopic appearance of a patient's retina. They allow the physician to identify retinal changes on follow-up or share the patient's condition with colleagues. It is mostly used for follow-up of glaucoma and diabetic retinopathy. Glaucoma is a condition which damages optic nerve over time. Physician can identify subtle changes in the optic nerve with serial fundus photographs and can recommend appropriate therapy to the patient.

It can document macular edema, newly occurred micro aneurysms and neovascularisation clearly. Detecting the macular edema may be easier with stereo fundus photographs..

3.2. Fundus Fluorescein Angiography (FFA)

FFA changed the diagnosis of macular and choroidal pathologic lesions in a revolutionary way. Although retina can be examined by slit lamp biomicroscopy, FFA provides valuable additive information to the practitioner. Fluorescein dye was first synthesized by Adolf von Baeryer in 1871 [65]. However, it was used as a diagnostic tool in 1960s by MacLean and Maumenee [66]. Modernization of fundus camera features, invention of special camera filters, improved optics, high resolution digital cameras and better understanding of biologic properties of fluorescein have changed FFA to a sophisticated valuable diagnostic tool in ophthalmology.

Fluorescein is used in ophthalmology as hydrocarbon salt of sodium with molecular formula $C_{20}H_{10}O_5Na_2$ (Figure 12) [67]. Molecular weight of fluorescein is 376.67 daltons and it is highly water soluble. Fluorescein has the ability to give off longer wavelength light after being exposed to a specific wavelength light. Excitation wavelength is 465 to 490 nm and fluorescence wavelength is 520-530 nm [68].

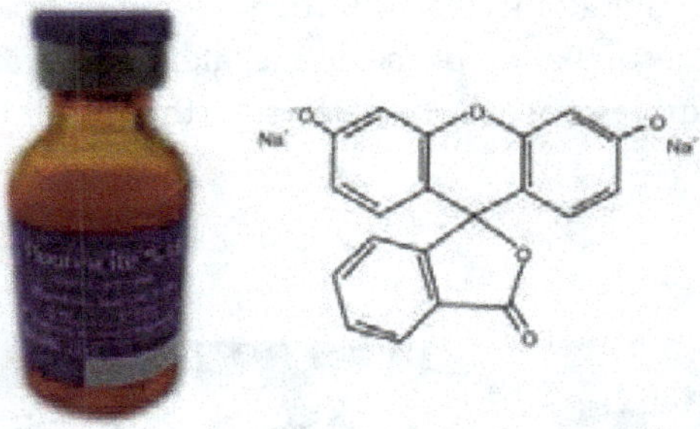

Figure 12. Marked form and chemical structure of sodium fluorescein.

Molecular weight is too large to pass through the RPE cells to pass through the RPE cells (Outer blood-retina barrier) and large choroidal vessels. But it is small enough to diffuse easily through the capillaries except central nervous system and retina (inner blood retina barrier) and these features makes it ideal for visualizing vessels [69]. Special feature for diagnostic purposes in ophthalmology is able to leak from disrupted blood-retina barrier areas. After injecting the fluorescein from antecubital vein, 80-85% of fluorescein binds to plasma proteins especially albumin [67, 69]. Unlike bound fluorescein, free fluorescein is able to absorb and emit light. Fluorescein is eliminated by glomerular filtration in the kidney and metabolized by liver [70].

The risks of angiography have been well described in literature [70, 71]. Mild reactions due to fluorescein angiograph are nausea, emesis, pruritus and vasovagal symptoms. The incidence of these reactions can be as low as 0,6% or as high as 15% [67, 69]. Most of the adverse effects are rapidly onset after injection and normally resolves approximately in 1,5 hours [71]. Severe reactions such as laryngeal edema, broncho spasm, anaphylaxis, shock, myocardial infarction, cardiac arrest and convulsion can be seen [72]. These reactions may even be fatal (1 in 222,000) [73]. Absolute contraindications include first trimester of pregnancy [74]. Relative contraindications are second and third trimesters of pregnancy, congestive cardiac, renal and hepatic failures [69].

After administration of fluorescein several phases can be seen in retinal circulation. Understanding the normal phases is essential for correct interpretation of FFA. These phases of FFA are shown in Figure 13. After administration of dye, fluorescence can be visualized in optic nerve and choroid within 10-15 seconds. But this interval can be changed by many factors such as injection site and circulation speed [75].

After initial appearance of dye in the choroid, arterial filling occurs 1-3 seconds later. Complete filling of arteries should finish less than 1 second. Venous filling phase occurs slower than arterial phase. Laminar filling of veins with dye can be seen in all individuals 2-3 seconds after completion of arterial filling (arterio-venous phase). It is named as also laminar venous filling. Venous filling should be completed in 11 seconds after first appearing the dye in arteries (Venous phase). Recirculation phase starts at 30th second after injection of dye and lasts approximately 2 minutes. In this phase, vessels are filled for the second cycle. With the elimination of dye through the glomerular filtration, concentration of the dye in the blood stream declines during the recirculation phase. In the late phase of angiogram, no dye should be detected in the vessels. Fluorescence can be detected in the vessels in case of vascular leakage secondary to inflammation [75].

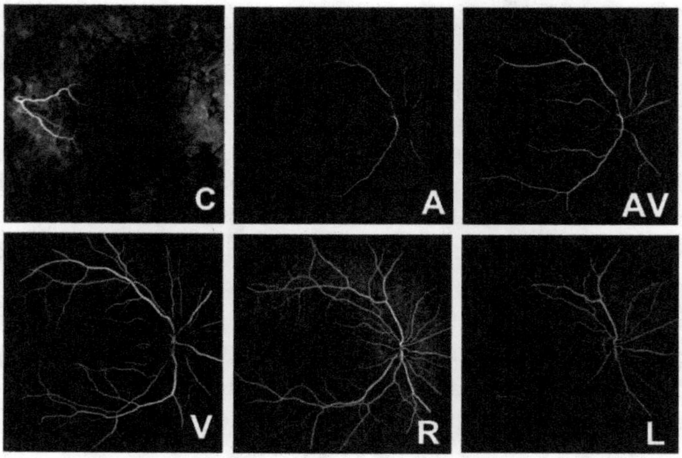

Figure 13. Phases of fluorescence angiography. C. Choroidal, A. Arterial, AV.Arteriovenous, V.Venous, R. Recirculation, L. Late phase.

Hypofluoresence can be detected in the FFA secondary to filling defects or blockage of fluorescence by an opaque medium. Filling defects can be seen by occlusion of small vessels in diabetes, radiation retinopathy, sickle cell disease or talc retinopathy. Capillary filling defects can be seen in diabetes and retinal vein and artery occlusion and Behcet's disease. Retinal arterial occlusion is observed as hypofluoresence in the retinal area distal to the site of the occlusion (Figure 15, A-B) [75].

Hyperfluorescence can be observed in 4 circumstances; leakage, staining, pooling and window defect. Window defect implies partial or total loss of blocking effect of RPE. It can be seen in geographic atrophy in macular degeneration and tear of the RPE. Neovascularisation in diabetic retinopathy, sickle cell retinopathy and choroidal neovascular membrane in AMD or myopic degeneration leads to leaking appearance. Microaneurysms in diabetes, Irvine-Gass syndrome, uveitis induced macular edema and arterial macroaneurysms are example of leakage due to the permeability loss of vessels [75]. Pooling means accumulation of the dye in fluid filled spaces. Examples of pooling appearance are central serous chorioretinopathy, pigment epithelial tear in AMD and intra ocular tumors. Staining is increased intensity of hyperfluorescence in a lesion. Examples of staining are disciform scars, regressed neovascular tissue, myopic degeneration and gyrate atrophy (Figure 14, C-F).

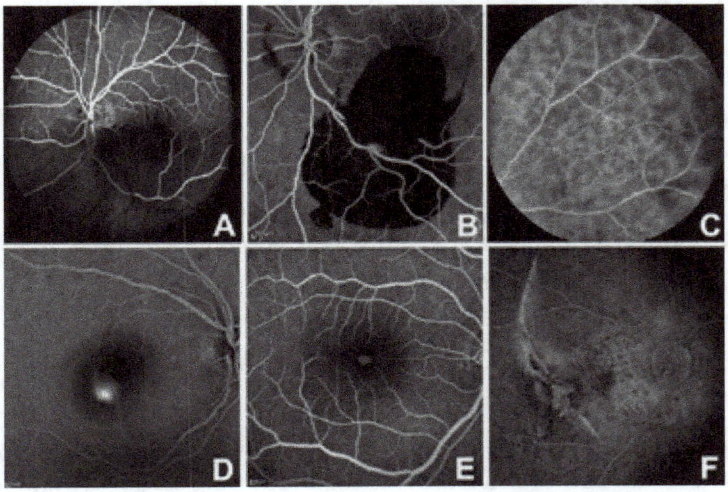

Figure 14. Sample FFA images A. Filling defect due to the occlusion of major artery, B. Blockage of fluorescence in intravitreal hemorrhage C. Leakage in behcet uveitis. D. Pooling in SSR, E. Window defect in macular hole, F. Late staining in choroidal scar.

3.3. Indocyanine green angiography

Investigations for visualizing the choroidal vasculature introduced the indocyanine green (ICG) angiography into the ophthalmology. It was first introduced into medicine in 1957 for measuring the cardiac output [76, 77]. In 1986 Hayashi et. al improved new filter combinations with sufficient sensitivity [78]. Indocyanine green is a water soluble dye and molecular weight is 775 daltons. Molecular formula is C43H47N2NaO6S2 [79] (Figure 15). It absorbs near-infrared light the range of 790-805 nm. Emission spectrum is in the range of 770-880 nm, peak at 835 nm. Indocyanine green bounds to plasma proteins with 98% but unlike fluorescein, 80% of indocyanine green bounds to the globulins such as A1-lipoprotein [79]. Therefore indocyanine dye cannot escape from choroidal vasculature and allows visualizing of the choroidal vasculature. ICG diffuses through the choroidal stroma slowly and stains in the choroid during the 12 minutes after injection.

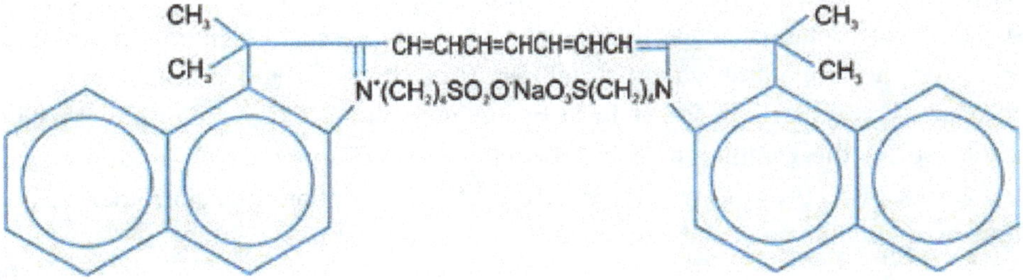

Figure 15. Molecular structure of indocyanine green

Standard dosage of ICG is 25 mg which is dissolved in 5 ml solvent. It should be injected rapidly through the antecubital vein. It is taken up by liver and secreted into the bile without metabolic alteration. It is a safer dye than fluorescein. Adverse reactions are rare. Nausea, vomiting and pruritus can be seen in 0.15% of patients. Isolated vasovagal type reactions and anaphylactic shock have been reported in the literature [80-82].

Image acquisition from ICG done by the near infrared laser or light through the excitation filter. Excited ICG molecules emits slightly different wavelength of light. Before being captured by the camera, emitted light passes the barrier filter which blocks the light with a shorter wavelength than 825 nm. Therefore, the camera captures only the light which is emitted by ICG, not the projected light near infrared spectrum [79].

Digital image capturing and processing systems made it easy to capture, view and store the acquired images. The Charge coupled device captures the ICG angiography images and converts to digital data. SLO systems provide high capturing sensitivity and allow simultaneous capturing with fluorescein angiography and ICG angiography. SLO systems use infrared diode laser (795 nm) to excite the ICG. The use of wide angle lenses allows instantaneous imaging of large fundus areas.

ICG angiography is widely used in the detection and follow-up of AMD related lesions. Serous pigment epithelial detachment is an ovoid or circular detachment of retina pigment epithelium and seen as blockage of normal choroidal vessels in ICG. Choroidal neovascularization (CNV) is a choroidal capillary proliferation through a break in the bruch membrane. Classic CNV can be detected as an area of bright hyperfluorescence but it can be better delineated by fluorescence angiography. Occult CNV without serous pigment epithelial detachment can be seen as early vascular hyperfluorescence and late staining of abnormal vessels. Occult CNV with serous pigment epithelial detachment reveals as early vascular hyperfluoresence and late staining of the CNV [83, 84]. Hot spot or focal CNV is seen as well delineated and no more than one disc diameter in size with ICG angiography.

Polipoidal choroidal vasculopathy is an abnormality of the choroidal circulation. it is seen as distinct network of vessels in choroid at the early phases. Retinal angiomatous proliferation is characterized by dilated retinal vessels, retinal hemorrhages and exudates. In ICG, it reveals as focal areas of intense hyperfluorescence (hot spot) and late extension of leakage which corresponds to intraretinal neovascularization. Central serous chorioretinopathy is a collection of fluid under the retina and makes visual distortion. It is detected in ICG angiography as multifocal areas of hyperfluorescence in early and late phases. ICG angiography is a valuable diagnostic tool in the evaluation of intraocular tumors. Pigmented choroidal melanomas absorb and block ICG fluorescence. It can be used for differentiation of choroidal melanomas from non-pigmented intra ocular tumors [79].

ICG angiography also can provide valuable information about intraocular inflammatory conditions.

3.4. Scanning Laser Ophthalmoscope (SLO)

SLO is a tool which can be used for FFA, ICG angiography, autoflourescence detection and acquiring OCT images with modification. Combination of low powered laser illumination and confocal imaging technique provides high contrast and detailed images. Using very narrow and exact wavelength laser allows more efficient excitation than filtered flash illumination of the fundus camera. Due to the monochromatic laser, captured images are in gray scale.

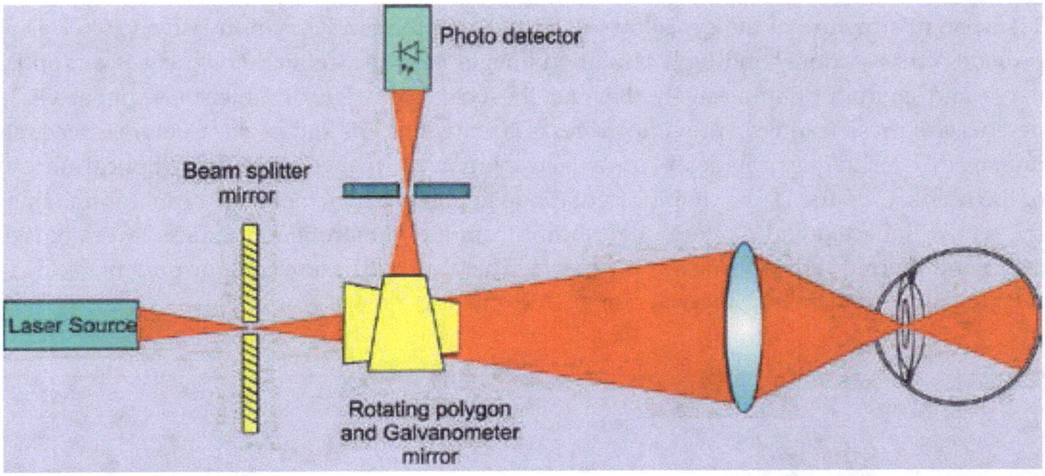

Figure 16. Working scheme of scanning laser opthalmoscope

SLO imaging principle basically starts with the pre-shaped laser beam which is focused to the retina. Pre-shaped laser beam passes through the 2mm aperture of a beam splitter mirror. Beam is deflected horizontally by a rotating polygon mirror to form a line scan. Galvanometric mirror is deflected vertically to form a two dimensional raster. Two dimensional raster laser beams are focused to a single point at the patient's lens which refocuses it onto the retina. The light reflected from the retina travels the same path and rescanned by two scanning mirrors. Beam separator collects the reflected light and focuses it onto the photo detector (Figure 16). Photo detector converts the reflected light to the images and transmits to the computer for processing and recording. Advantage of SLO is reduced scattered light in the reflected light. Reduced scattered light results with improved image contrast.

There are two types of SLO-based device available in the market. These are Heidelberg Retinal Tomography (HRT) and Heidelberg Retinal Angiography (HRA). HRT is designed to acquire images from especially optic nerve and macula. It provides quantitative three dimensional imaging of the posterior segment. HRA uses 670nm laser diode and confocal aperture to acquire images. HRT II has 15-degree scan area. Image resolution is 384x384 pixels. Scan depth ranges between 1 to 4 mm. Sixteen images are captured at each 1 mm. After acquiring images, bundled software allows the analysis of retinal thickness and optic nerve topography [85].

HRA is a confocal SLO designed for simultaneous FA, ICG angiography and autoflourescence imaging. Blue laser (488nm) is used for exciting fluorescein and near infrared laser (795nm) is used for exciting indocyanine green dye. Barriers for acquiring emitted light are 500nm for FA and 810nm for ICG angiography. The field of range starts from 10°x10° to as much as 150°x 150° with the contact lens attachment [86]. Another firm 'Optos' also combined the scanning laser ophthalmoscope with OCT [87].

3.5. Optical Coherence Tomography (OCT)

Transparent structure of the eye allows us visualizing the fundus non-invasively. OCT also provides cross sectional and high resolution images of retina, retina nerve fiber layer, optic nerve and choroid non-invasively. Beyond the posterior segment, anterior segment OCT devices also present and can provide images of cornea, lens, iris and angle structures. Spectral domain (SD) technique provides 5-7μm axial resolution which means an in-vivo optical biopsy of the retina. OCT uses super luminescent diode to obtain a coherent laser beam for imaging the retina. Reflected and scattered light beam from the vitreoretinal interface, layers of the retina and choroid allows acquisition of images. There are two basic technique present for OCT imaging; time-domain and spectral domain techniques.

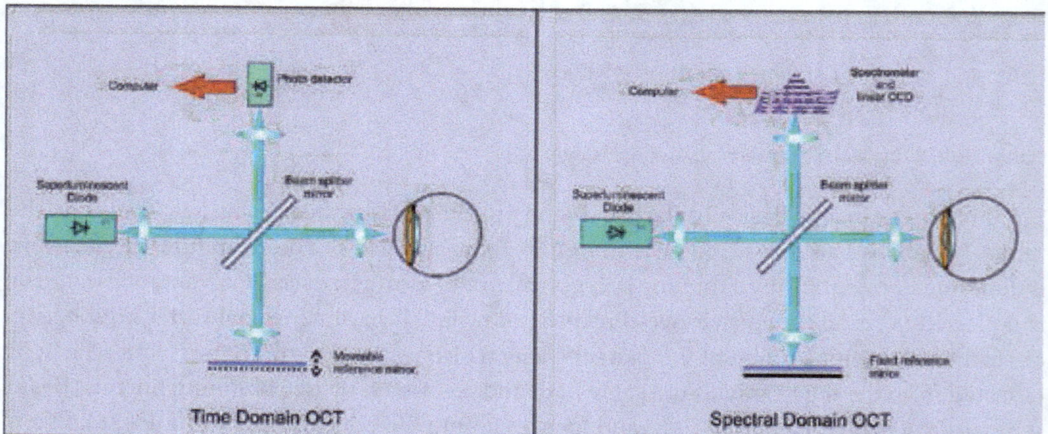

Figure 17. Comparison of time domain and spectral domain OCT working principle

Time-domain technique emits laser beam by super luminescent diode. The beam is splitted into two different paths by a beam splitter. First beam is sent to ocular media, other beam is sent to the movable mirror. Reflected light from the ocular media and movable mirror are combined on the same path and a partial interference is created. Photo detector and the computer measure the interference amplitude and calculate the depth information for each A-scan. To create a B scan image, A-scan sequences are repeated for different directions. Obtained image quality depends on the count of A-scan in each direction (Vertical, horizontal, oblique) and absorption rate of the projected light by tissue. Time-domain devices can provide 400 A scans per second with a maximal axial resolution of 8-10μm (Figure 17). High quality images require longer time to create. Therefore time is the major limitation of this technique. Time-domain technique cannot visualize deeper layers such as choroid due to the light scattering feature of the RPE and low signal-noise ratio [88](Figure 18 A).

In SD-technique, the light source is the same as in time-domain technique. There is also a reference mirror, but it is fixed unlike time-domain technique. This technique uses spectrometer and linear CCD for analyzing interferences between sample beam and reference beam. Fourier transform equation is used for calculating interference information. Absence of movable mirror speeds up the image acquisition up to 50 times. This technique enables to obtain large numbers of A-scans that allows creating high resolution images. SD devices can provide 20.000-52.000 A-scan per second with a 5-7μm resolution [89](Figure 18 B). Such a speed reduces the eye movement artifacts. Obtaining large numbers of images in a short period of time allows 3D reconstruction of the examined area.

One of the newer techniques in OCT imaging modalities is swept-source OCT (SS-OCT). It uses a different form of fourier analysis and employs tunable frequency swept laser source. Unlike spectral OCT measurements, interference is detected with photo detectors instead of spectrometer. Axial scan rate of SS-OCT is 100.000 to 236.000 per second with 11μm tissue resolution [90-92]. Prototype OCT systems using longer wavelength light are also present. Using longer wavelength light provides better penetration of deep tissues and allows visualizing of the choroid and opaque media in better detail [93]. Another new technology is Doppler OCT which detects the precise location of vascular abnormalities using cross sectional imaging. It can evaluate blood flow and volume of retinal and choroidal vasculature [94].

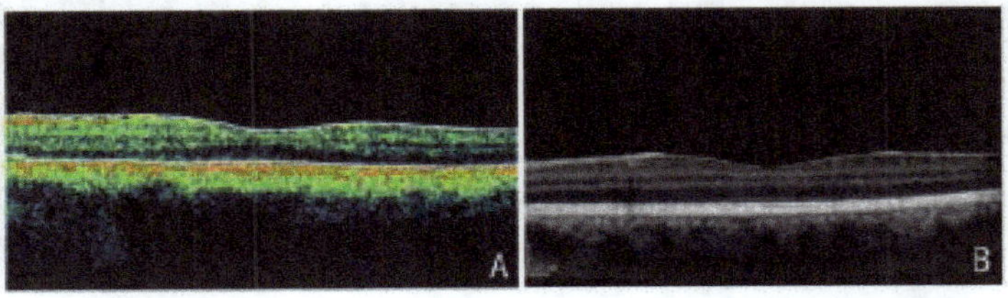

Figure 18. A. Macular cross-section acquired by time domain OCT, B. Macular cross-section image acquired by spectral-domain OCT

Automated retinal thickness measurements calculated by OCT devices are used for monitoring disease progression and response to therapies such as AMD, diabetic macular edema and vein occlusions. Accurate measurement of the retinal thickness helps physician for clinical decision regarding treatment in these conditions. Determining the retinal nerve fiber layer profile with OCT provides valuable information in detecting and management of glaucoma patients. OCT helps in diagnosing and classification of the macular holes. The determined size and configuration by OCT helps predicting the surgery outcomes [95, 96]. It allows evaluation of the vitreoretinal interface in epiretinal membrane and vitreoretinal traction [97]. OCT contributed to better understanding the AMD and helped monitoring the progression and therapeutic response to the intravitreal injections [98]. It is a valuable tool for early diagnosis, analysis and monitoring of diabetic retinopathy with high repeatability and resolution [99]. OCT provides quantitative assessment of retinal thickness in diabetic retinopathy [100].

3.6. Ocular ultrasonography

Ultrasound is a safe, non-invasive, widely used diagnostic tool in medical imaging. It has an important role in ophthalmological diagnosis. Ultrasound produces two-dimensional cross-sectional views of the eye and orbit. It has especially important role for imaging intraocular lesions in the presence of anterior segment opacities. Ultrasound devices produce acoustic sound waves above the audible range of 20KHz to visualize ocular and orbital tissues. Acoustic sound is created by a piezoelectric crystal which is a transducer for converting electric energy into the ultrasound. A short acoustic wave generated by a piezoelectric crystal is sent to the examining tissue. Some of the ultrasound waves are reflected back to the probe. Probe converts returned echoes into electrical signal and image of the tissue is created with processing and combining every electrical signal (Figure 19).

Currently ophthalmic ultrasound devices use 8-100 MHz frequency echoes. In other fields 2-6 MHz frequency is mostly used. Higher frequencies provide increased resolution but decreased pentrance. Eye is a superficially located tissue and has low absorptive properties which make the use of high frequencies practical.

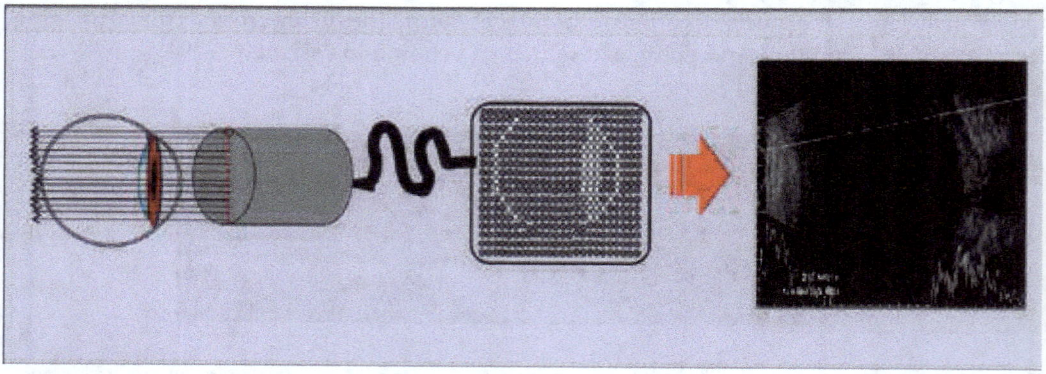

Figure 19. Working principle of ultrasonography

First report of ultrasound applied in ophthalmology belongs to Munth and Hughes who reported A-scan ultrasonography of intraocular tumors in 1956 [101]. B-scan images of the specific ocular diseases and tumors has been described two year later after the initial publication [102]. Most frequently used ultrasound imaging modes are A-scan, B-scan, ultrasound biomicroscopy, color doppler ultrasonography and three dimensional ultrasonography. Ultrasound biomicroscopy has been discussed in detail above.

Ocular ultrasonography is frequently used for evaluating intra ocular tissue integrity, searching and diagnosing intraocular foreign bodies, assessment of intraocular or peri-ocular lesions and examining trauma patients. It is frequently used in the presence of opaque media such as cataract, corneal pathologies, etc. It can be used for determining intralesional characteristics or ecographic nature of a visible mass or foreign body.

A-scan imaging is a one dimensional display of echo strength over time. Vertical height corresponds to echo intensity. There are two types of A-scan present in opthalmological use; biometric A-scan and standardized diagnostic A-scan. Biometric A-scan is used for axial length measurement and corneal pachymetry in evaluation of ocular hypertension and calculation of intraocular lens power [103]. It uses 10-12 MHz frequency and has linear amplification curve. Standardized A-scan is used with 8MHz probe. It is used to determine and differentiate abnormal intraocular tissues. Retina consists highly dense ocular structures such as sclera and choroid which produces 100% echo spikes.

B-scan is the two dimensional view of the combined multiple A-scan echoes. Unlike A-scan, every spike is encoded as a bright dot and every dot brightness changes with the strength of the echo. B-scan images are highly accurate representations of ocular structures and provide shape, location and extensive information. Most of the ophthalmic ultrasound devices use 10MHz frequency for B-scan imaging. The evaluation and differentiation of intraocular lesions are one of the primary indications for ultrasonography. Combined use of B-scan and A-scan provides more reliable information for evaluating ocular lesions. Simultaneously viewing kinetic properties of echo amplitudes (A scan) with B-scan provides more accurate evaluation of intraocular lesions such as choroidal melanomas [104].

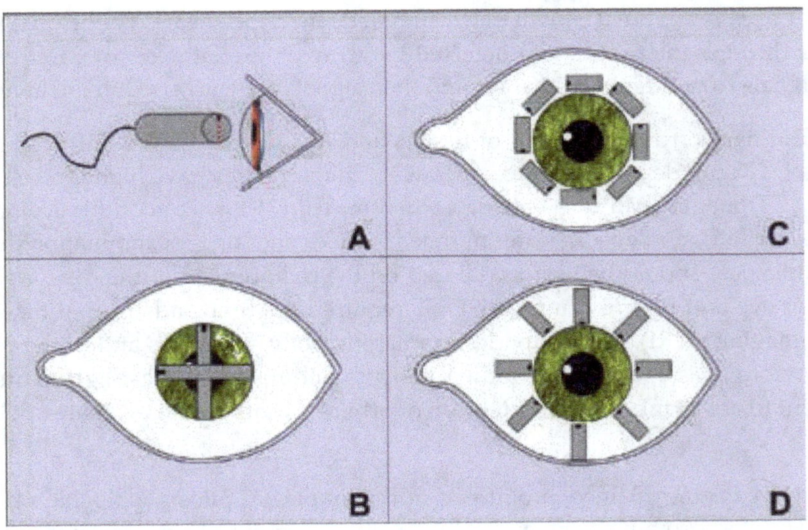

Figure 20. B-scan orientations A. External view of axial scan probe orientation B. Axial scan orientation, C. Transverse scan orientation, D. Longitudinal scan orientation

B-scan probe can be applied to the eye in axial, transverse and longitudinal orientation. Axial scan can be obtained by placing the probe across the visual axis through the cornea and lens. It is the easiest and mostly used orientation but sound attenuates due to the lens. This limits

its diagnostic use (Figure 20). Longitudinal scan can be obtained by placing the probe on sclera to visualize the specific clock hour anterior-posterior cross section. Transverse B-scan also can be obtained by placing the probe on the sclera parallel to the limbus. It provides antero-posterior dimension of the lesion. These two methods is not affected by the attenuation effect of the lens. It provides lateral dimension of the lesion.

Color-doppler ultrasonography allows evaluating B-scan image of the eye and blood flow simultaneously. If the flow moves toward the transducer it is coded with red color. The blood flow that moves away from the transducer is coded with blue color. It provides valuable information about vasculature of orbital tumors, carotid disease, central retinal artery and vein occlusions and non-arteritic ischemic optic neuropathy [105-107].

Ophthalmic 3D ultrasonography uses multiple consecutive two-dimensional B-scan images to create three-dimensional blocks with the help of bundled software. Specially designed transducer probe rapidly scans the eye in trans-scleral orientation and software creates the 3D image. It is useful for calculating the volume of the intraocular lesions [108].

3.7. Computerized Tomography (CT)

Computed tomography is a useful imaging tool in the evaluation of most orbital and ocular lesions. It allows us to detect location, extent and configuration of the lesion. It also provides tissue mass composition and helps planning of an appropriate surgical approach to minimize morbidity. Computed tomography works slightly different than conventional X-ray imaging methods. CT uses x-rays but it emits a thin collimated fan shaped beam. The beam is attenuated as it passes through the tissues and detected by array of special detectors. Detectors create electrical signals from attenuated X-rays and then signals are converted to the images.

CT provides images from thin slices of tissues and it is devoid of superimposition. Spatial resolution of CT scan depends on slice thickness. Thinner slices have higher resolution. Slice thickness of CT imaging can vary between 1-10 mm. Thin slices are good for ocular use but it requires higher radiation dose, greater number of slices and longer examination time. Therefore, slice thickness should be balanced based on the requirement of the case. Optimal slice thickness for eye and orbit is 2 mm [109]. CT requires less time and cheaper than magnetic resonance imaging (MRI). CT is superior in imaging bony structures and in the presence of blood. Therefore, it is excellent in trauma patients. Iodinated contrast agents are used for enhancement to detect intracranial extension of orbital tumors and to evaluate optic chiasmal lesions.

CT is indicated in unexplained propitosis, opthalmoplegia, pitosis, palpable orbital mass, preseptal cellulites, orbital trauma and orbital signs of paranasal sinus diseases. One should request CT imaging only when absolutely indicated because of X-ray exposure.

3.8. Magnetic Resonance Imaging (MRI)

MRI has complex working principle but it has one of the largest diagnostic potential in medicine. It is especially used for imaging neural tissue visualization and has substantial advantage to other imaging methods. MRI creates images with the help of magnetic field and radio waves. It is based on the ability of a small number of protons within the body to absorb and emit radio wave energy when the body or tissue is exposed to strong magnetic field. Soft tissue contrast ratios of MRI are superior to other imaging modalities. Differences in the density of protons in different tissues are provides discriminating one from other. Different tissues absorb and release radio wave energy at different characteristic rates.

Various pulse sequence techniques are used in MRI imaging but most popular ones are T1 and T2-weighted images. T1 images measures ability of protons in a tissue to exchange energy with the surrounding environment or how fast the tissue is magnetized. T2 images measures how quickly the tissue loses its magnetization. In T1 images, fat appears as bright and water appears dark. Reverse view is present in T2 images. T1 images are used especially for viewing anatomy. T2 images are more valuable for detecting pathology. Contrast materials enhance recognition of primary pathology by demonstrating areas of breakdown of the blood-brain barrier.

MRI uses non-ionizing radiation. It can generate images through the entire body. It can visualize the tissue in sagittal, coronal and axial planes. It can visualize vascular tissues with or without contrast material. Beyond the advantages, it is relatively expensive and not widely available. Claustrophobia may be a problem for some patients. Cardiac pacemakers or implanted ferromagnetic foreign bodies are contraindications for MRI.

3.9. Angiography

There are three type of angiography imaging techniques. These are digital subtraction angiography, CT-angiography and MR-angiography. Digital subtraction angiography uses X-rays and iodine based intra-arterial contrast material. It subtracts the structures other than the vascular system, such as bone and muscles. It is still the gold standard method for imaging intra- and extra-cranial vasculature and in the diagnosis of cerebral aneurysms.

CT-angiography uses X rays and iodine based contrast agent. After bolus injection of the contrast agent from antecubital vein, high speed CT scan is performed. It provides images of three dimensional view of surface anatomy with color and blood vessel anatomy without color. It needs shorter examination times that MR-angiography and superior image resolution. Implanted magnetic foreign body is not a contraindication. It is safer and faster than digital subtraction angiography. It can outline surgical anatomy finer than MR-angiography.

No requirement of ionizing radiation and iodinated contrast agent are the main advantages of MR angiography over CT scan.

4. Conclusion

Imaging modalities has changed greatly in recent years. Especially newest OCT technologies promise better understanding and diagnosing of the disease. Advances in laser technologies and optical systems also have enhanced image quality and resolution in most of the imaging techniques. Newest digital technologies enable more easily reproducible information and facilities telemedicine applications. Examination in Ophthalmology starts with imaging the eye either with inspection or a sophisticated tool. Caution should be taken no to skip the basic techniques and principles while evaluating the patients. Otherwise we can spend valuable time and money with sophisticated tests unnecessarily.

Author details

Umit Yolcu[1*], Omer Faruk Sahin[2] and Fatih C. Gundogan[3]

*Address all correspondence to: umit_yolcu@hotmail.com

1 Siirt Military Hospital, Ophthalmology, Siirt, Turkey

2 Etimesgut Military Hospital, Ophthalmology, Ankara, Turkey

3 GATA Medical School, Ophthalmology, Ankara, Turkey

References

[1] Nema HV, Nema N. Diagnostic Procedures in Ophthalmology. New Delhi2009.

[2] González J, Benavides C. Atlas of Slit Lamp: (ocular Biomicroscopy): Imagen y Comunicación Multimedia; 2004.

[3] Guthoff RF, Zhivov A, Stachs O. In vivo confocal microscopy, an inner vision of the cornea - a major review. Clinical & experimental ophthalmology. 2009;37(1):100-17.

[4] Petran M, Hadravsky M. Tandem scanning microscope--a new tool for three-dimensional microanatomy. Progress in clinical and biological research. 1989;295:551-8.

[5] Bohnke M, Masters BR. Confocal microscopy of the cornea. Progress in retinal and eye research. 1999;18(5):553-628.

[6] Bohnke M, Masters BR. Long-term contact lens wear induces a corneal degeneration with microdot deposits in the corneal stroma. Ophthalmology. 1997;104(11):1887-96.

[7] Xiao GQ CT, Kino GS. Real-time confocal scanning optical microscope. Applied Physics Letters. 1988;53(8):716–18.

[8] Davidovits P, Egger MD. Scanning laser microscope. Nature. 1969;223(5208):831.

[9] Davidovits P, Egger MD. Scanning laser microscope for biological investigations. Applied optics. 1971;10(7):1615-9.

[10] Webb RH, Hughes GW, Delori FC. Confocal scanning laser ophthalmoscope. Applied optics. 1987;26(8):1492-9.

[11] Stave J, Zinser G, Grummer G, Guthoff R. [Modified Heidelberg Retinal Tomograph HRT. Initial results of in vivo presentation of corneal structures]. Der Ophthalmologe : Zeitschrift der Deutschen Ophthalmologischen Gesellschaft. 2002;99(4):276-80.

[12] Erie JC, McLaren JW, Patel SV. Confocal microscopy in ophthalmology. American journal of ophthalmology. 2009;148(5):639-46.

[13] Jalbert I, Stapleton F, Papas E, Sweeney DF, Coroneo M. In vivo confocal microscopy of the human cornea. The British journal of ophthalmology. 2003;87(2):225-36.

[14] Masters BR, Thaer AA. In vivo human corneal confocal microscopy of identical fields of subepithelial nerve plexus, basal epithelial, and wing cells at different times. Microscopy research and technique. 1994;29(5):350-6.

[15] Mustonen RK, McDonald MB, Srivannaboon S, Tan AL, Doubrava MW, Kim CK. Normal human corneal cell populations evaluated by in vivo scanning slit confocal microscopy. Cornea. 1998;17(5):485-92.

[16] Patel S, McLaren J, Hodge D, Bourne W. Normal human keratocyte density and corneal thickness measurement by using confocal microscopy in vivo. Investigative ophthalmology & visual science. 2001;42(2):333-9.

[17] Patel SV, McLaren JW, Camp JJ, Nelson LR, Bourne WM. Automated quantification of keratocyte density by using confocal microscopy in vivo. Investigative ophthalmology & visual science. 1999;40(2):320-6.

[18] Vanathi M, Tandon R, Sharma N, Titiyal JS, Pandey RM, Vajpayee RB. In-vivo slit scanning confocal microscopy of normal corneas in Indian eyes. Indian journal of ophthalmology. 2003;51(3):225-30.

[19] Hara M, Morishige N, Chikama T, Nishida T. Comparison of confocal biomicroscopy and noncontact specular microscopy for evaluation of the corneal endothelium. Cornea. 2003;22(6):512-5.

[20] Vincent AL, Patel DV, McGhee CN. Inherited corneal disease: the evolving molecular, genetic and imaging revolution. Clinical & experimental ophthalmology. 2005;33(3):303-16.

[21] Zhivov A, Stachs O, Kraak R, Stave J, Guthoff RF. In vivo confocal microscopy of the ocular surface. The ocular surface. 2006;4(2):81-93.

[22] Knappe S, Stave J, Guthoff RF. [Epidemic keratoconjunctivitis. In vivo images of corneal structures with the confocal Rostocker laser scanning microscope (RLSM)]. Der Ophthalmologe : Zeitschrift der Deutschen Ophthalmologischen Gesellschaft. 2005;102(8):798-801.

[23] Scheimpflug T. Der photoperspektrograph und seine anwendung. Photogr Korr. 1906;43:516–31.

[24] Drews RC. Depth of Field in Slit Lamp Photography. An Optical Solution Using the Scheimpflug Principle. Ophthalmologica Journal international d'ophtalmologie International journal of ophthalmology Zeitschrift fur Augenheilkunde. 1964;148:143-50.

[25] Niesel P. [Slit-lamp photography of lens for measurement purposes]. Ophthalmologica Journal international d'ophtalmologie International journal of ophthalmology Zeitschrift fur Augenheilkunde. 1966;152(5):387-95.

[26] Brown N. Slit-image photography. Transactions of the ophthalmological societies of the United Kingdom. 1970;89:397-408.

[27] Brown N. Quantitative slit-image photography of the lens. Transactions of the ophthalmological societies of the United Kingdom. 1972;92:303-7.

[28] OCULUS, Optikgeräte, G.m.b.H. http://www.pentacam.com/sites/index.php (accessed in 29 august 2013).

[29] Ziemer, Ophthalmic, Systems, AG. http://galilei.ziemergroup.com/key-features-g4.html (accesed in 29 august 2013).

[30] Holladay JT. Corneal topography using the Holladay Diagnostic Summary. Journal of cataract and refractive surgery. 1997;23(2):209-21.

[31] Belin MW, Ambrosio R, Jr. Corneal ectasia risk score: statistical validity and clinical relevance. Journal of refractive surgery. 2010;26(4):238-40.

[32] Huang D, Swanson EA, Lin CP, Schuman JS, Stinson WG, Chang W, et al. Optical coherence tomography. Science. 1991;254(5035):1178-81.

[33] Izatt JA, Hee MR, Swanson EA, Lin CP, Huang D, Schuman JS, et al. Micrometer-scale resolution imaging of the anterior eye in vivo with optical coherence tomography. Archives of ophthalmology. 1994;112(12):1584-9.

[34] Maeda N. Optical coherence tomography for corneal diseases. Eye & contact lens. 2010;36(5):254-9.

[35] Yasuno Y, Madjarova VD, Makita S, Akiba M, Morosawa A, Chong C, et al. Three-dimensional and high-speed swept-source optical coherence tomography for in vivo investigation of human anterior eye segments. Optics express. 2005;13(26):10652-64.

[36] Dada T, Sihota R, Gadia R, Aggarwal A, Mandal S, Gupta V. Comparison of anterior segment optical coherence tomography and ultrasound biomicroscopy for assessment of the anterior segment. Journal of cataract and refractive surgery. 2007;33(5): 837-40.

[37] Jancevski M, Foster CS. Anterior segment optical coherence tomography. Seminars in ophthalmology. 2010;25(5-6):317-23.

[38] Goldsmith JA, Li Y, Chalita MR, Westphal V, Patil CA, Rollins AM, et al. Anterior chamber width measurement by high-speed optical coherence tomography. Ophthalmology. 2005;112(2):238-44.

[39] Doors M, Cals DW, Berendschot TT, de Brabander J, Hendrikse F, Webers CA, et al. Influence of anterior chamber morphometrics on endothelial cell changes after phakic intraocular lens implantation. Journal of cataract and refractive surgery. 2008;34(12):2110-8.

[40] Mohamed S, Lee GK, Rao SK, Wong AL, Cheng AC, Li EY, et al. Repeatability and reproducibility of pachymetric mapping with Visante anterior segment-optical coherence tomography. Investigative ophthalmology & visual science. 2007;48(12): 5499-504.

[41] Lai MM, Tang M, Andrade EM, Li Y, Khurana RN, Song JC, et al. Optical coherence tomography to assess intrastromal corneal ring segment depth in keratoconic eyes. Journal of cataract and refractive surgery. 2006;32(11):1860-5.

[42] Choi CY, Youm DJ, Kim MJ, Tchah H. Changes in central corneal thickness of preserved corneas over time measured using anterior segment optical coherence tomography. Cornea. 2009;28(5):536-40.

[43] Lim LS, Aung HT, Aung T, Tan DT. Corneal imaging with anterior segment optical coherence tomography for lamellar keratoplasty procedures. American journal of ophthalmology. 2008;145(1):81-90.

[44] Wylegala E, Nowinska A. Usefulness of anterior segment optical coherence tomography in Descemet membrane detachment. European journal of ophthalmology. 2009;19(5):723-8.

[45] Hong JP, Kim TI, Chung JL, Huang D, Cho HS, Kim EK. Analysis of deposit depth and morphology in granular corneal dystrophy type 2 using fourier domain optical coherence tomography. Cornea. 2011;30(7):729-38.

[46] Wylegala E, Dobrowolski D, Nowinska A, Tarnawska D. Anterior segment optical coherence tomography in eye injuries. Graefe's archive for clinical and experimental ophthalmology = Albrecht von Graefes Archiv fur klinische und experimentelle Ophthalmologie. 2009;247(4):451-5.

[47] Konstantopoulos A, Kuo J, Anderson D, Hossain P. Assessment of the use of anterior segment optical coherence tomography in microbial keratitis. American journal of ophthalmology. 2008;146(4):534-42.

[48] Pavlin CJ, Harasiewicz K, Sherar MD, Foster FS. Clinical use of ultrasound biomicroscopy. Ophthalmology. 1991;98(3):287-95.

[49] Pavlin CJ, Harasiewicz K, Foster FS. Ultrasound biomicroscopy of anterior segment structures in normal and glaucomatous eyes. American journal of ophthalmology. 1992;113(4):381-9.

[50] Pavlin CJ, Sherar MD, Foster FS. Subsurface ultrasound microscopic imaging of the intact eye. Ophthalmology. 1990;97(2):244-50.

[51] Dada T, Gadia R, Sharma A, Ichhpujani P, Bali SJ, Bhartiya S, et al. Ultrasound biomicroscopy in glaucoma. Survey of ophthalmology. 2011;56(5):433-50.

[52] Arun D, Hayden BC, Pavlin CJ. Ophthalmologic Ultrasound, An Issue of Ultrasound Clinics, 1e (The Clinics: Radiology): Saunders; 2008.

[53] Pavlin CJ, Foster FS. Ultrasound biomicroscopy in glaucoma. Acta ophthalmologica Supplement. 1992(204):7-9.

[54] Potash SD, Tello C, Liebmann J, Ritch R. Ultrasound biomicroscopy in pigment dispersion syndrome. Ophthalmology. 1994;101(2):332-9.

[55] Pavlin CJ, Easterbrook M, Harasiewicz K, Foster FS. An ultrasound biomicroscopic analysis of angle-closure glaucoma secondary to ciliochoroidal effusion in IgA nephropathy. American journal of ophthalmology. 1993;116(3):341-5.

[56] Yamamoto T, Sakuma T, Kitazawa Y. An ultrasound biomicroscopic study of filtering blebs after mitomycin C trabeculectomy. Ophthalmology. 1995;102(12):1770-6.

[57] Milner MS, Liebmann JM, Tello C, Speaker MG, Ritch R. High-resolution ultrasound biomicroscopy of the anterior segment in patients with dense corneal scars. Ophthalmic surgery. 1994;25(5):284-7.

[58] Pavlin CJ, Easterbrook M, Hurwitz JJ, Harasiewicz K, Eng P, Foster FS. Ultrasound biomicroscopy in the assessment of anterior scleral disease. American journal of ophthalmology. 1993;116(5):628-35.

[59] Gentile RC, Pavlin CJ, Liebmann JM, Easterbrook M, Tello C, Foster FS, et al. Diagnosis of traumatic cyclodialysis by ultrasound biomicroscopy. Ophthalmic surgery and lasers. 1996;27(2):97-105.

[60] Berinstein DM, Gentile RC, Sidoti PA, Stegman Z, Tello C, Liebmann JM, et al. Ultrasound biomicroscopy in anterior ocular trauma. Ophthalmic surgery and lasers. 1997;28(3):201-7.

[61] Deramo VA, Shah GK, Baumal CR, Fineman MS, Correa ZM, Benson WE, et al. Ultrasound biomicroscopy as a tool for detecting and localizing occult foreign bodies after ocular trauma. Ophthalmology. 1999;106(2):301-5.

[62] Pavlin CJ, McWhae JA, McGowan HD, Foster FS. Ultrasound biomicroscopy of anterior segment tumors. Ophthalmology. 1992;99(8):1220-8.

[63] THE, OPHTHALMIC, PHOTOGRAPHERS', SOCIETY, INC. Fundus Photography Overview. Available from: http://www.opsweb.org/?page=fundusphotography (accesed in 29.08.2013).

[64] Optos PLC D, Scotland KY11 8GR UK. Available from: http://www.optos.com/en/Products/Retinal-imaging-products/Ultra-widefield-imaging/ (accesed in 31.12.2013).

[65] Baeryer Av. Uber ein neue Klasse van farbstoffen. Der Deutschen Chem Ges. 1871(4): 555.

[66] Maclean AL, Maumenee AE. Hemangioma of the Choroid. Transactions of the American Ophthalmological Society. 1959;57:171-94.

[67] Anand R. Fluorescein angiography. Part 1: Technique and normal study. Journal of ophthalmic nursing & technology. 1989;8(2):48-52.

[68] Brancato R, Trabucchi G. Fluorescein and indocyanine green angiography in vascular chorioretinal diseases. Seminars in ophthalmology. 1998;13(4):189-98.

[69] Cavallerano AA. Ophthalmic fluorescein angiography. Optometry clinics : the official publication of the Prentice Society. 1996;5(1):1-23.

[70] Bloome MA. Fluorescein angiography: risks. Vision research. 1980;20(12):1083-97.

[71] Jennings BJ, Mathews DE. Adverse reactions during retinal fluorescein angiography. Journal of the American Optometric Association. 1994;65(7):465-71.

[72] Kelley JS. Fluorescein angiography: techniques and toxicity. International ophthalmology clinics. 1977;17(2):25-33.

[73] Yannuzzi LA, Rohrer KT, Tindel LJ, Sobel RS, Costanza MA, Shields W, et al. Fluorescein angiography complication survey. Ophthalmology. 1986;93(5):611-7.

[74] Halperin LS, Olk RJ, Soubrane G, Coscas G. Safety of fluorescein angiography during pregnancy. American journal of ophthalmology. 1990;109(5):563-6.

[75] J. Fernando Arevalo. Fluorescein Angiography: General Principles and Interpretation. Retinal Angiography and Optical Coherence Tomography: Springer; 2009.

[76] Ó. G. Björnsson RM, and V. S. Chadwick. Physicochemical studies of indocyanine green (ICG): absorbance/concentration relationship, pH tolerance and assay precision in various solvents. Experientia. 1982;38(12):1441–2.

[77] Engel E, Schraml R, Maisch T, Kobuch K, Konig B, Szeimies RM, et al. Light-induced decomposition of indocyanine green. Investigative ophthalmology & visual science. 2008;49(5):1777-83.

[78] Hayashi K, Hasegawa Y, Tokoro T. Indocyanine green angiography of central serous chorioretinopathy. International ophthalmology. 1986;9(1):37-41.

[79] Klais CM, Ober MD, Yannuzzi LA. Indocyanine Green Angiography: General Aspects and Interpretation. In: Arevalo JF, editor. Retinal Angiography and Optical Coherence Tomography: Springer; 2009.

[80] Benya R, Quintana J, Brundage B. Adverse reactions to indocyanine green: a case report and a review of the literature. Catheterization and cardiovascular diagnosis. 1989;17(4):231-3.

[81] Gilmore DM, Khullar OV, Jaklitsch MT, Chirieac LR, Frangioni JV, Colson YL. Identification of metastatic nodal disease in a phase 1 dose-escalation trial of intraoperative sentinel lymph node mapping in non-small cell lung cancer using near-infrared imaging. The Journal of thoracic and cardiovascular surgery. 2013;146(3):562-70.

[82] Wolf S, Arend O, Schulte K, Reim M. Severe anaphylactic reaction after indocyanine green fluorescence angiography. American journal of ophthalmology. 1992;114(5): 638-9.

[83] Orth DH, Patz A, Flower RW. Potential clinical applications of indocyanine green choroidal angiography--preliminary report. Eye, ear, nose & throat monthly. 1976;55(1):15-28, 58.

[84] Bischoff PM, Flower RW. Ten years experience with choroidal angiography using indocyanine green dye: a new routine examination or an epilogue? Documenta ophthalmologica Advances in ophthalmology. 1985;60(3):235-91.

[85] Heidelberg, Engineering, Inc. http://www.heidelbergengineering.com/us/products/hrt-glaucoma-module/hrt-product-specifications/ (accesed in 29.08.2013).

[86] Heidelberg, Engineering, Inc. http://www.heidelbergengineering.com/us/wp-content/uploads/2106_Product%20Lit_HRA%20wBluePeak_Product%20Sheet_v2.pdf (accesed in 29.08.2013).

[87] Optos. plc. http://www.optos.com/en-US/Products/Retinal-imaging-products/OCT-imaging/ (accesed in 31.12. 2013).

[88] Adhi M, Duker JS. Optical coherence tomography--current and future applications. Curr Opin Ophthalmol. 2013;24(3):213-21.

[89] Leitgeb R, Hitzenberger C, Fercher A. Performance of fourier domain vs. time domain optical coherence tomography. Optics express. 2003;11(8):889-94.

[90] Grulkowski I, Liu JJ, Potsaid B, Jayaraman V, Lu CD, Jiang J, et al. Retinal, anterior segment and full eye imaging using ultrahigh speed swept source OCT with vertical-cavity surface emitting lasers. Biomedical optics express. 2012;3(11):2733-51.

[91] Srinivasan VJ, Huber R, Gorczynska I, Fujimoto JG, Jiang JY, Reisen P, et al. High-speed, high-resolution optical coherence tomography retinal imaging with a frequency-swept laser at 850 nm. Optics letters. 2007;32(4):361-3.

[92] Huber R, Adler DC, Srinivasan VJ, Fujimoto JG. Fourier domain mode locking at 1050 nm for ultra-high-speed optical coherence tomography of the human retina at 236,000 axial scans per second. Optics letters. 2007;32(14):2049-51.

[93] Povazay B, Bizheva K, Hermann B, Unterhuber A, Sattmann H, Fercher A, et al. Enhanced visualization of choroidal vessels using ultrahigh resolution ophthalmic OCT at 1050 nm. Optics express. 2003;11(17):1980-6.

[94] Wang Y, Lu A, Gil-Flamer J, Tan O, Izatt JA, Huang D. Measurement of total blood flow in the normal human retina using Doppler Fourier-domain optical coherence tomography. The British journal of ophthalmology. 2009;93(5):634-7.

[95] Haouchine B, Massin P, Tadayoni R, Erginay A, Gaudric A. Diagnosis of macular pseudoholes and lamellar macular holes by optical coherence tomography. American journal of ophthalmology. 2004;138(5):732-9.

[96] Hillenkamp J, Kraus J, Framme C, Jackson TL, Roider J, Gabel VP, et al. Retreatment of full-thickness macular hole: predictive value of optical coherence tomography. The British journal of ophthalmology. 2007;91(11):1445-9.

[97] Barak Y, Ihnen MA, Schaal S. Spectral domain optical coherence tomography in the diagnosis and management of vitreoretinal interface pathologies. Journal of ophthalmology. 2012;2012:876472.

[98] Fung AE, Lalwani GA, Rosenfeld PJ, Dubovy SR, Michels S, Feuer WJ, et al. An optical coherence tomography-guided, variable dosing regimen with intravitreal ranibizumab (Lucentis) for neovascular age-related macular degeneration. American journal of ophthalmology. 2007;143(4):566-83.

[99] Goebel W, Kretzchmar-Gross T. Retinal thickness in diabetic retinopathy: a study using optical coherence tomography (OCT). Retina. 2002;22(6):759-67.

[100] Sanchez-Tocino H, Alvarez-Vidal A, Maldonado MJ, Moreno-Montanes J, Garcia-Layana A. Retinal thickness study with optical coherence tomography in patients with diabetes. Investigative ophthalmology & visual science. 2002;43(5):1588-94.

[101] Mundt GH, Jr., Hughes WF, Jr. Ultrasonics in ocular diagnosis. American journal of ophthalmology. 1956;41(3):488-98.

[102] Baum G, Greenwood I. The application of ultrasonics locating techniques to ophthalmology; theoretic considerations and acoustic properties of ocular media. I. Reflective properties. American journal of ophthalmology. 1958;46(5 Part 2):319-29.

[103] Şahin ÖG. Central corneal thickness, axial length, intraocular pressure and visual field indices in patients with ocular hypertension. Gulhane Medical Journal. 2010;52(4):266-9.

[104] Ossoinig KC. Ruling out posterior segment lesions with echography. International ophthalmology clinics. 1978;18(2):117-20.

[105] Lieb WE, Cohen SM, Merton DA, Shields JA, Mitchell DG, Goldberg BB. Color Doppler imaging of the eye and orbit. Technique and normal vascular anatomy. Archives of ophthalmology. 1991;109(4):527-31.

[106] Lieb WE, Shields JA, Cohen SM, Merton DA, Mitchell DG, Shields CL, et al. Color Doppler imaging in the management of intraocular tumors. Ophthalmology. 1990;97(12):1660-4.

[107] Baxter GM, Williamson TH. Color Doppler flow imaging in central retinal vein occlusion: a new diagnostic technique? Radiology. 1993;187(3):847-50.

[108] Romero JM, Finger PT, Rosen RB, Iezzi R. Three-dimensional ultrasound for the measurement of choroidal melanomas. Archives of ophthalmology. 2001;119(9): 1275-82.

[109] Naik MN, Tourani KL, Sekhar GC, Honavar SG. Interpretation of computed tomography imaging of the eye and orbit. A systematic approach. Indian journal of ophthalmology. 2002;50(4):339-53.

2

Tonometry

Felicia Ferreri, Rosa Minniti, Alessandra Polimeni,
Lucia Zavettieri, Giuseppina Ferreri,
Paolo Ferreri and Pasquale Aragona

1. Introduction

Tonometry is a diagnostic method which, through the use of different tools, allows the evaluation of the pressure existing inside the human eye.

An elevated intraocular pressure (IOP) is the main risk factor for the development of glaucoma, an ocular disease, that if not properly treated, causes irreversible damage to the optic nerve, leading to blindness.

The aim of tonometry is to detect the IOP that is measured in millimeters of mercury (mmHg); it is performed through the interaction with the ocular structures and in particular with the cornea. The human cornea is a curved structure with an increasing thickness from the center to the periphery and with different radius of curvature in the anterior and posterior faces. From the histological point of view, the cornea has five layers, which, from inside out are:

1. Endothelium: the inner layer made from a layer of hexagonal cells that act as a barrier modulating the penetration of substances within the corneal structure from the aqueous humor;

2. Descemet's membrane: made by collagen;

3. Stroma: it is characterized by particular cells, keratocytes, and by collagen lamellae, arranged in parallel and covered with a mucopolysaccharide substance;

4. Bowman layer: a dense acellular cluster;

5. Epithelium: the outer layer made from non-keratinized cells.

Recently, it has been identified with the electron microscope, another layer, the layer of Dua, localized in the posterior stroma, close to the Descemet's membrane. [1] The cornea, is wetted in the most external part by the tear film that consists of two layers: the mucous-aqueous and the lipid layers. Cornea and tear film play a key-role in assessing the IOP; in fact, all the clinical instruments used to measure the IOP interact with these structures, being the value of IOP obtained studing the corneal deformation resultant from the strength applied on the anterior part of the eye. Therefore tonometry is based on the biomechanical characteristics of cornea, namely the elastic and viscoelastic characteristics, and thus IOP and corneal properties are closely interdependent [2].The ease of corneal deformability is called corneal hysteresis (CH), which is calculated as the difference in air pressures between force-in applanation (P1) and force-out applanation (P2), or (P1 – P2). Studies have shown that CH is altered in various disease.

Measurement of CH also provides a more complete characterization of the contribution of corneal resistance to intraocular pressure measurements than central corneal thickness (CCT) alone [3]. However, corneal hysteresis values can be produced by various combinations of corneal thickness, rigidity, intraocular pressure, and hydration. All these factor interfere with the evaluation of the IOP.

2. Tonometry

The history of the tonometry begins in 1622, when, for the first time, Richard Banister estimated the increase of intraocular pressure (IOP) by finger pressure on the bulb (digital eye pressure) and, for several centuries, this remained the only common and simple method to evaluate IOP.

In fact, in several studies, the digital eye pressure is described as a method to assess the IOP in uncooperative patients.

Nowadays, there is a rating scale for the digital eye pressure

Nt	Normal Tension
T+	Increased Tension
T+1	Appreciable tension
T+2	Manifests tension
T+3	Hardness wooden
T-	Hypotonia
T-1	Appreciable hypotonia
T-2	Manifested hypotonia
T-3	Bulb very soft

Afterwards, several instruments were created to obtain an IOP value, in terms of pressure brought to the cornea needed to achieve the applanation of its curvature.

The tonometry can be distinguished in base at the type of corneal deformation obtained in:

- Schiötz tonometry of known weight
- Applanation tonometry to force variable
- Applanation tonometry to force constant

2.1. Schiötz tonometry of known weight

It was the first tonometer able to give reproducible results, simple and inexpensive to be used in clinical practice,being invented in 1905 by the Norwegian ophthalmologist Hjalmar Schiötz. Schiötz tonometry studies lOP by measuring the indentation of the cornea produced by a known weight applied on the corneal surface. It also measures the facility of aqueous outflow calculating the rate at which the pressure declines with time, being this related to the ease with which the aqueous leaves the eye. The decline in lOP over time can be used to determine outflow facility in micronL/min/mmHg through a series of mathematical calculations.

The Schiötz tonometer (Fig.1) is constituted by a piston, applied directly to the cornea, that moves vertically within a scale. The test is performed with the patient in the supine position. Although the test can be performed in an examination chair that reclines. The right position of the base of the scale applied on the cornea allows, to the piston and the weights fitted, to slide, until the intraocular pressure opposes to the applied force; this is indicated on the linear scale on the instrument and the resulting value is converted to millimeters of mercury by a table called "nomogram of Friedenwald" (Fig.2). Each unit of the scale indicates 1/20 mm of the cornea and evaluate the extent of the corneal deformation caused by a weighted force applied from the outside [4].The Schiötz tonometer does not require the use of the slit lamp, it is simple to use, but the IOP value obtained can be biased since repeated measurements may reduce the IOP value while the supine position is known to increase IOP [5].

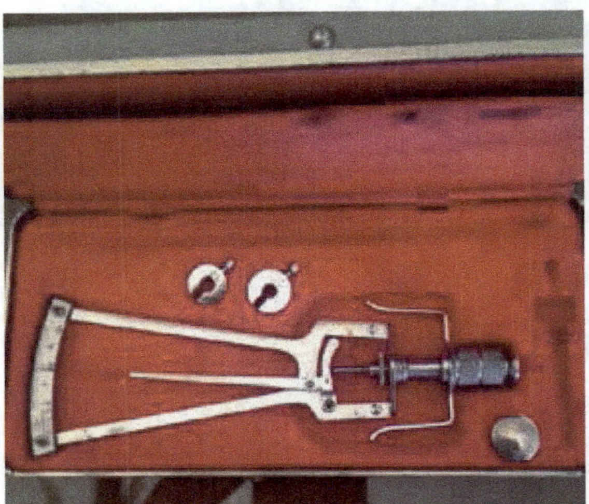

Figure 1. Schiötz tonometer of known weight

The values of IOP obtained with this tool depend on several factors: the elastic properties of the eye, aqueous humor formation and removal, scleral rigidity [6],, high myopia and ocular blood volume changes. Others factors may cause an erroneous result: calibration problems, patient position, squeezing of the eyelids during the measurement, just to name a few although these errors affect the outcome of other tonometers also to some extent. These problems reduce the accuracy and reproducibility of the Schiötz tonometry for an individual patient [7]. In general, Schiötz tonometer finds its best use as a research tool for the investigation of pharmacokinetics and is rarely used clinically.

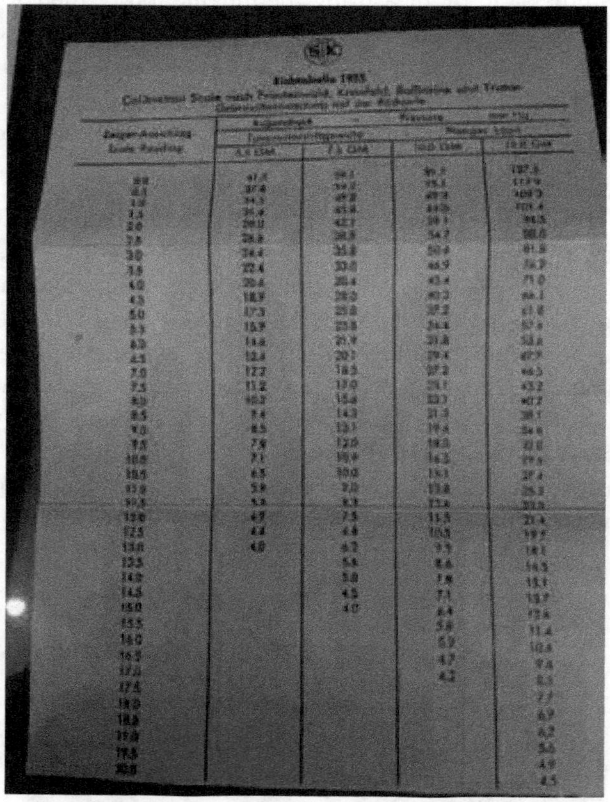

Figure 2. Nomogram of Friedenwald

2.2. Applanation tonometry to force variable

There are different type of Applanation tonometry to force variable

- Goldmann Tonometer
- Perkins Tonometer
- Draeger Tonometer

- Mackay-Marg Tonometer
- Tonopen
- Pneumatic applanation tonometer.

2.3. Goldmann applanation tonometer (GAT) (Fig.3)

This instrument is based on an interesting physical principle: the "Imbert –Flick principle", which states that the pressure inside an ideal, dry, infinitely thin, and a perfect sphere is equal to that applied to obtain the applanation of its surface. However, the human eye is not an ideal sphere, since it is not thin-walled and dry, and this produces two confounding forces:

- a force produced by the corneal rigidity (because the cornea is not infinitely thin and is usually toriodal),which is directed towards the outside of the globe;
- a force produced by the surface tension of the tear film (because the eye is not dry), which is directed towards the globe.

Goldmann estimated that a circular area of flattening, of the size of 3.06 mm of diameter applied on the cornea, is sufficient to avoid the influence of sclera and corneal rigidity and surface tension, allowing a realistic measurement of the IOP. The applanating force required to flatten this area, is directly proportional to the intraocular pressure. Specifically, the force (measured in dynes) multiplied by 10 is equal to the intraocular pressure (measured in millimeters of mercury).

The GAT is mounted on the slit lamp to produce a magnified image, and when it touches the tear film and the cornea, a circle appears as to the observer. Staining the ocular surface with fluorescein and using a cobalt blue light in the slit lamp allow obtaining a better observation of the tear film(Fig.4). The final image looks like two semicircles of exactly 3.06 mm in diameter, displaced by the presence of a prism in the head of the instrument, giving the applanation pressure when the half circles just overlap at the central end. The semicircles move with the ocular pulse, and the endpoint is reached when the inner edges of the semicircles touch each other at the midpoint of their excursion(Fig.5). At this point, the IOP value is reported, in millimeters of mercury, on the instrument dial used to modulate the pressure. This measurement is safe, easy to use and relatively accurate in most clinical situations [8].

The GAT remains the gold-standard to assess the IOP, because it is relatively unaffected by ocular rigidity.

An excessive amount of fluorescein results in wide mires and an inaccurately high reading, whereas an inadequate amount of fluorescein leads to artificially low readings.

Marked corneal astigmatism causes an elliptical fluorescein pattern, and the clinician should rotate the prism to obtain an accurate reading [9].

The accuracy of GAT is reduced in certain situations

- Corneal edema: the increased corneal thickness gives falsely high values.

- Soft corneal lens: give falsely low values.
- Scleral rigidity modifications: in the scleral buckling procedures the IOP may appear inappropriately low [10].
- The central corneal thickness (CCT): The IOP value is most accurate with a CCT of 520 micron [11].

Applanation tonometry measurements are not accurate, if CCT is increased or decreased compared to the reference values. Increased CCT may give an artificially high IOP measurement; decreased CCT, an artificially low reading [12].

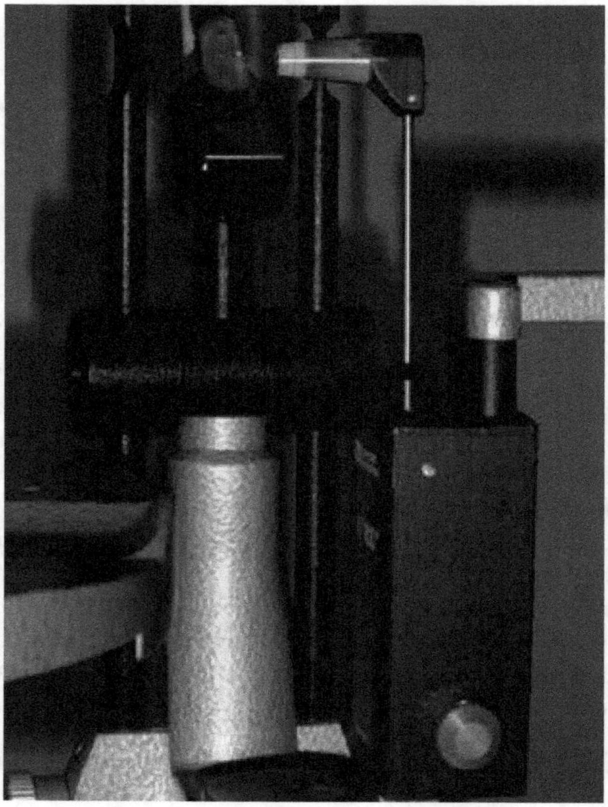

Figure 3. GAT

However, because the relationship of measured IOP and CCT is not linear, it is important to remember that the biomechanical properties of an individual cornea may vary, resulting in changes of the relative stiffness or rigidity of the cornea and altering the measurement. Currently, there is no validated correction factor for the effect of CCT on the GAT [13].

The GAT has some disadvantages [14]:

- The IOP assessment is subjective
- It 's always required the sitting position of the patient
- It is possible to transmit infections if the prism head is not disinfected before each measurement
- The pulsations of the eye can lead to excessive movements of the semicircles
- The amplitude of the semicircles, after application of fluorescein, can influence the readings of IOP
- Repeated or prolonged contact between the cornea and the tonometer may damage the corneal epithelium, resulting in a not reliable assessment of IOP
- The characteristics of the cornea (thickness, astigmatism, corneal surface regularity, viscoelastic properties) may make it difficult or incorrect the reading of the IOP values
- Excessive pressure on the eye, caused by squeezing of the eyes of the patient or by the force applied by the operator on the lid to keep the eyelids open, may induce incorrect readings
- Possible incorrect results due to an altered calibration of the tonometer

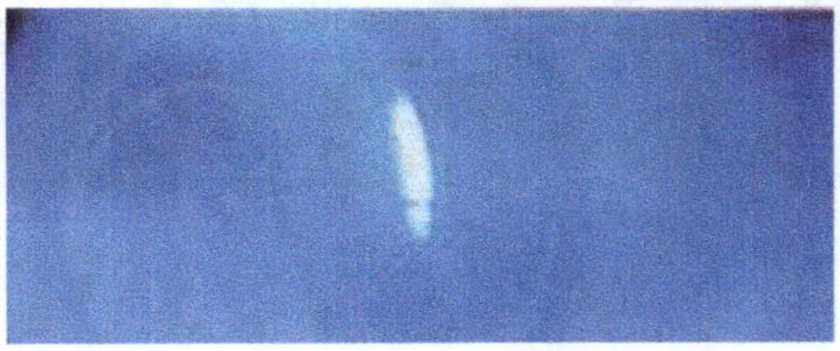

Figure 4. Semicircles

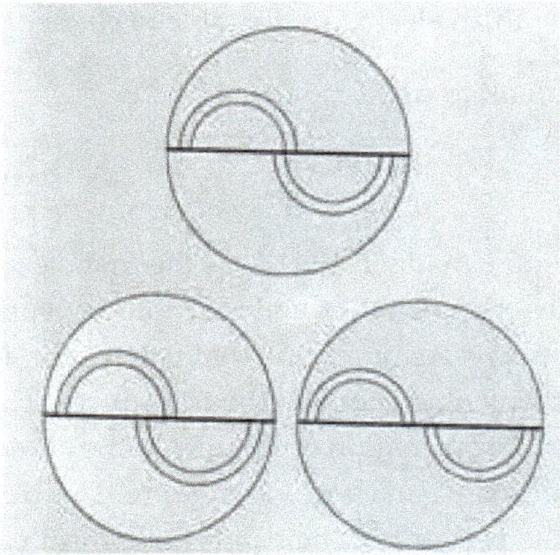

Figure 5. Semicircles readings

2.4. Perkins tonometer

The Perkins tonometer (Fig. 6) is a counterbalanced applanation tonometer that is portable and can be used with the patient either upright or supine [15].

It is similar to the GAT in using a split-image device and fluorescein stained ocular surface. However, the values of IOP are not well correlated with that obtained by Goldmann tonometer [16].

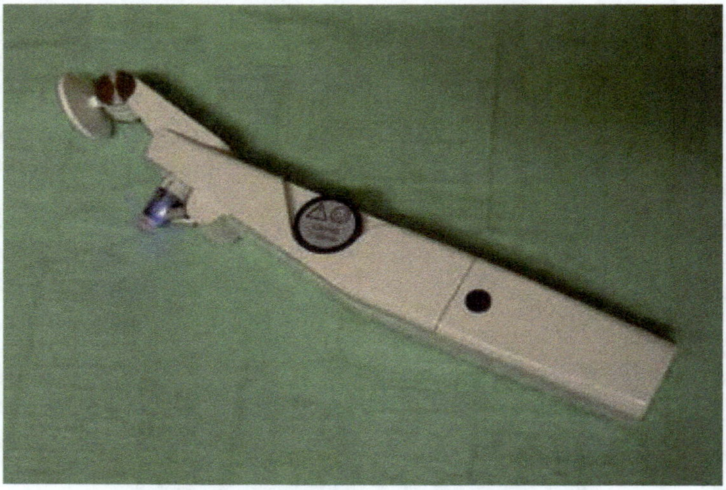

Figure 6. Perkins tonometer

2.5. Draeger tonometer

Portable version, supplied with an electric motor, able to change the applied force.

Less common and more difficult to use

2.6. Mackay-Marg tonometer

The Mackay-Marg model(Fig.7), made in 1959, was the first electronic tonometer and can be said to combine the principles of applanation and indentation. It uses a free-floating transducer to detect the transmitted pressure. An outer ring that flattens the adjacent cornea, reducing its influence on the IOP measurement, surrounds the transducer. The mobile tip that protrudes from a probe has a diameter of applanation of 1.5 mm on the corneal surface and, therefore, it is less affected by corneal thickness and corneal curvature. This device can be used in children and non-cooperative patients because of their portability and ease of use, in irregular and edematous corneas, even in the presence of LAC [17]; it gives values slightly higher compared to those obtained with the GAT [18].

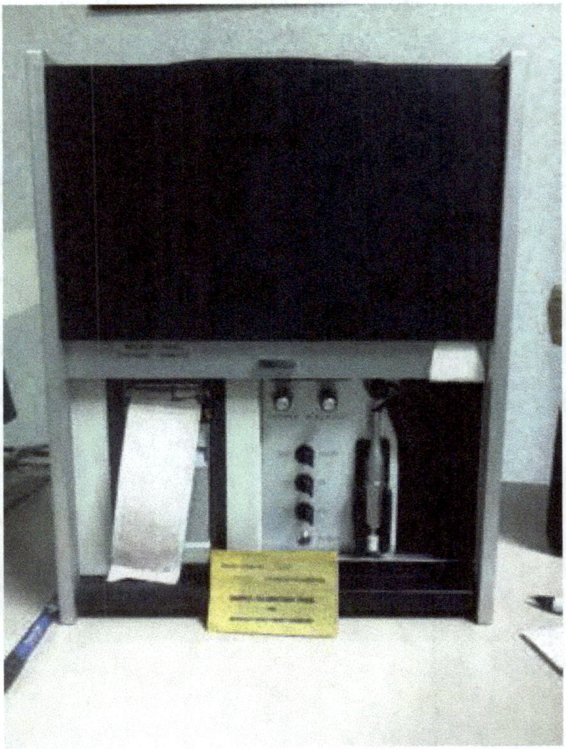

Figure 7. MACKAY-MARG TONOMETER

3. Tonopen (Fig.:8)

It is based on the principle of the MACKAY-MARG tonometer. The values of IOP are converted into an electronic signal that is processed by a microprocessor. The area of applanation is smaller than that of GAT [19].

The instrument performs 4-10 measurements and calculates the average value, giving even higher percentages of reliability for values of 24 mmHg or higher, with a good correlation with the GAT [20].

The values below to 24 mm Hg are overestimated of about 2 mmHg compared to those of GAT.

The advantages of Tonopen are:

- It can be used in irregular corneas
- it allows to perform tonometry on patients in any position
- Easy to use

The disadvantages are that in presence of important corneal irregularities it gives unreliable results.

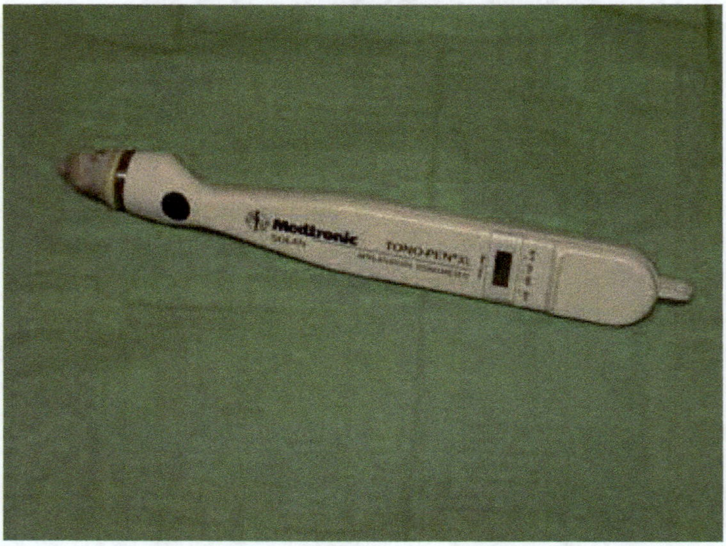

Figure 8. Tonopen

4. Pneumatic applanation tonometer (Fig.9)

The pneumatic tonometer, or pneumotonometer, has a pressure-sensing device that consists of a gas-filled chamber covered by a Silastic diaphragm. The gas in the chamber escapes through an exhaust vent.

As the diaphragm touches the cornea, the gas vent decreases in size and the pressure in the chamber rises.

Because this instrument perform an applanation on only a small area of the cornea, it is especially useful in the presence of corneal scars or edema [21].

The Ocular Blood Flow Analyzer (BFA) is a particular pneumotonometer. It performs the measurements of the IOP, 200 times per second and it records, with great precision, the amplitude of the eye pulse. It is based on the combination of a pneumatic system and an electronic system. A piston is moved by an air-flow until arriving in contact with the cornea, the force required to obtain the cornea applanation is given by the compressed air.

The air can freely exit the tool when far away from the cornea while when the probe is placed on the eye the airflow will be hampered to exit, so creating a proportional pressure. The IOP value is given as the force necessary to obtain the cornea applanation; the values are higher than that obtained by the GAT [22]. Furthermore it is known that its values are influenced by physiological variations in central corneal thickness ([23] and corneal curvature [24] and the values are also not reliable if the cornea is significantly pathological

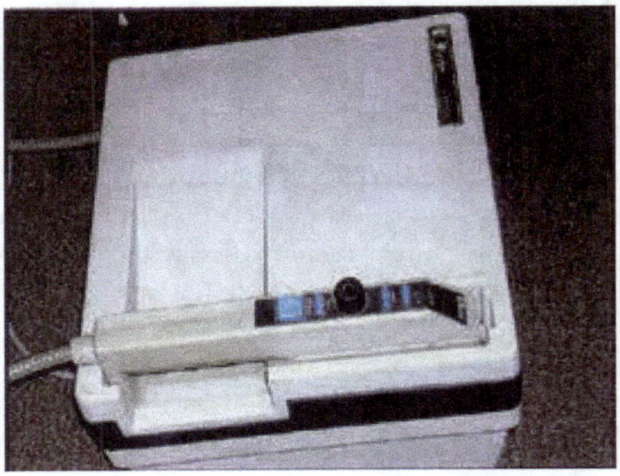

Figure 9. Pneumatic Applanation Tonometer.

5. Applanation tonometry to force variable

5.1. The Non-Contact Tonometries (NCT)

These instruments are based on two processes:

The applanation is obtained by a jet of compressed air that it is properly positioned on the cornea and checked optically ;

The applanation time is assessed by the maximum reflection of a beam incident at an angle of 45° and the speed with which it is obtained corresponds to the IOP.

The influence of corneal thickness is variable. There would be an overestimation for hypotension and underestimation for hypertension [25]

The instruments are often used in large-scale glaucoma-screening programs or by nonmedical health care providers.

5.2. Pascal dynamic contour tonometer (PDCT) (Fig. 10)

This tool entered the market recently and is based on the method of dynamic tonometry. While for the static tonometry, the tool deforms the corneal surface, and this deformation is correlated with the IOP, the dynamic tonometry is based not on the deformation itself, but on the fact that the instrument puts the applanation force on the cornea with a well-defined speed. The relationship between the time and the speed with which the deformation is achieved correlates with the value of IOP. The static IOP assessment is replaced by the concept of dynamic corneal deformation speed and inertial mass. The profiled tip of the tonometer, called SensorTip, has a radius of curvature of 10.5 mm and the contact surface has a diameter of 7.5 mm which determines a line profile with the corneal surface and the tear film. The tip is mounted on a movable arm (cantilever) which is placed on the cornea giving a force equivalent to a gram and constantly kept by a spring mechanism.

A piezo-electric tip with a diameter of 1.2 mm is placed on the center of the contact surface, generates an electrical signal proportional to the IOP.

In conclusion, the PDCT eliminates most of the systematic errors due to individual changes of corneal characteristics, which, instead, influence all types of applanation tonometers. The advantage of measuring the real pressure in combination with the ability to record the dynamic fluctuations of the pressure gives the opportunity to diagnose and classify different types of glaucoma [26]

Indeed, it is important to underline that with the PDCT tonometer is possible to obtain an accurate definition of the pressure fluctuation due to the heartbeat (ocular pulse amplitude-OPA)

In fact, the PDCT seems to be the most accurate method for measuring the ocular pulse amplitude.

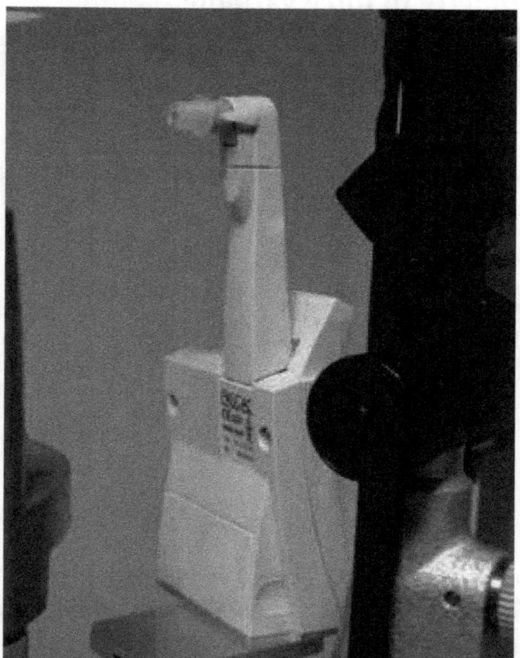

Figure 10. PDCT

5.3. Icare rebound tonometers (Fig.11)

The rebound technology is based on the rebound measuring principle, in which a very light-weight probe is used to make a momentary contact with the cornea.

In the rebound technology, motion parameters of the probe are recorded during the measurement. An induction based coil system is used for measuring the motion parameters. An advanced algorithm, combined with the state of the art software, analyzes deceleration and the contact time of the probe while it touches the cornea. Deceleration and the contact time of the probe change as a function of IOP. In simple terms, the higher the IOP, the faster the probe decelerates and the shorter the contact time.

The Icare rebound tonometer does not require any maintenance calibration, the anaesthesia is not needed since the touch of the probe is so gentle that the measurement is barely noticed by the patient [27].

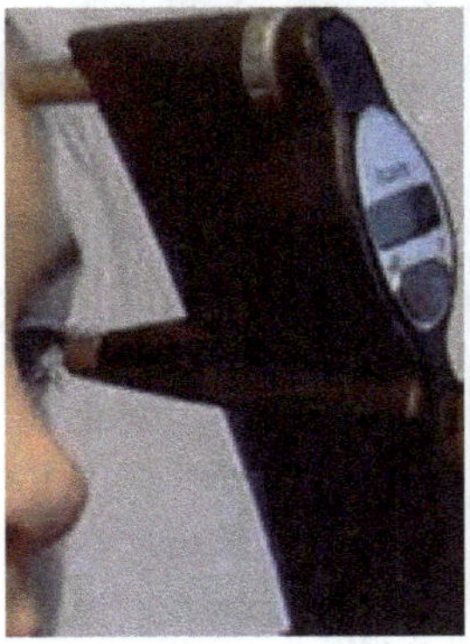

Figure 11. Icare

5.4. The self-tonometers (Fig.13)

The Proview phosphene tonometer is based on an entoptic phenomenon called phosphene (flash of light); that is a feeling of light obtained from the retina by non-luminous stimuli. It looks like a pen, but inside it is present in a small, flat probe, an internal spring and a graduated scale for the values of IOP.

The patient can measure the IOP several times a day, with a device safe, easy to use and inexpensive. The measurement is carried out through the upper lid, does not require either anesthesia or fluorescein stain, it is portable, does not require batteries or electrical outlets.

The patient puts the instrument on the upper eyelid, at the root of the nose, and he presses until he sees a phosphene, and the IOP is recorded.

There is not a corneal applanation, and then tonometry can be performed on the abnormal corneas or after ocular surgery [28].

The Proview may be useful for perform a self-tonometry, but it needs to be calibrated with the GAT to have a good correlation between the values obtained by the two instruments [29]

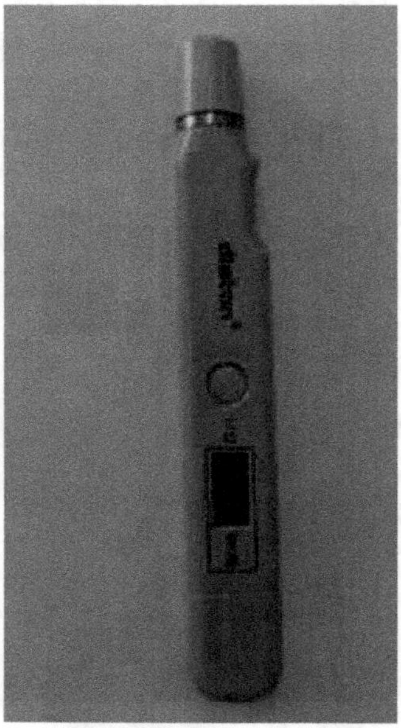

Figure 12. Self Tonometer

5.5. iCare tonometer

This tool is ideal for all patients treated with anti-glaucoma medications.

iCare tonometer is used in the diagnosis, follow-up and screening of intraocular pressure.

The iCare is an handheld tonometer, which is based on the impact-induction principle also known as rebound tonometry [31] The main advantages of this device include its quick and simple use, and that local anesthesia and slitlamp are not needed.

iCare tonometer has shown good reproducibility [31]and correlation with GAT and other tonometers in healthy and glaucomatous eyes. [31,32,33,34] Although iCare was designed not to be influenced by corneal properties, studies have shown that CCT and other corneal structural characteristics affect iCare IOP readings [32,33,34,35,36]

6. Sensory system lenses

This system consists of a soft contact lens attached to a micro-voltage detection unit connected to the external recording tool. It is still a prototype and several physiological parameters such as the tear film and eyelid movements need to be evaluated.

Another type of lens is the tonometric gonioscopic Smart Lens.

The values obtained are overestimated compared to those obtained with the Goldmann of approximately 4-5 mmHg.

6.1. The continuous measurement tonometry

Based on methods that allow evaluating the IOP through the application of a sensor to lens applied on the cornea, during the day, or to an intra-ocular lens (IOL). The latter system allows to obtain continuous values of IOP, without interference of the corneal thickness and curvature. This sensor, made of silicone, is applied on the IOL and has a plate shape divided into 4 parts where there are some cavities that generate a specific electrical voltage. The intraocular pressure fluctuations change the silicone structure and consequently the generate voltage. The chip present on the lens transforms the electric pulses into digital signals that are sent to a tool, called Photodisc, constituted by radio waves and a coil. The receiver is inserted in special glasses and is connected to a portable display. The values of IOP are sent to the photodisc and then displayed on the external display expressed in mmHg [37]

Conclusion Tonometry is the fastest, simple, and popular way to assess the IOP, which is the main risk factor for the glaucoma disease. The GAT is considered, the gold-standard for the assessment of IOP. Over the centuries it has been tried to develop accurate tonometers, searching for the true IOP value, and not altered from the biomechanical characteristics of the human eye. The way to the pursuit of the best tonometer is still long, but certainly the evolution of technology in ophthalmology will permit to develop more and more sophisticated and accurate tools to defeat the "thief of sight": glaucoma.

Author details

Felicia Ferreri[1], Rosa Minniti[1], Alessandra Polimeni[1], Lucia Zavettieri[1], Giuseppina Ferreri[1], Paolo Ferreri[2] and Pasquale Aragona[1]

1 Institute of Ophthalmology, University of Messina, Italy

2 Institute of Ophthalmology, University of Bari, Italy

References

[1] Dua HS, Faraj LA, Said DG, Gray T, Lowe J. Human corneal anatomy redefined: a novel pre-Descemet's layer (Dua's layer). Ophthalmology. 2013 Sep;120(9):1778-85.

[2] Shah S, Laiquzzaman M, Bhojwani R, Mantry S, Cunliffe I: Assessment of the biomechanical properties of the cornea with the ocular response analyzer in normal and keratoconic eyes. Invest Ophthalmol Vis Sci 2007, 48(7):3026-3031.

[3] Touboul D, Roberts C, Kerautret J, Garra C, Maurice-Tison S, Saubusse E, Colin J: Correlations between corneal hysteresis, intraocular pressure, and corneal central pachymetry. Journal of cataract and refractive surgery 2008, 34(4):616-622.

[4] .Moses RA, Grodzki WJ. Theory and calibration of the Schiötz tonometer. VII. Experimental results of tonometric measurements: scale reading versus indentation volume. Invest Ophthalmol. 1971 Sep;10(9):716-23.

[5] Friedenwald Js.: Jun;52:543-7

[6] Pemberton JW.: Schiötz-applanation disparity following retinal detachment surgery.Arch Ophthalmol. 1969 Apr;81(4):534-7.

[7] Friedenwald Js.: Some problems in the calibration of tonometers. Am J Ophthalmol. 1948 Aug;31(8):935-44.

[8] Goldmann H, Schmidt T. Applanation tonometry. Ophthalmologica. 1957 Oct;134(4): 221-42.

[9] Holladay JT, Allison ME, Prager TC.Goldmann applanation tonometry in patients with regular corneal astigmatism. Am J Ophthalmol. 1983 Jul;96(1):90-3.

[10] Johnson MW, Han DP, Hoffman KE. The effect of scleral buckling on ocular rigidity. Ophthalmology. 1990 Feb;97(2):190-5.

[11] Ehlers N, Bramsen T, Sperling S.: Applanation tonometry and central corneal thickness. Acta Ophthalmol. 1975 Mar;53(1):34-43.

[12] Doughty MJ, Jonuscheit S.: Effect of central corneal thickness on Goldmann applanation tonometry measures-a different result with different pachymeters. Graefes Arch Clin Exp Ophthalmol. 2007 Nov;245(11):1603-10.

[13] Kohlhaas M, Boehm AG, Spoerl E, Pürsten A, Grein HJ, Pillunat LE :Effect of central corneal thickness, corneal curvature, and axial length on applanation tonometry. Arch Ophthalmol. 2006 Apr;124(4):471-6.

[14] Whitacre MM, Stein R.:Sources of error with use of Goldmann-type tonometers. Surv Ophthalmol. 1993 Jul-Aug;38(1):1-30

[15] Dunn JS, Brubaker RF: Perkins applanation tonometer. Clinical and laboratory evaluation. Arch Ophthalmol. 1973 Feb;89(2):149-51

[16] Arora R, Bellamy H, Austin M. Applanation tonometry: a comparison of the Perkins handheld and Goldmann slit lamp-mounted methods. Clin Ophthalmol. 2014 Mar 26;8:605-10.

[17] Kaufman HE, Wind CA, Waltman SR: Validity of Mackay-Marg electronic applanation tonometer in patients with scarred irregular corneas. Am J Ophthalmol. 1970 Jun;69(6):1003-7.

[18] Moses Ra, Marg E, Oechsli R. Evaluation of the basic validity and clinical usefulness of the Mackay-Marg tonometer.Invest Ophthalmol. 1962 Feb;1:78-85.

[19] Hessemer V, Rössler R, Jacobi KW: Tono-Pen, a new tonometer. Int Ophthalmol. 1989 Jan;13(1-2):51-

[20] Deuter CM, Schlote T, Hahn GA, Bende T, Derse M.: Measurement of intraocular pressure using the Tono-Pen in comparison with Goldmann applanation tonometry- a clinical study in 100 eyes. Klin Monbl Augenheilkd. 2002 Mar;219(3):138-42.

[21] West CE, Capella JA, Kaufman HE.Measurement of intraocular pressure with a pneumatic applanation tonometer. Am J Ophthalmol. 1972 Sep;74(3):505-9.

[22] Pianka O Geyer O : Comparison of the pneumatonometry with applanation tonometry. Inv Ophthalmology Vis Sci 1998; 39: 4309

[23] Doughty MJ, Zaman ML Human corneal thickness and its impact on intraocular pressure measures: a review and meta-analysis approach. Surv Ophthalmol. 2000 Mar-Apr;44(5):367-408.

[24] Gunvant P, Baskaran M, Vijaya L, Joseph IS, Watkins RJ, Nallapothula M, Broadway DC, O'Leary DJ.Effect of corneal parameters on measurements using the pulsatile ocular blood flow tonograph and Goldmann applanation tonometer.Br J Ophthalmol. 2004 Apr;88(4):518-22.

[25] Shields MB. The non-contact tonometer. Its value and limitations. Surv Ophthalmol. 1980 Jan-Feb;24(4):211-9.

[26] Ku JY, Danesh-Meyer HV, Craig JP, Gamble GD, McGhee CN. Comparison of intraocular pressure measured by Pascal dynamic contour tonometry and Goldmann applanation tonometry.Eye (Lond). 2006 Feb;20(2):191-8.

[27] Fernandes P1, Díaz-Rey JA, Queirós A, Gonzalez-Meijome JM, Jorge J. Comparison of the ICare rebound tonometer with the Goldmann tonometer in a normal population. Ophthalmic Physiol Opt. 2005 Sep;25(5):436-40

[28] Groenhoff S, Draeger J, Deutsch C, Wiezorrek R, Hock B.: Self-tonometry: technical aspects of calibration and clinical application. Int Ophthalmol. 1992 Sep;16(4-5): 299-303.

[29] Avarez TL Gollance SA The Proview Phosphene tonometer fails to measure ocular pressure accurately in clinical practice,Ophthalmology 2004 Jun;111(6):1077-85

[30] Witte V, Glass Ä, Beck R, Guthoff R.Evaluation of the self-tonometer Icare ONE in comparison to Goldmann applanation tonometry.Ophthalmologe. 2012 Oct;109(10): 1008-13.

[31] Kontiola AI. A new induction-based impact method for measuring intraocular pressure. Acta Ophthalmol Scand. 2000;78:142–145.

[32] Martinez-de-la-Casa JM, Garcia-Feijoo J, Castillo A, Garcia-Sanchez J. Reproducibility and clinical evaluation of rebound tonometry. Invest Ophthalmol Vis Sci. 2005;46:4578–4580.

[33] Nakamura M, Darhad U, Tatsumi Y, Fujioka M, Kusuhara A, Maeda H, et al. Agreement of rebound tonometer in measuring intraocular pressure with three types of applanation tonometers. Am J Ophthalmol. 2006;142:332–334.

[34] Martinez-de-la-Casa JM, Garcia-Feijoo J, Vico E, Fernandez-Vidal A, Benitez del Castillo JM, Wasfi M, et al. Effect of corneal thickness on dynamic contour, rebound, and Goldmann tonometry. Ophthalmology. 2006;113:2156–2162.

[35] Brusini P, Salvetat ML, Zeppieri M, Tosoni C, Parisi L. Comparison of ICare tonometer with Goldmann applanation tonometer in glaucoma patients. J Glaucoma. 2006;15:213–217.

[36] Chui W, Lam A, Chen D, Chiu R. The influence of corneal properties on rebound tonometry. Ophthalmology. 2008;115:80–84.

[37] Mottet B, Aptel F, Romanet JP, Hubanova R, Pépin JL, Chiquet C. 24-hour intraocular pressure rhythm in young healthy subjects evaluated with continuous monitoring using a contact lens sensor. Jama Ophthalmol 2013 Dec;131(12):1507-16

3

Dry Eye — An Insight into Meibomian Gland Dysfunction

Vikas Tah, Kamran Saha, James Myerscough, Muhammad Ahad, Jason Ho, Pranev Sharma, Farihah Tariq and Stephen Tuft

1. Introduction

The term 'Dry Eyes' was first coined in 1950 by the Ophthalmologist Andrew De Roeth (1893–1981): a dacryologist who introduced the term dry eye. For decades it was thought dry eyes was limited to a reduction in the aqueous phase of the tear film. It was as recent as 1995 that dry eyes was eventually recognised as a multifaceted ocular pathology which was due to decreased tear production and increased tear evaporation [1]. In this chapter we will focus on the latter, specifically looking at meibomian gland dysfunction.

An estimate of the prevalence of dry eyes is difficult given that many sufferers may be asymptomatic or dismissive of subjective questionnaires of their symptoms if mild. Various studies estimate the prevalence as between 7.4% to 33.7% [2-3]. The epidemiology of dry eye depends on the mode of diagnosis, population surveyed and study cited.

Large American epidemiological studies estimate symptomatic dry eyes to affect 7% of women and 4% of men over the age of 50 years in the United States [4]. Similar data is seen in Australian studies [3]. The far eastern studies report the largest proportion of dry eye sufferers with Taiwan having the highest at 33.7% [5] followed by Japan and Indonesia [6].

2. Meibomian gland dysfunction

The meibomian glands, named after the German physician Meibom in 1966, are specialised sebaceous glands within the eyelids. They number 20-5 on the lower lids and up to 50 on the upper lid. Meibomian glands are responsible for secretion of a lipid rich mixture call meibum onto the tear surface through small openings found on the lid margin. A single gland consists of a central duct linked to multiple acini via ductules. Meibum is loaded into acini and released into the central duct where it moves to the openings on the lid margin and ocular surface. The glands undergo constant renewal and are delicate owing to their holocrine nature.

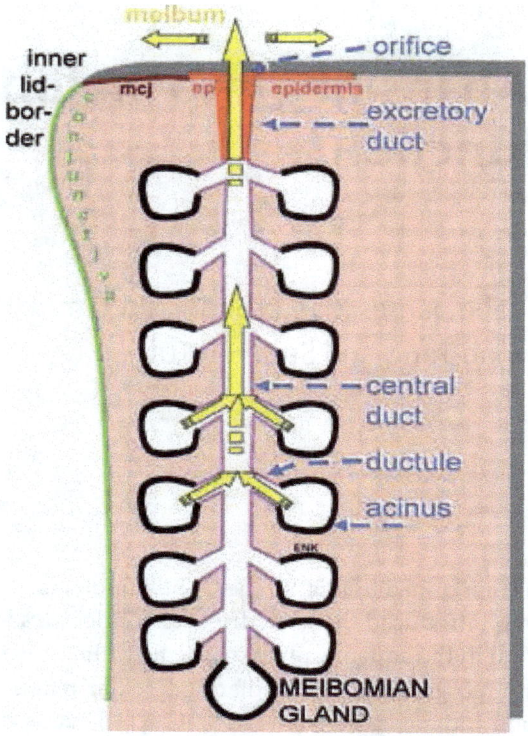

Scheme 1. Diagram courtesy of International Workshop on Meibomian Gland Dysfunction

It is widely thought that reduced meibum quality and quantity in addition to hyperkeratinisation of the ductal epithelium are the main reasons for meibomian gland dysfunction (MGD). Hyperkeratinised ducts and thicker meibum secretions lead to obstruction of the ducts. A progressive increase in pressure from continuous meibum secretion causes widening of the duct, acinar atrophy with cornification of duct epithelia. Ultimately there is reduced meibum secretion and gland drop out causing an unstable tear film. [7]

The tear film lubricates the ocular surface, which is vital to its maintaining its function and well being. It also forms a vital role in light refraction in the air-tear-cornea interface. Tear film is structured into 3 primary layers: The inner layer comprises mucin and a layer of glycocalyx that is synthesised by the conjunctiva and epithelial cells. The lacrimal gland primarily secretes the middle aqueous layer. The outermost lipid layer is secreted by the meibomian gland. This superficial layer stabilises the tear film by preventing its evaporation. Meibomian gland dysfunction is the most common cause of evaporative dry eye. Left untreated dry eye initially causes irritating ocular surface symptoms and signs that can threaten visual impairment, cause corneal perforation and blindness.[8]

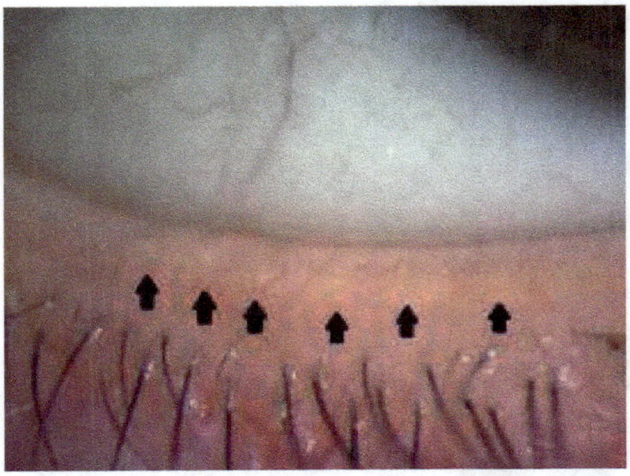

(courtesy of Stoke Mandeville Hospital)

Figure 1. Lower lid meibomian glands

Broadly meibomian gland dysfunction can be defined as *a chronic, diffuse abnormality of the meibomian glands commonly characterized by terminal duct obstruction and/or qualitative/quantitative changes in the glandular secretion. It may result in alteration of the tear film, symptoms of eye irritation, clinically apparent inflammation, and ocular surface disease[9-10].*

3. Aetiology

Meibomian gland dysfunction can affect many different groups.

Age is a major risk factor for the development of MGD. It is more common in the elderly. Studies in humans seem to mirror the effects in animals [9]. Decreased acinar proliferation, atrophy and altered localisation of the lipogenesis factor PPARγ (regulates meibomian differentiation and secretion) are seen in mice. Elderly patients have been noted to have a higher rate of meibomian glad dropout [10-11] with half as many functioning glands between 20 to 80 years of age. Human cadaveric studies show gland orifice metaplasia and narrowing [12-13] with hyperkeratinisation and lipogranulomatous inflammatory changes. Additionally meibum composition changes with age yielding a reduced volume and increased viscosity [10-14].

Androgens are known to be integrally involved in differentiation of sebaceous glands all over the body and have been shown to promote genes essential for meibomian function [13-14] Furthermore, complete androgen insensitivity syndrome has been shown to have altered meibomian glands and composition of lipid secretions that resulted in clinically apparent signs and symptoms of MGD [15-16].

Confusingly, chronic blepharitis has been suggested as a cause for MGD. Whilst MGD itself is a cause of chonic blepharitis, there is considerable overlap with other causes of chronic blepharitis that may accentuate MGD. One study showed 74% (42 of 57) chronic blepharitis sufferers had evidence of meibomian gland loss on meibography whereas 20% (4) of matched normal patients had any dropout. More detailed understanding is needed regarding the overlap of MGD with chronic blepharitis [18-19].

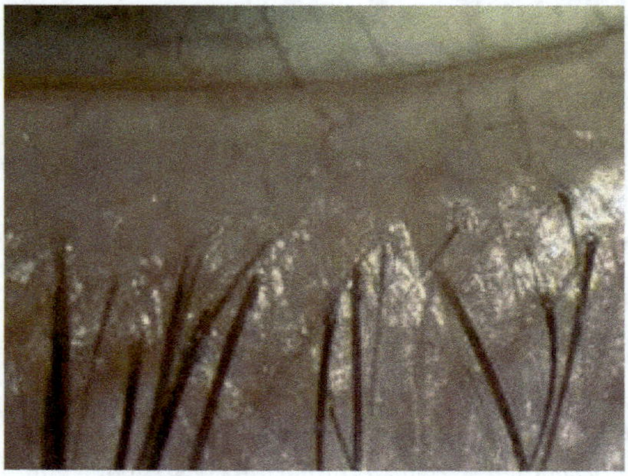

Figure 2. Lower lid meibomian glands and dropout in an elderly patient (courtesy of S Tuft)

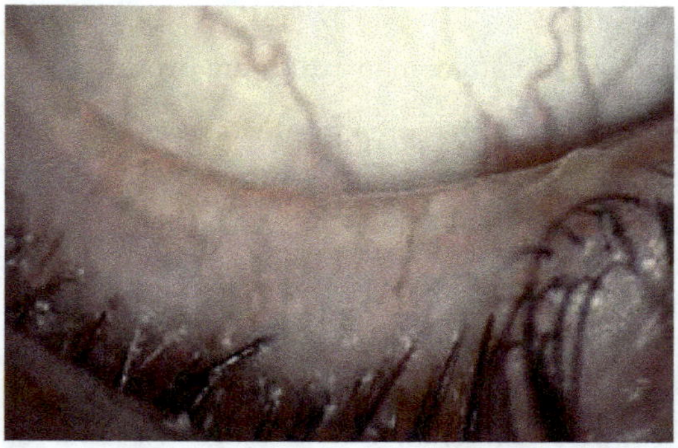

Figure 3. Meibum secretions of elderly patient showing increased plugging and viscosity (courtesy of S Tuft)

Demodex mites are the most common ectoparasites found in human skin. Of this species *D.brevis* is thought to be the most pertinent in MGD [20]. Current thinking is that the mite burrows deep into sebaceous and meibomian glands to feed on sebum and meibum respectively, as this forms as its main food source. Its chitinous exoskeleton causes a granulomatous reaction which ultimately leads to a mechanical blockage of the gland. *D.brevis* has been found in the centre of granulomatous meibomian glands surrounded by histocytes, epithelioid cells, fibroblasts and plasma cells which may thus offer a potential explanation for refractory and recurrent chalazia in some patients. [21]

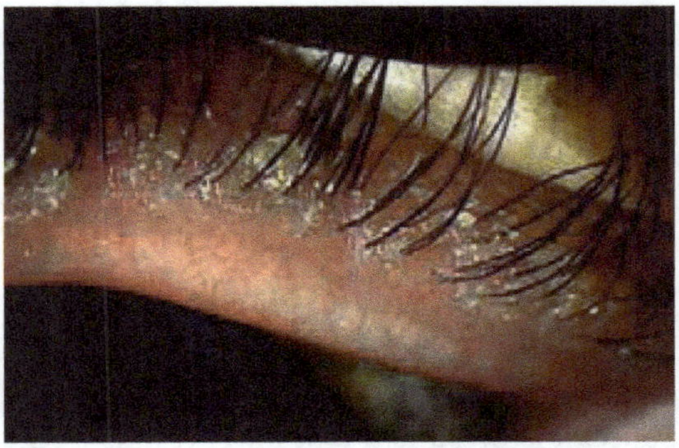

Figure 4. Desmodex infested lashes with meibomian gland dysfunction

Contact lens wear can increase the risk of MGD. Studies utilising meibography have shown that contact lenses alter meibomian gland morphology with greater rates of dropout than non-contact lens wearers. The duration and type of contact lens was weakly associated with this. By inserting and removing contact lenses, desquamated epithelial cells have been shown to obstruct the duct orifice leading to stagnation and atrophy [22-23]. While some studies show a statistically significant increase in MGD in contact lens wearers [22-24] others did not show significant differences [25-26]. It is important however to bear in mind these studies defined meibomain gland dysfunction differently. Damage to stem cells at the limbus is likely to be different based on duration on contact lens wear and may help account for the differences.

Environment may play a role in MGD. It is likely that factors such as temperature, humidity and visual undertaking have an accentuating impact rather than develop MGD. For example, concentrated computer use may be associated with reduced blink rate, exacerbating symptoms of MGD. One study of 70 patients found 74% of video display terminal users had MGD [27]. Decreased conjunctival temperature has been suggested to cause obstructive MGD through increased meibum viscosity [28-29].

Various medical conditions have been associated with MGD. Polycystic ovary syndrome (PCOS), where there is often insulin resistance and hyperinsulinaemia can result in increased androgen synthesis. Androgen receptors have been found in meibomian glands with a possible effect on function [30-33]. Twenty two (22)% of PCOS patients had MGD compared to 13% of normals in one study [34].

Dyslipidaemia appears to be associated with MGD. Patients with moderate to severe MGD have a higher incidence of dyslipidemia with respect to elevated total cholesterol than the general population [35-36]. Higher meibomian cholesterol ester levels are associated with MGD in humans [37].

Sjorgen's syndrome has been shown to have a higher incidence of MGD. One study found a higher incidence of MGD in MGD related dry eye to other causes of dry eye. The actual association, whether causative or a consequence of dry eye is not established and further study is needed [38-39]

Multiple medications have been implicated as possible risk factors for MGD. Studies looking at the acne treatment isotretinoin, 13-cis retinoic acid, have found that this resulted in altered meibum secretion, atrophy of the gland, reduced tear break up time and dry eye symptoms [40-41]. Other studies have looked at medication under the umbrella category of dry eye, not specially MGD. There may however be some overlap with MGD. Included in this category are antihistamines. One study has shown that treatment of allergic conjunctivitis with once daily loratidine resulted in signs of ocular dryness [42-43].

Post-menopausal hormone therapy has been associated with MGD [44-47] although the pathophysiology is not fully understood. Whilst established that sex hormone levels change from pre-to post-menopause, it is presumed that PMH results in changes to meibum gland secretions that can lead to MGD. Higher estrogen levels post-menopausally have been implicated in reduced tear function [45]. The largest of the studies, looking at 3500 patients from the Blue Mountain Study has shown a statistically significant 60% higher prevalence of dry eye in PMH users. A longer duration of use has been associated with longer symptoms [44].

Anitidepressant use has been associated with a higher risk of evaporative dry eye symptoms. Often many such medications simply have visual blurring only as a side effect without any mention of dry eye disease [48-51].

Omega 3 oils have been shown to have a beneficial effect on MGD whilst omega 6 oils have an opposite effect. Both are essential for growth and development. The omega 3 oils are found naturally in Mediterranean diets, flaxseed and cod liver oil [52]. Omega 6 oils are found typically in Northern European diets containing high red meat and less of the above [52]. The most detailed study to date showed a reduction in meibum thickness, dry eye signs and tear break up time in those with a high omega 3 to omega 6 ratio [53], agreeing with previous findings [52, 54. 55]. These oils compete for an enzyme involved in the inflammatory pathwaytherefore it is the ratio of omega 3 and 6 that is crucial. The ideal omega 6:3 ratio is 4:1 but typical Northern European and American diets are in the realm of 14:1 A higher omega 6 to 3 ratio results in overproduction of pro-inflammatory PGE2 from omega 6 and underproduction of anti-inflammatory PGE1 and PGE3 via omega 3 that induces MGD [53].

4. Presentation

Meibomian gland dysfunction is the leading cause of evaporative dry eye. As such patients will present with dry eye symptoms.

Most patients with MGD are likely to be asymptomatic. The vast majority will not experience any symptoms unless it is moderate in nature or exacerbated by other causes of evaporative dry eye. Burning, irritation, redness, watering or intermittent visual blur are frequently described. It is important to ask what time of day this occurs to try to distinguish from other causes of dry eye. Blepharitis is typically worse in the morning with redness, crusting, puffiness, itchy lids or a 'gritty sensation' within the eyes.

5. Clinical assessment

There are different ways to assess meibomian gland dysfunction. Whilst a slit lamp is certainly beneficial and the commonest form of assessment, one can simply use a direct ophthalmoscope for those in primary care settings. Though it does not give as detailed a view the principles are the same as for slit lamp examination. The key is to observe the meibomian glands and ocular surface. With the ophthalmoscope one needs to place on high magnification to view the state of the meibomian glands which are located posterior to the greyline Often orifices can be seen to be plugged, or pouting. Surrounding tissue can be erythematous with telangiectatic vessels. Misdirected eyelashes can also be a sign of eyelid inflammatory changes. A good clinical examination will also include eversion of the eyelids which will often show white, hard deposits called concretions on the tarsal conjunctiva, follicles or granulomatous changes from previous chalazia. The ocular surface should also be assessed. Important to evaporative dry eyes is assessment of the tear film break up (TFBUT). This is done by instilling fluorescein sodium 2% (although 0.25% is an acceptable alternative) and asking the patient to blink a few times. The patient should then be asked to keep their eyes open and careful note of the time taken for vacuoles to appear in the tear film. A normal time frame is 10-15 seconds. The ocular surface should also be noted for punctate epithelial erosions which can be wide-spread or mainly inferior. In severe cases mucous filaments have been noted on the cornea. Abrasions can also be seen in those with associated in-turned eyelashes. The conjunctiva can be injected to varying degrees. As MGD is almost always bilateral, a unilateral presentation must alert the clinician of the possibility of basal cell carcinoma or meibomian cell carcinoma.

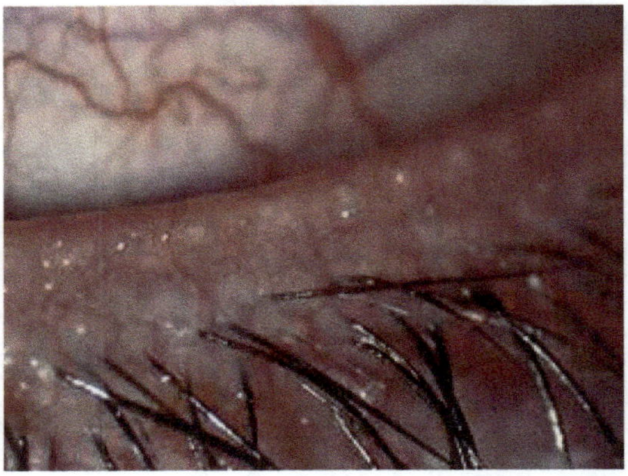

Figure 5. Thickened meibomian secretions i

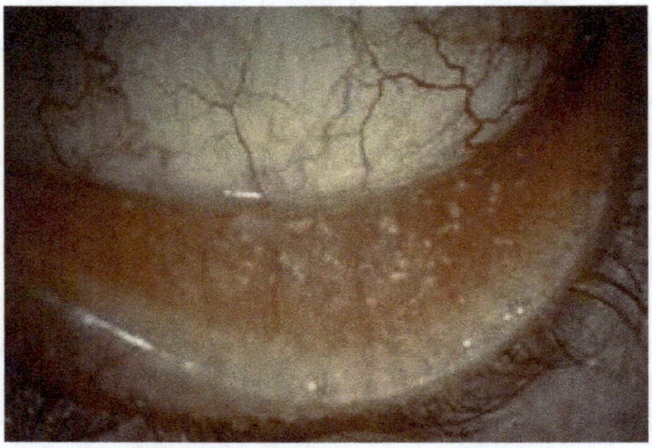

Figure 6. Concretions on the lower lid (courtesy of S Tuft)

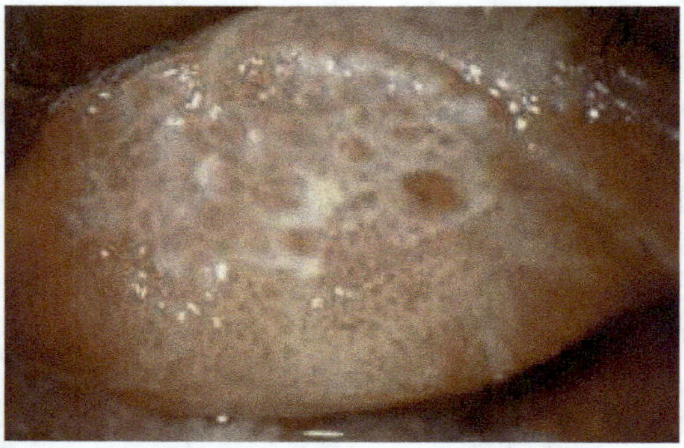

Figure 7. Follicles and sebaceous material (courtesy of S Tuft)

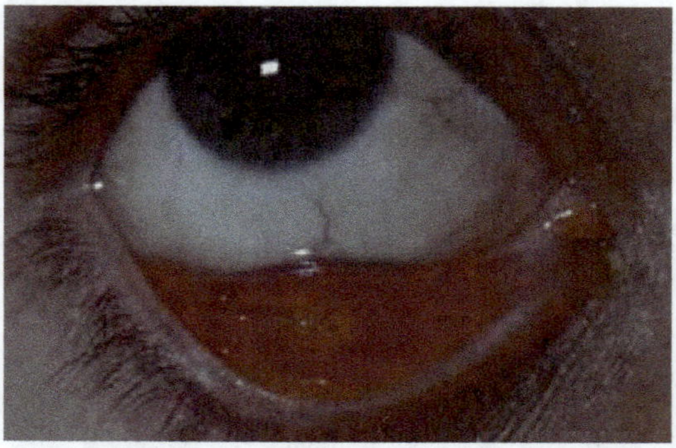

Figure 8. Chalazion on lower lid (courtesy of S Tuft)

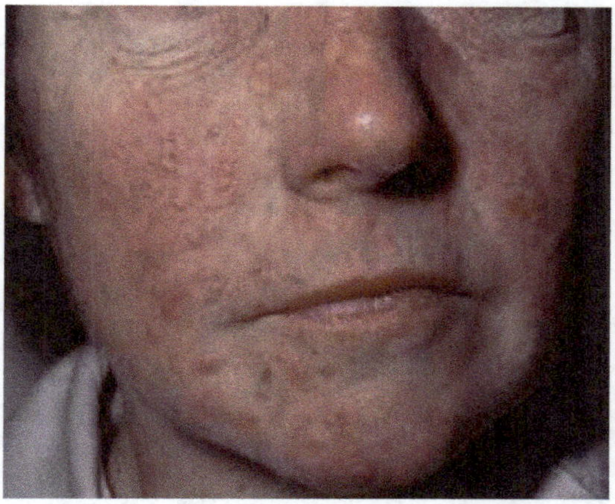

Figure 9. Rosacea above is associated with meibomian gland dysfunction (courtesy of S Tuft)

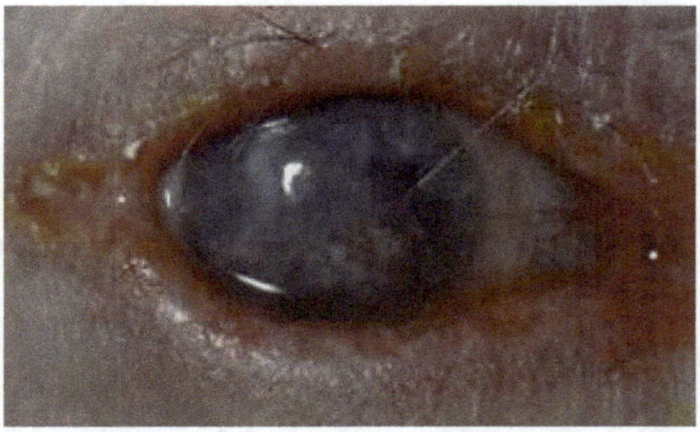

Figure 10. Trichiatic lashes resulting in corneal damage (courtesy of S Tuft)

There is no universal classification system of MGD. Different approaches have been used. The International Workshop Meibomian Gland subcommittee have recommended categorisation into 4 subtypes, although this is not universally applied.

1. MGD alone Asymptomatic Symptomatic (noncicatricial, cicatricial)
2. MGD with associated with ocular surface damage
3. MGD-related evaporative dry eye
4. MGD associated with other ocular disorders.

Alternatively, clinical measurement has been described. This is based on lid signs and meibum quality. Meibum can be graded on the Oxford score scale 0-3 (0=clear, 1=cloudy, 2=cloudy/particulate and 3=toothpaste like) [107].

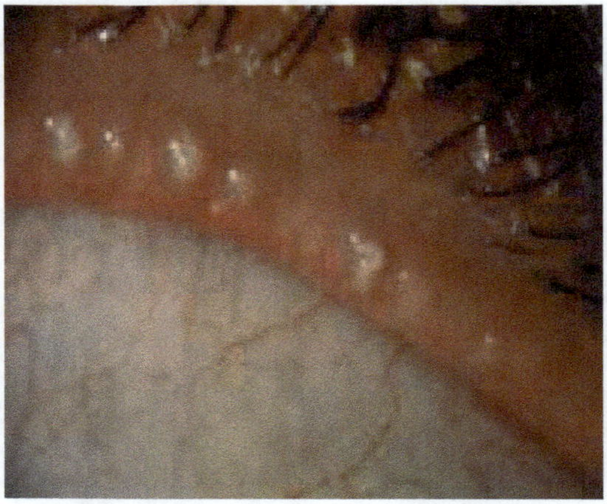

Figure 11. cloudy and particulate meibum: Oxford scale 2

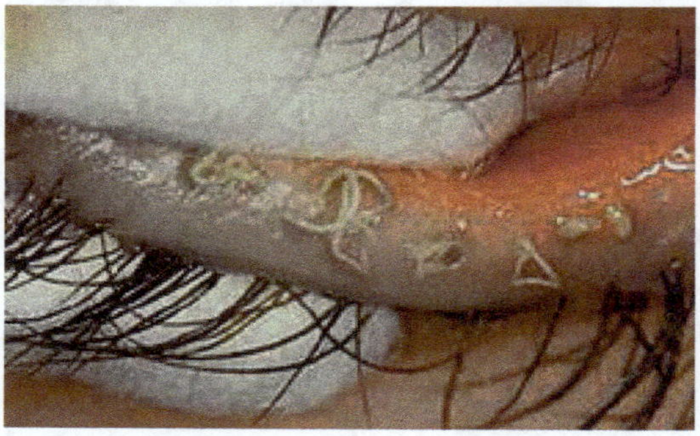

Figure 12. Toothpaste like meibum: Oxford score 3

5.1. Differential

A common misnomer is that MGD and posterior blepharitis are interchangeable terms [56-58]. Some previous literature has used the terms as such. MGD though, is one cause of posterior blepharitis (inflammation of the lid margins) and must be distinguished from other causes based on the anatomical structures of the posterior lid. Other causes include conjunctivitis (allergic or infective) and dermatological (acne rosacea or sebhorreic dermatitis).

Anterior blepharitis is another differential. This refers to inflammation anterior to the gray line, particularly around the lashes. The gray line anatomically subdivides the anterior and posterior lamellae of the lid. Anterior blepharitis can result in scurf on lashes, collarettes at the lash base and vascular changes of the eyelids.

5.2. Treatment principles

Typically treatment is predominantly based on the general term 'lid hygeine', ocular lubricants and antibiotics. There are more recent advances in the field and these are described further below.

Lid hygeine as a method varies across different centres [59]. Currently there is no standardised method. Commonly patients are told to either to place a warm compress over the lids at least twice daily or massage the lids for 10 minutes during each session. Compresses alone have been shown to cause transient visual blurring [60-61]. Active massage is encouraged. MGD secretions have been shown to have higher melting (35 C) points relative to normal (32C) [62-63]. The warmness melts the pathological meibum within the glands and active massage helps to unblock the glands. The authors feel that cotton wool whilst more gentle on the eye is often not firm enough to dislodge meibum that a flannel or towel is able to do. Lid hygeine is made more efficient by encouraging active massage just under the lashes themselves so the patient can directly affect the glands themselves. This needs to be demonstrated to patients directly. By pressing the lateral canthus firmly, traction can be provided and using a flannel the pulp of the finger swept gently over the inner aspect of the upper and lower lids. This needs to be balanced against any possible damage to the ocular and careful explanation and assessment of patient technique needs to be balanced against this [64-65]. The use of mild baby shampoo over the lids has also been advocated as part of lid hygeine. Ultimately patients need to be educated that lid hygiene is the basis upon which MGD will be controlled and that compliance is crucial in not only reducing symptoms but preventing recurrence.

Physical expression of the meibomian glands has been described [66-67]. Methods vary from gentle lid palpation to forceful squeezing of the lids. Use of a finger on the outer lid and a rigid object on the inner aspect like a metal paddle have been reported [68]. Often considerable force is needed to express pathological meibum and transient visual blurring owing to corneal distortion has been reported [60-61]. We believe that the risks involved and potential discomfort from this outweigh any benefit and do not recommend this.

Ocular lubricants are helpful to provide symptomatic relief. They help to alleviate symptoms experienced secondary to evaporative dry eye and do not treat the MGD itself. It is important for patients to realise that they are not a cure but give temporary respite. Ocular lubricants are helpful in bolstering the tear film volume, spreading of tears [69] and providing a layer over the cornea that reduced the possibility of corneal erosion from friction of the lid moving over the cornea by blinking [70-71]. The ocular lubricants may also help wash away pro-inflammatory molecules and dilute the concentration of inflammatory cytokines in tears. This has not been tested and remains a speculative theory presently.

Much research has been based around the contents of ocular lubricants. Preservatives can cause discomfort and toxicity to the corneal epithelium. Frequently used preservatives like benzylalkonium chloride and polyquaternium have been shown to decrease goblet cell density and thus affect tear film stability [72-77]. There is no evidence nor consensus on frequency of usage. It should be based on an individual level. Preservative free drops are recommended in severe dry eye where high frequency drops are required. More recently so called vanishing preservatives such as sodium perborate or sodium chlorite have been incorporated into artificial tears. There is a lack of data to date to suggest whether these have the intended less preservative toxicity than the traditional preservatives mentioned.

Lipid supplemented tears have been shown of benefit in MGD [79-84]. Patients have reported reduced symptoms with an increased tear break up time and thicker lipid layer of the tear film. Castor oil drops have been shown to reduce tear break up time in a randomised control trial [84]. Temporary visual blurring has been reported in older studies that used ointments but more recent formulations have not been shown to have this problem [84]

Leading from this is the viscosity of the ocular lubricant. The greater the viscosities the more benefit in bulking tear film thickness and volume in dry eyes [85-87] as well as increased transit time on the eye. This needs to be counterbalanced against visual blurring and inconvenience.

Antibiotics are often used in MGD. The exact pathogenesis of bacteria remains not entirely understood. However the presence of bacterial flora on the lid surface, notably staphylococcus epidermidis, staph aureus, propion acnes amongst others is known. It may be the case that the keratinisation of the meibum and abnormal lipids provide prime conditions for normal bacterial flora to produce enzymes such as lipases and exotoxins resulting in proinflammatory changes. Thus an antibiotic would need to be effective against common flora.

Macrolides are commonly used. Studies have shown that they exert many anti-inflammatory effects. Neutrophil activity is affected by downregulating adhesion protein expression [88]. Phagocytosis and chemotaxis are affected through this. A reduction in proinflammatory cytokines has been demonstrated [89-90].

Tetracyclines have multiple helpful anti-inflammatory properties, including influencing neutrophil chemotaxis and proliferation of lymphocytes [91-92]. Matrix metalloproteinases and inflammatory cytokines like IL1 are suppressed as are anti-angiogenesis properties [93-94]. Collagenase 2 (matrix metalloproteinase P8) is directly suppressed by doxycycline specifically. They have been established for treatment of acne rosacea. Lipase production of the typical bacterial flora such as S epidermidis is suppressed. The lipases are responsible for production of pro-inflammatory free fatty acids that can detstabilise the tear film and directly alter meibum composition. The tetracyclines as a group have varying lipophillicity that alters individual drug pharmacokinetics. The international workshop on meibomian gland dysfunction recommend the use of doxycycline and minocycline [96]. These have been shown to be clinically effective at lower doses relative to tetracycline, which is poorly lipophilic and has been found at lower relative concentrations in tears after 5 days [97-100]. Typically doxycycline or monocycline are given at 100mg dosage for 2 months.

Dietary modification have been popular treatments amongst patients. Omega 3 rich foods as can be found in flax seed or cod-liver oil have been shown to have improved meibum scores, tear break up time and surface signs [100-102]. Omega 6 rich foods such as red meat have a counter effect and should be discouraged [101].

Surgical management is reserved for complications from MGD. Typically this would occur where the MGD is severe. Chalazia can be treated with incision and curettage where they are inflamed and affecting vision. Eyelid cicatrisation may cause trichiatic lashes that can commonly undergo epilation or electrolysis. Lid laxity, ectropion or entropion may be treated surgically.

Recently, devices have been created to be worn by patients to help with lid hygiene. These include blepharitis goggles, which aim to provide heat and moisture via steam to unclog blocked meibomian glands [103-104].LipiFlow® Thermal Pulsation System is similar but provides heat therapy and physical pressure to express the meibomian glands [105]. These variables can be adjusted accordingly, and seems to offer more favourable outcomes over 12 months than typical lid hygiene and lubricating drops [105]. The evidence base for such devices is currently limited further studies on outcomes and potential side effects are needed.

5.3. Primary care setting

It is understandably difficult to make an unambiguous diagnosis of meibomian gland dysfunction without a slit lamp in primary care or on the ward.

However through careful history of symptoms and possible risk factors mentioned earlier, along with a direct ophthalmoscope on high magnification, an informed judgment can be made. Use of the direct ophthalmoscope does require practice to look at anterior surface structures in detail. Most hand held ophthalmoscopes have a cobalt blue mode, meaning that with available fluroscein drops an evaluation of the tear break up time and state of the corneal surface can be undertaken.

Where MGD is suspected, we would recommend starting lid hygiene, taking care to assess whether the patient is capable of performing this safely without damage to anterior structures. If there is suspicion of anterior surface structure damage from unsafe hygiene measures or possible other causes we recommend referral without starting lid hygiene. Prescribing suitable preservative free lubricating eye drops is recommended before ophthalmic referral.

6. Conclusion

Meibomian gland dysfunction is the most common ocular sign encountered in patients and cause of evaporative dry eye. Whilst awareness of the condition improves and research continues to be undertaken, a universal consensus on the definition, pathophysiology, signs and management is still being awaited. This is needed to allow for earlier detection and optimal structured treatment for MGD. Further questions do need to be answered regarding meibomian gland dysfunction too. Owing to a lack in consensus over definition and clinical tests performed in studies there is difficulty comparing results in different studies. The International Workshop for Meibomian Gland Dysfunction have suggested future research aim to prioritise a specific validated questionnaire for symptoms, a standard grading system of signs and validated outcomes for MGD [106]. It is hoped this will provide greater clarity in diagnosing, understanding the extent and severity of disease. Ultimately this would allow the most suitable treatment to be started improving the level of patient care in meibomian gland dysfunction.

Author details

Vikas Tah[1,2*], Kamran Saha[2], James Myerscough[3], Muhammad Ahad[1], Jason Ho[2], Pranev Sharma[4], Farihah Tariq[5] and Stephen Tuft[2]

1 Stoke Mandeville Hospital, UK

2 Moorfields Eye Hosptial London, UK

3 Colchester University Hospital NHS Foundation Trust, UK

4 Chelsea and Westminister Hospital, UK

5 Raigmore Hospital Inverness, UK

References

[1] CLAO J. 1995 Oct;21(4):221-32. Report of the National Eye Institute/Industry workshop on Clinical Trials in Dry Eyes. Lemp MA.

[2] Ophthalmology. 2003 Jun;110(6):1096-101. Prevalence of dry eye among an elderly Chinese population in Taiwan: the Shihpai Eye Study. Lin PY, Tsai SY, Cheng CY, Liu JH, Chou P, Hsu WM.

[3] Ophthalmology. 1998 Jun;105(6):1114-9. The epidemiology of dry eye in Melbourne, Australia. McCarty CA, Bansal AK, Livingston PM, Stanislavsky YL, Taylor HR.

[4] Am J Ophthalmol. 2003 Aug;136(2):318-26. Prevalence of dry eye syndrome among US women. Schaumberg DA, Sullivan DA, Buring JE, Dana MR.

[5] Results of a population-based questionnaire on the symptoms and lifestyles associated with dry eye. Shimmura S, Shimazaki J, Tsubota K. Br J Ophthalmol. 2002 Dec; 86(12):1347-51.

[6] Prevalence and risk factors associated with dry eye symptoms: a population based study in Indonesia. Lee AJ, Lee J, Saw SM, Gazzard G, Koh D, Widjaja D, Tan DT.

[7] The international workshop on meibomian gland dysfunction: report of the subcommittee on anatomy, physiology, and pathophysiology of the meibomian gland. Knop E, Knop N, Millar T, Obata H, Sullivan DA. Invest Ophthalmol Vis Sci. 2011 Mar 30;52(4):1938-78. doi: 10.1167/iovs.10-6997c. Print 2011 Mar. Review. No abstract available.

[8] Research in dry eye: report of the Research Subcommittee of the International Dry Eye WorkShop(2007). [No authors listed] Ocul Surf. 2007 Apr;5(2):179-93. Review. PMID:17508121

[9] Aging and dry eye disease. Ding J, Sullivan DA. Exp Gerontol. 2012 Jul;47(7):483-90. doi: 10.1016/j.exger.2012.03.020. Epub 2012 Apr 28. Review. PMID:22569356

[10] Norn, M., 1987. Expressibility of meibomian secretion. Relation to age, lipid precorneal film, scales, foam, hair and pigmentation. Acta Ophthalmol. 65, 137–142.

[11] Arita, R., Itoh, K., Inoue, K., Amano, S., 2008. Noncontact infrared meibography to document age-related changes of the meibomian glands in a normal population. Ophthalmology 115, 911–915

[12] Hykin, P.G., Bron, A.J., 1992. Age-related morphological changes in lid margin and meibomian gland anatomy. Cornea 11, 334–342

[13] Sullivan, B.D., Evans, J.E., Dana, M.R., Sullivan, D.A., 2006. Influence of aging on the polar and neutral lipid profiles in human meibomian gland secretions. Arch. Ophthalmol. 124, 1286–1292.

[14] Schirra, F., Richards, S.M., Liu, M., Suzuki, T., Yamagami, H., Sullivan, D.A., 2006. Androgen regulation of lipogenic pathways in the mouse meibomian gland. Exp. Eye Res.

[15] Krenzer, K.L., Dana, M.R., Ullman, M.D., Cermak, J.M., Tolls, D.B., Evans, J.E., Sullivan, D.A., 2000. Effect of androgen deficiency on the human meibomian gland and ocular surface. J. Clin. Endocrinol. Metab. 85, 4874–4882

[16] Sullivan, B.D., Evans, J.E., Cermak, J.M., Krenzer, K.L., Dana, M.R., Sullivan, D.A., 2002a. Complete androgen insensitivity syndrome: effect on human meibomian gland secretions. Arch. Ophthalmol. 120, 1689–1699.

[17] Sullivan, B.D., Evans, J.E., Dana, M.R., Sullivan, D.A., 2002b. Impact of androgen deficiency on the lipid profiles

[18] Mathers WD, Shields WJ, Sachdev MS, Petroll WM, Jester JV. Meibomian gland dysfunction in chronic blepharitis. Cornea. 1991;10:277–285

[19] The international workshop on meibomian gland dysfunction: report of the subcommittee on the epidemiology of, and associated risk factors for, MGD. Schaumberg DA, Nichols JJ, Papas EB, Tong L, Uchino M, Nichols KK. Invest Ophthalmol Vis Sci. 2011 Mar 30;52(4):1994-2005. doi: 10.1167/iovs.10-6997e. Print 2011 Mar. Review. No abstract available.

[20] Corneal manifestations of ocular demodex infestation. Clinical treatment of ocular demodecosis by lid scrub with tea tree oil. Gao YY, Di Pascuale MA, Elizondo A, Tseng SC Cornea. 2007 Feb; 26(2):136-43.

[21] Am J Ophthalmol. 1985 Sep 15;100(3):482-3.Desmodectic mites and chalazion. English FP, Cohn D, Groeneveld ER.

[22] Korb DR, Henriquez AS. Meibomian gland dysfunction and contact lens intolerance. J Am Optom Assoc. 1980;51:243–251

[23] Henriquez AS, Korb DR. Meibomian glands and contact lens wear. Br J Ophthalmol. 1981;65:108–111

[24] Ong BL, Larke JR. Meibomian gland dysfunction: some clinical, biochemical and physical observations. Ophthalmic Physiol Opt. 1990;10:144–148

[25] Prevalence of Meibomian gland dysfunction. Hom MM, Martinson JR, Knapp LL, Paugh JR Optom Vis Sci. 1990 Sep; 67(9):710-2.

[26] Relation between contact lens wear and Meibomian gland dysfunction. Ong BL Optom Vis Sci. 1996 Mar; 73(3):208-10.

[27] Meibomian gland dysfunction and ocular discomfort in video display terminal workers.

[28] Fenga C, Aragona P, Cacciola A, Spinella R, Di Nola C, Ferreri F, Rania L Eye (Lond). 2008 Jan; 22(1):91-5.

[29] Nagymiha´lyi A, Dikstein S, Tiffany JM. The influence of eyelid temperature on the delivery of meibomian oil. *Exp Eye Res*. 2004;78(3):367-370

[30] Baudouin C. The pathology of dry eye. *Surv Ophthalmol*. 2001;45:211–220.

[31] McCulley JP, Shine WE. The lipid layer of tears: Dependent on meibomian gland function. *Exp Eye Res*. 2004;78:361–365.

[32] Sutphin JE, Chodosh J, Dana MR, et al. Normal physiology of the ocular surface. In: Liesegang TJ, Skuta GL, Cantor LB, eds. *Basic and Clinical Science Course External Disease and Cornea*. San Francisco: American Academy of Ophthalmology; 2005: 47–52.

[33] Sullivan DA, Sullivan BD, Ullman MD, et al. Androgen influence on the meibomian gland. *Invest Ophthalmol Vis Sci*. 2000;41:3732–3742.

[34] Curr Eye Res. 2008 Feb;33(2):133-8. Meibomian gland alterations in polycystic ovary syndrome. Yavas GF, Ozturk F, Kusbeci T, Ermis SS, Yilmazer M, Cevrioglu S, Aktepe F, Kose S.

[35] Association of dyslipidemia in moderate to severe meibomian gland dysfunction. Dao AH, Spindle JD, Harp BA, Jacob A, Chuang AZ, Yee RW. Am J Ophthalmol. 2010 Sep;150(3):371-375.e1. doi: 10.1016/j.ajo.2010.04.016

[36] Ophthal Plast Reconstr Surg. 2013 Mar-Apr;29(2):101-3. doi: 10.1097/IOP.0b013e31827a007d. Associations between the grade of meibomian gland dysfunction and dyslipidemia. Bukhari AA.

[37] Shine WE, McCulley JP. The role of cholesterol in chronic blepharitis. *Invest Ophthalmol Vis Sci* 1991;32: 2272–2280.

[38] Meibomian gland dysfunction in patients with Sjögren syndrome. Shimazaki J, Goto E, Ono M, Shimmura S, Tsubota K Ophthalmology. 1998 Aug; 105(8):1485-8.

[39] Tear evaporation rates in Sjögren syndrome and non-Sjögren dry eye patients. Goto E, Matsumoto Y, Kamoi M, Endo K, Ishida R, Dogru M, Kaido M, Kojima T, Tsubota K Am J Ophthalmol. 2007 Jul; 144(1):81-85

[40] Ocular side effects associated with 13-cis-retinoic acid therapy for acne vulgaris: clinical features, alterations of tearfilm and conjunctival flora. Egger SF, Huber-Spitzy V, Böhler K, Raff M, Scholda C, Barisani T, Vecsei VP. Acta Ophthalmol Scand. 1995 Aug; 73(4):355-7.

[41] Ocular side effects of isotretinoin therapy.[J Am Optom Assoc. 1988] Caffery BE, Josephson JE J Am Optom Assoc. 1988 Mar; 59(3):221-4.

[42] Prevalence of and risk factors for dry eye syndrome.[Arch Ophthalmol. 2000] Moss SE, Klein R, Klein BE Arch Ophthalmol. 2000 Sep; 118(9):1264-8.

[43] An open-label, investigator-masked, crossover study of the ocular drying effects of two antihistamines, topical epinastine and systemic loratadine, in adult volunteers with seasonal allergic conjunctivitis.Ousler GW 3rd, Workman DA, Torkildsen GL. Clin Ther. 2007 Apr; 29(4):611-6.

[44] Dry eye in post-menopausal women using hormone replacement therapy.[Maturitas. 2007] Erdem U, Ozdegirmenci O, Sobaci E, Sobaci G, Göktolga U, Dagli S Maturitas. 2007 Mar 20; 56(3):257-62.

[45] W.D. Mathers, D. Strovall, J.A. Lane, M.B. Zimmerman Menopause and tear function: the influence of prolactin and sex hormones on human tear production Cornea, 17 (4) (1998), pp. 353–358

[46] B.E. Klein, R. Klein, L.L. Ritter Is there evidence of estrogen effect on age-related lens opacities? The Beaver Dam Eye Study Arch Ophthalmol, 112 (1994), pp. 85–91

[47] Chia EM, Mitchell P, Rochtchina E, Lee AJ, Maroun R, Wang JJ. Prevalence and associations of dry eye syndrome in an older population: The Blue Mountains Eye Study. Clin Exp Ophthalmol. 2003;31:229–232

[48] Schaumberg DA, Dana R, Buring JE, Sullivan DA. Prevalence of dry eye disease among US men: estimates from the Physicians' Health Studies. Arch Ophthalmol. 2009;127:763–768

[49] Long-term incidence of dry eye in an older population. Moss SE, Klein R, Klein BE Optom Vis Sci. 2008 Aug; 85(8):668-74.

[50] Wilkes S Bupropion. Drugs Today (Barc) 2006;42 (10) 671-681 PubMed

[51] Hudson JIPerahia DGGilaberte IWang FWatkin JGDetke MJ Duloxetine in the treatment of major depressive disorder: an open-label study. *BMC Psychiatry* 2007;743 PubMed

[52] Omega-3 Dietary Supplementation in Dry Eye and Blepharitis Trans Am Ophthalmol Soc / Vol 106 / 2008 338

[53] Calder PC. N-3 Polyunsaturated fatty acids and inflammation: from molecular biology to the clinic. Lipids 2003;38:343-352

[54] Simopoulos AP. The Mediterranean diets: what is so special about the diet of Greece? The scientific evidence. J Nutr 2001;131:3065-3073S.

[55] Am J Clin Nutr. 2005 Oct;82(4):887-93. Relation between dietary n-3 and n-6 fatty acids and clinically diagnosed dry eye syndrome in women. Miljanović B, Trivedi KA, Dana MR, Gilbard JP, Buring JE, Schaumberg DA.

[56] Meibomian keratoconjunctivitis. McCulley JP, Sciallis GF Am J Ophthalmol. 1977 Dec; 84(6):788-93.

[57] McCulley JP, Dougherty JM, Deneau DG. Classification of chronic blepharitis. Ophthalmology. 1982;89:1173–1180

[58] Luchs J. Efficacy of topical azithromycin ophthalmic solution 1% in the treatment of posterior blepharitis. Adv Ther. 2008;25:858–870

[59] The international workshop on meibomian gland dysfunction: report of the subcommittee on management and treatment of meibomian gland dysfunction. Geerling G, Tauber J, Baudouin C, Goto E, Matsumoto Y, O'Brien T, Rolando M, Tsubota K, Nichols KK. Invest Ophthalmol Vis Sci. 2011 Mar 30;52(4):2050-64. doi: 10.1167/iovs.10-6997g. Review

[60] Warm compress induced visual degradation and Fischer-Schweitzer polygonal reflex. Solomon JD, Case CL, Greiner JV, Blackie CA, Herman JP, Korb DR Optom Vis Sci. 2007 Jul; 84(7):580-7.

[61] Goto E, Monden Y, Takano Y, et al. Treatment of non-inflamed obstructive meibomian gland dysfunction by an infrared warm compression device. Br J Ophthalmol. 2002;86:1403–1407

[62] Assessment of meibomian gland function in dry eye using meibometry. Yokoi N, Mossa F, Tiffany JM, Bron AJ. Arch Ophthalmol. 1999 Jun; 117(6):723-9

[63] Review Meibomian secretions in chronic blepharitis. McCulley JP, Shine WE Adv Exp Med Biol. 1998; 438():319-26.

[64] Smith GT, Dart J. External eye disease. In: Jackson TL, editor. ed. Moorfields Manual of Ophthalmology. Philadelphia: Mosby Elsevier; Chap 4:2008

[65] Ehler J, Shah ChP. Wills Eye Manual. Philadelphia: Lippincott Williams & Wilkins; 2008

[66] Krenzer, K.L., Dana, M.R., Ullman, M.D., Cermak, J.M., Tolls, D.B., Evans, J.E., Sullivan, D.A., 2000. Effect of androgen deficiency on the human meibomian gland and ocular surface. J. Clin. Endocrinol. Metab. 85, 4874–4882

[67] Sullivan, B.D., Evans, J.E., Cermak, J.M., Krenzer, K.L., Dana, M.R., Sullivan, D.A., 2002a. Complete androgen insensitivity syndrome: effect on human meibomian gland secretions. Arch. Ophthalmol. 120, 1689–1699.

[68] Mastrota K. The meibomian Mastrota paddle. Rosenberg, TX: Cynacon/Ocusoft, Inc., 2006. Available at http://www.ocusoft.com/for-eye-care-professionals/surgical/misc-surgical-instruments/mastrota-meibomian-paddle.html Accessed: July 16, 2010

[69] Rheology of tear film lipid layer spread in normal and aqueous tear-deficient dry eyes. Yokoi N, Yamada H, Mizukusa Y, Bron AJ, Tiffany JM, Kato T, Kinoshita S Invest Ophthalmol Vis Sci. 2008 Dec; 49(12):5319-24

[70] Lid-wiper epitheliopathy and dry-eye symptoms in contact lens wearers. Korb DR, Greiner JV, Herman JP, Hebert E, Finnemore VM, Exford JM, Glonek T, Olson MC CLAO J. 2002 Oct; 28(4):211-6.

[71] Prevalence of lid wiper epitheliopathy in subjects with dry eye signs and symptoms. Korb DR, Herman JP, Blackie CA, Scaffidi RC, Greiner JV, Exford JM, Finnemore VM Cornea. 2010 Apr; 29(4):377-83

[72] Labbe A, Pauly A, Liang H, et al. Comparison of toxicological profiles of benzalkonium chloride and polyquaternium-1: an experimental study. J Ocul Pharmacol Ther. 2006;22:267–278

[73] Fraunfelder FW. Corneal toxicity from topical ocular and systemic medications. Cornea. 2006;25:1133–1138. [PubMed]

[74] Debbasch C, Brignole F, Pisella PJ, Warnet JM, Rat P, Baudouin C. Quaternary ammoniums and other preservatives' contribution in oxidative stress and apoptosis on Chang conjunctival cells. Invest Ophthalmol Vis Sci. 2001;42:642–652. [PubMed]

[75] Furrer P, Mayer JM, Plazonnet B, Gurny R. Ocular tolerance of preservatives on the murine cornea. Eur J Pharm Biopharm. 1999;47:105–112. [PubMed]

[76] Palmer RM, Kaufman HE. Tear film, pharmacology of eye drops, and toxicity. Curr Opin Ophthalmol. 1995;6:11–16. [PubMed]

[77] Lapalus P, Ettaiche M, Fredj-Reygrobellet D, Jambou D, Elena PP. Cytotoxicity studies in ophthalmology. Lens Eye Toxic Res. 1990;7:231–242. [PubMed]

[78] Burstein NL. Corneal cytotoxicity of topically applied drugs, vehicles and preservatives. Surv Ophthalmol. 1980;25:15–30

[79] Low-concentration homogenized castor oil eye drops for noninflamed obstructive meibomian gland dysfunction. Goto E, Shimazaki J, Monden Y, Takano Y, Yagi Y, Shimmura S, Tsubota K Ophthalmology. 2002 Nov; 109(11):2030-5.

[80] Topical omega-3 and omega-6 fatty acids for treatment of dry eye. Rashid S, Jin Y, Ecoiffier T, Barabino S, Schaumberg DA, Dana MR Arch Ophthalmol. 2008 Feb; 126(2):219-25.

[81] Rieger G. Lipid-containing eye drops: a step closer to natural tears. Ophthalmologica. 1990;201:206–212. [PubMed]

[82] Tiffany JM. Lipid-containing eye drops. Ophthalmologica. 1991;203:47–49. [PubMed]

[83] Korb DR, Scaffidi RC, Greiner JV, et al. The effect of two novel lubricant eye drops on tear film lipid layer thickness in subjects with dry eye symptoms. Optom Vis Sci. 2005;82:594–601. [PubMed]

[84] Craig JP, Purslow C, Murphy PJ, Wolffsohn JS. Effect of a liposomal spray on the pre-ocular tear film. Cont Lens Anterior Eye. 2010;33:83–87

[85] Dynamic distribution of artificial tears on the ocular surface. Wang J, Simmons P, Aquavella J, Vehige J, Palakuru J, Chung S, Feng C Arch Ophthalmol. 2008 May; 126(5):619-25.

[86] Simmons PA, Vehige JG. Clinical performance of a mid-viscosity artificial tear for dry eye treatment. Cornea. 2007;26:294–302

[87] Khanal S, Tomlinson A, Pearce EI, Simmons PA. Effect of an oil-in-water emulsion on the tear physiology of patients with mild to moderate dry eye. Cornea. 2007;26:175–181.

[88] Sanz MJ, Nabah YN, Cerda-Nicolas M, et al. Erythromycin exerts in vivo anti-inflammatory activity downregulating cell adhesion molecule expression. *Br J Pharmacol.* 2005;144:190–201.

[89] Bosnar M, Bosnjak B, Cuzic S, et al. Azithromycin and clarithromycin inhibit lipopolysaccharide-induced murine pulmonary neutrophilia mainly through effects on macrophage-derived granulocyte-macrophage colony-stimulating factor and interleukin-1beta. *J Pharmacol Exp Ther.* 2009;331:104–113.

[90] Yamaryo T, Oishi K, Yoshimine H, Tsuchihashi Y, Matsushima K, Nagatake T. Fourteen-member macrolides promote the phosphatidylserine receptor-dependent phagocytosis of apoptotic neutrophils by alveolar macrophages. *Antimicrob Agents Chemother.* 2003;47:48 –53.

[91] Sanchez J, Somolinos AL, Almodovar PI, Webster G, Bradshaw M, Powala C. A randomized, double-blind, placebo-controlled trial of the combined effect of doxycycline hyclate 20-mg tablets and metronidazole 0.75% topical lotion in the treatment of rosacea. *J Am Acad Dermatol.* 2005;53:791–797.

[92] Sneddon IB. A clinical trial of tetracycline in rosacea. *Br J Dermatol.* 1966;7

[93] Li DQ, Lokeshwar BL, Solomon A, Monroy D, Ji Z, Pflugfelder SC. Regulation of MMP-9 production by human corneal epithelial cells. *Exp Eye Res.* 2001;73:449–459.8:649–652.

[94] Sobrin L, Liu Z, Monroy DC, et al. Regulation of MMP-9 activity in human tear fluid and corneal epithelial culture supernatant. *Invest Ophthalmol Vis Sci.* 2000;41:1703–1709.

[95] Beardsley RM, De Paiva CS, Power DF, Pflugfelder SC. Desiccating stress decreases apical corneal epithelial cell size–modulation by the metalloproteinase inhibitor doxycycline. *Cornea.* 2008;27: 935–940.

[96] The international workshop on meibomian gland dysfunction: report of the subcommittee on management and treatment of meibomian gland dysfunction. Geerling G, Tauber J, Baudouin C, Goto E, Matsumoto Y, O'Brien T, Rolando M, Tsubota K, Nichols KK. Invest Ophthalmol Vis Sci. 2011 Mar 30;52(4):2050-64.

[97] Ta CN, Shine WE, McCulley JP, Pandya A, Trattler W, Norbury JW. Effects of minocycline on the ocular flora of patients with acne rosacea or seborrheic blepharitis. *Cornea.* 2003;22:545–548.

[98] Aronowicz JD, Shine WE, Oral D, Vargas JM, McCulley JP. Short term oral minocycline treatment of meibomianitis. *Br J Ophthalmol.* 2006;90:856–860.

[99] Hoeprich PD, Warshauer DM. Entry of four tetracyclines into saliva and tears. *Antimicrob Agents Chemother.* 1974;5:330–

[100] Pinna A, Piccinini P, Carta F. Effect of oral linoleic and gammalinolenic acid on meibomian gland dysfunction. *Cornea.* 2007; 26:260–264

[101] Miljanovic B, Trivedi KA, Dana MR, Gilbard JP, Buring JE, Schaumberg DA. Relation between dietary n-3 and n-6 fatty acids and clinically diagnosed dry eye syndrome in women. *Am J Clin Nutr.* 2005;82:887–893.

[102] Macsai MS. The role of omega-3 dietary supplementation in blepharitis and meibomian gland dysfunction (an AOS thesis). *Trans Am Ophthalmol Soc.* 2008;106:336–356.

[103] http://www.spectrum-thea.co.uk/apps/content/html/ViewContent.aspx?fid=31

[104] http://www.butterflies-eyecare.co.uk/Blephasteam-Blephasteam.html

[105] *Current Eye Research, 37(4), 272–278, 2012*A Single LipiFlow® Thermal Pulsation System Treatment Improves Meibomian Gland Function and Reduces Dry Eye Symptoms for 9 Months Jack V. Greiner DO, PhD1,2

[106] Invest Ophthalmol Vis Sci. 2011 Mar 30;52(4):1922-9. doi: 10.1167/iovs.10-6997a. The international workshop on meibomian gland dysfunction: executive summary. Nichols KK, Foulks GN, Bron AJ, Glasgow BJ, Dogru M, Tsubota K, Lemp MA, Sullivan DA.

[107] Meibomian gland disease. Classification and grading of lid changes. Bron AJ, Benjamin L, Snibson GR. Eye (Lond). 1991;5 (Pt 4):395-411. Review.

4

Keratitis — A Clinical Approach

Patricio A. Pacheco

1. Introduction

Any inflammatory reaction of the cornea of the eye is known as keratitis. The concept originates from the Greek word "κέρας-(kerat)" that means "horn" and "itis" which represents the classical suffix in medicine for inflammation. Since early civilization, the cornea was considered to be "strong as a horn". Its highly complex, almost indestructible, collagen conformation gives it strong physical properties that made the ancients to name it like that.

Keratitis is a frequent clinical condition. A correct initial diagnosis and treatment are critical in limiting the amount of residual damage and scarring left to the cornea, as the preservation of its transparent property is critical in the recovery and maintenance of useful vision in any ffected patient.

he present chapter a description of the clinical findings in different forms of keratits, intend ıstrate ophthalmic practitioners with the different potential diagnosis associated to this on and through this, to orientate them in the useful investigations that will lead to the iagnosis.

and physiology

ve layers: a superficial one called "epithelial", an intermediate one or al named "endothelial" and two limiting membranes: Bowman's and h of these layers is conformed by different structures and types of cells properties and different responses when affected by disease, this ers produces an inflammatory response that is typical to each layer, an orientate to the primarily affected site.

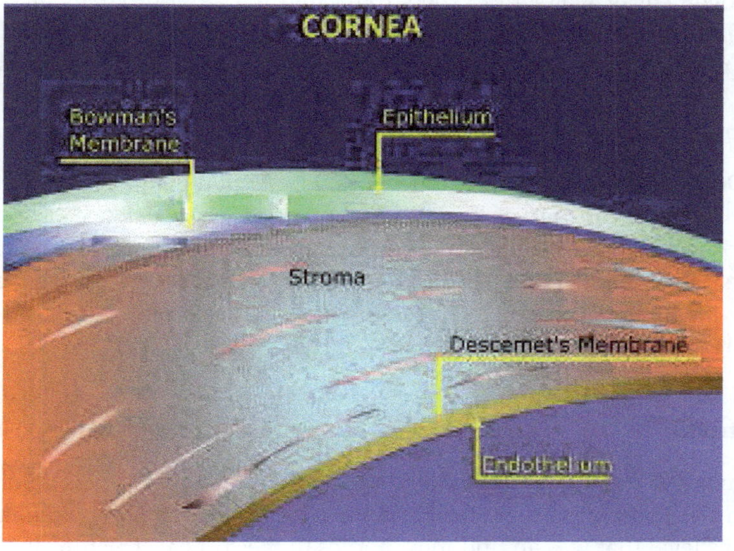

Figure 1. Corneal layers

The epithelial layer is formed by a stratified, squamous and non-keratinized epithelium that comprises a single layer of basal columnar cells attached by hemi-desmosomes to the underlying basement membrane followed by two to three rows of epithelial wing cells and two external layers of squamous surface cells which surface area is increased by microplicae and microvilli that facilitates the attachment of the mucin layer of the tear film. After a lifespan of approximately twenty-four hours the superficial cells are often shed into the tear film. The epithelial stem cells are located in the limbal region (this is the area between the cornea and the sclera), within the palisades of Vogt mainly located in the superior and inferior limbus. The indemnity of the corneal stem cells is essential for the maintenance of a healthy corneal epithelium and they also act as a barrier, preventing conjunctival epithelium from growing on to the clear cornea.

The stromal layer makes up to 90% of the corneal thickness, it is composed of regularly orientated collagen type I and V fibrils layers whose space is maintained by proteoglycan ground substance (chondroitin and keratan sulphate) with interspread modified fibroblast cells (keratocytes). The superficial portion of the stroma is called the Bowman membrane that constitutes an acellular portion of the stroma. It is, in part, the congruent and precise distribution of the collagen fibers of the stromal layer that permits the structure of the cornea to be transparent, letting the spectrum of visible light to pass through into the inner structures of the eye to finally allowing us to see.

The endothelial layer consists of a single layer of hexagonal cells that sits on a fine basal membrane made of a latticework of collagen fibers named the Descemet membrane. This layer and its indemnity is also crucial in keeping the transparency of the cornea by reducing the amount of water in the corneal stroma through an active membrane channels mechanism that allows the movement of water from the stroma into the anterior chamber of the eye. The endothelial cells cannot regenerate as they are arrested in the G1 phase of the cell cycle; the normal adult cell density is about 2500 cells/mm^2, this amount of cells decreases at a rate of 0.6% per year. When the cell density falls to about 500 cells/mm^2, corneal edema develops and then corneal transparency is reduced.

In 2013, the Dua's layer was described for the first time. In a paper published by Dua et al., experimental and electron microscopy studies revealed the existence of a thin layer (15 microns) of corneal collagen between the corneal stroma and the Descemet membrane. This layer has physical properties that are different to the stromal layer and the Descemet membrane, having the highest resistance to pressure among the corneal layers. Its discovery has implications in corneal surgical procedures.

Macrophages and dendritic antigen presenting cells are present mainly in the epithelium and the anterior stroma. Small numbers of macrophages are also present in the posterior stroma.

The sensory innervation of the cornea derives from the trigeminal nerve (V_1) and it is mainly distributed in the sub-epithelial region and anterior stroma as sub-epithelial plexus, it is therefore at this level that we can find most nerves in the corneal structure.

3. Keratitis: Clinical history

A detailed clinical history is crucial in the diagnosis keratitis. Demographic aspects like age, sex, ethnicity and occupation are always needed and can orientate to certain specific associated pathologies or risk factors. The use of contact lenses is important to note in detail including the type of lenses, length of use, cleaning systems used and daily routines (i.e. tap water washing, swimming, etc). History of any recent injury to the eye or systemic disease that might relate to corneal compromise is also needed. History of recent infections, cold sores or flu can be helpful in orientating a diagnosis. The use of topical eye drops or any other medication needs to be recorded as the use of topical steroids, anesthetics, etc can be significant as a risk factor for infections and anatomical/ functional changes of the corneal surface.

4. Keratitis: Anatomical classification

Keratitis can be classified on the portion of the cornea affected. It is important to note that perhaps most of the cases have more than one layer involved and in some cases all three are compromised, however this classification can help the diagnosis of more pure forms of keratitis.

Epithelial: when the most superficial layer of the cornea is affected, a characteristic epithelial defect or epithelial cellular infiltrate can be seen, fluorescein staining can help in the diagnosis, there are multiple sizes and possible shapes for both the defect and/or the infiltration. Some of the epithelial defects are pathognomonic as it is the dendriform seen in herpes simplex virus keratitis, it is therefore important to note the size, shape and depth of the defect in any epithelial form, as it will certainly help not only in the diagnosis but also in the assessment of the progression or recovery of the affected patient. In the case of the infiltrate, it is important to note the size, color and quality of the borders that can be of help in diagnosis and follow up. Any satellite lesions need also to be assessed as well as the upper and lower tarsal plates in search for any foreign bodies or other associated lesions like calcareous concretions, meibomian gland cysts, papillae or follicles. The epithelial form of keratitis is extremely painful and at times enlarged or infiltrated corneal nerves can be seen. Usually the anterior stroma is also affected with an inflammatory cellular infiltrate surrounding the epithelial lesions, it has in general poorly defined borders. Corneal pannus can be seen as a result of previous episodes of epithelial keratitis in some cases. Examples include herpetic epithelial keratitis, adenoviral keratoconjunctivitis, microbial corneal ulcers and contact lens related keratitis.

Stromal: this is the keratitis that has primarily a compromise of the corneal stroma. An associated epithelial defect may be or not detected at initial presentation. The main finding in this type of keratitis is an infiltration of the collagen layers in the stroma by inflammatory cells, this can be seen at any depth, it can be unifocal or multifocal, with many different shapes and sizes, but usually has a very well defined and regular edge. There is in general some degree of anterior chamber cell reaction and at times keratic precipitates can be seen. Thickening of the cornea is another way to appreciate the cellular infiltration seen in these cases. Examples are herpetic stromal keratitis, sclero-keratitis and fungal/atypical microorganisms' related keratitis.

Endothelial: the main structure affected in these cases is the endothelial layer. Characteristic features include keratic precipitates, descemet folds and almost invariably a significant anterior chamber cells reaction. Secondary diffuse corneal thickening at later stages can be seen as a result of impaired endothelial function. Examples include corneal graft rejection, herpetic endothelial keratitis, any form of kerato-uveitis, and post-traumatic/post-surgical endothelial damage.

5. Keratitis: Causes

The cornea is sometimes the target of one direct pathophysiological condition, others, the compromise is secondary to an external indirect event in the complex functional anatomical triad between the lids, the cornea and the tear film.

There are multiple different causes of keratitis; these can be grouped in three major groups including infectious, autoimmune/inflammatory, neoplastic and traumatic causes.

5.1. Infectious keratitis

As an important component of the anatomical anterior wall of the eye, the cornea is a structure highly exposed and vulnerable to external pathogens. The use of contact lenses constitutes an accumulative risk for developing infectious keratitis, as it is also any history of chronic corneal disease or the use of topical steroids. Any corneal epithelial disruption as seen sometimes in dry eye syndrome, severe blepharitis and injuries are able to cause disruptions of the epithelial barrier as seen in corneal abrasions, post-surgical procedures or corneal foreign bodies that can predispose to corneal infections. Sometimes it is the result of highly pathogenic microorganisms with high affinity to the epithelial cells the ones that can cause a direct involvement as it is frequently seen with the herpes virus family.

5.1.1. Viral

By far the most frequent cause of viral keratitis is the one caused by herpes viruses type 1 and 2, also varicella-zoster virus can sometimes be responsible in the context of herpes zoster ophthalmicus. The typical form of viral keratitis is epithelial, with a characteristic dendritiform epithelial defect and secondary infiltrate very easy to diagnose with fluorescein staining (Fig 2). The epithelial defect seen in herpes zoster infection is classically described as geographic rather than dendritiform. In less than 10% of the cases the compromise can be primarily stromal or endothelial that typically is associated with elevated intraocular pressure (Fig 3). A PCR for virology in a swab of the epithelial lesion usually confirms diagnosis. Recent history of herpes zoster or recurrent cold sores can also orientate the clinician. If PCR is not available, another way of confirming diagnosis is by performing antibodies serology (IgG / IgM) for HSV and VZV at the time of presentation, an elevated IgM would confirm the diagnosis of recent infection and an elevated IgG a recurrence. This form of keratitis leaves behind sometimes significant corneal scarring with pannus, this clinical finding, in the context of an atypical recurrent hypertensive stromal or endothelial keratouveitis, can help sometimes achieve the correct clinical diagnosis.

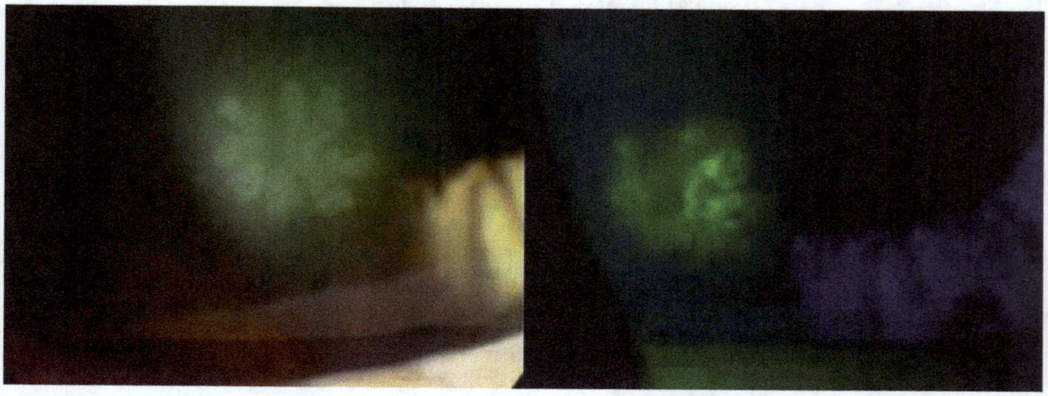

Figure 2. Herpes simplex virus epithelial keratitis as typical dendrite.

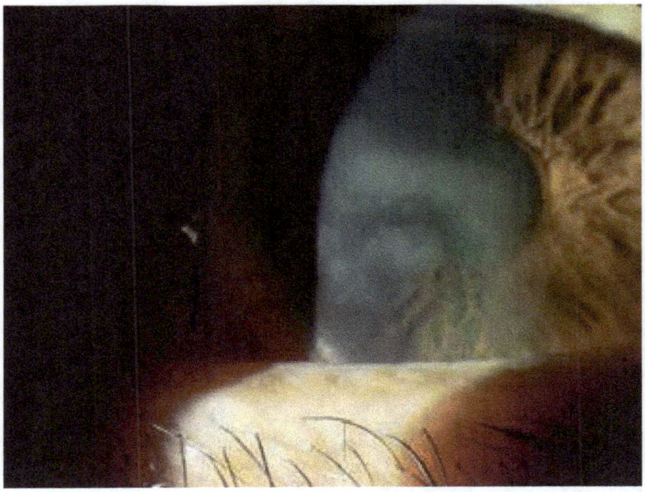

Figure 3. Herpes simplex virus stromal keratitis.

5.1.2. Bacterial

For bacteria to act as a pathogen in the cornea, it is necessary a disruption in the epithelial barrier like the ones seen in injuries (corneal foreign bodies and corneal abrasions) or a significant risk factor like contact lens wear or use of topical steroids. Almost any bacterium is able to cause keratitis, the most frequently involved are the ones that are the gram positive microorganisms found in the eyelids margin and skin (staphylococcus sp, streptococcus sp), sometimes gram negative bacteria like pseudomonas sp can be isolated. The typical keratitis caused by bacteria is epithelial and the presentation is acute; it usually has a well-defined epithelial defect surrounded by a stromal grayish infiltrate, which has a depth and extension proportional to the time of onset to presentation. Often a level of hypopyon and anterior chamber reaction are seen. The speed and extension of the compromise also depends on the pathogenicity of the bacteria involved, often being worse in the case of gram-negative microorganisms (Fig 4). Slow growth bacteria like streptococcus viridans can give the aspect of crystalline keratitis, as the invasion of the corneal stroma is very slow following the branching of the collagen layers. The diagnosis is usually confirmed by a corneal scrape of the lesion that can be sent for microbiological studies; in any ophthalmic setting it is crucial to perform a gram stain, blood agar, brain heart infusion (BHI) and cooked meat broth (CMB) cultures to be able to isolate the pathogen and determine the sensitivities to antibiotic therapy. The gram stain can give immediate initial information of the type of microorganism excluding other causes of keratitis. In contact lens wearers is important also to send for culture the contact lenses container and the last pair of lenses used.

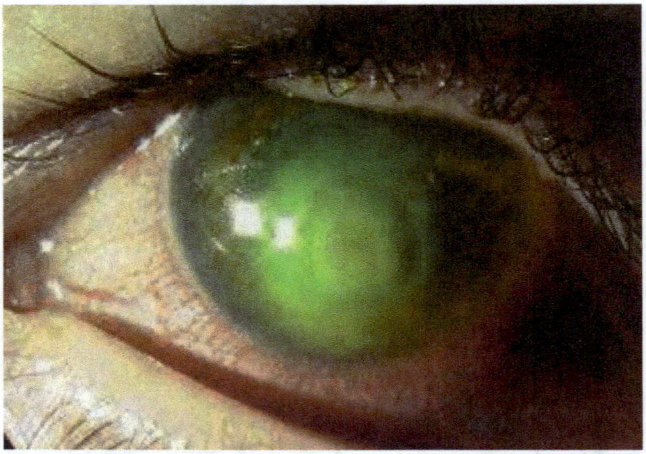

Figure 4. A patient with pseudomonas sp keratitis.

5.1.3. Fungal

It is a rare cause of keratitis in temperate climates but common cause of keratitis in tropical countries. It is difficult to treat. Usually occurs following trauma to the cornea especially the one caused by vegetable matter. Also contact lens wearing is emerging as a significant risk factor. The course is indolent sub-acute, it takes weeks for the patient to seek help as it does not cause significant discomfort in the early stages as fungi are slow in replicate. The clinical presentation is that of a stromal form of keratitis, an epithelial defect can or not be present, but usually is small compared to the amount of stromal infiltrate associated. The stromal infiltrate is always irregular in the borders and poorly defined, it has a 'fluffy' aspect and very white (Fig 5). In very advanced cases the infiltration of the stroma can be full thickness with associated anterior chamber whitish solid hypopyon. The diagnosis is often confirmed by a corneal scrape or a corneal biopsy sent for microbiological studies; the gram stain can be very useful in identifying hyphae, filaments or microorganisms very quickly, for the culture it is important to repeat the cultures described for bacteria (in case of mixed infection) and also a Sabouraud's media that is more specific for fungal growth.

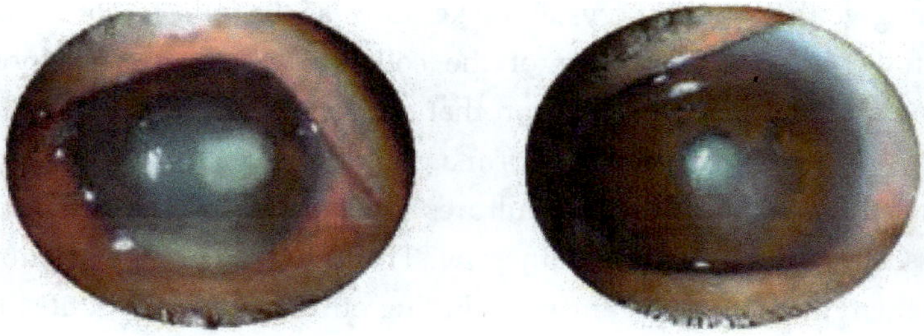

Figure 5. Fungal keratitis pre / post treatment.

5.1.4. *Acanthamoeba*

It is a rare cause of keratitis caused by one of the most common protozoa found in soil and water. In 90% of the cases a history of contact lens wear is found. Clinically this form of keratitis is combined with an epithelial and stromal component. The epithelial component is characteristically a large epithelial defect with abundant sub-epithelial infiltrate and enlargement of the corneal nerves that have been described as invaded by the pathogen at some stages of the disease, causing intense pain; this is perhaps the most painful form of keratitis, and this is regarded as a significant clinical finding at the time of diagnosing contact lens related keratitis. The stromal infiltrate is grey-whitish with irregular, multiple or single lesions, sometimes satellite areas can be seen (Fig 6 a & b). The diagnosis is confirmed by scrape or corneal epithelial biopsy sent for microbiological studies, it is important to repeat the gram and all the previously described medias (blood, BHI, CMB, Sabouraud's) and add the E. coli enriched non-nutrient agar media where this pathogen can be detected easily.

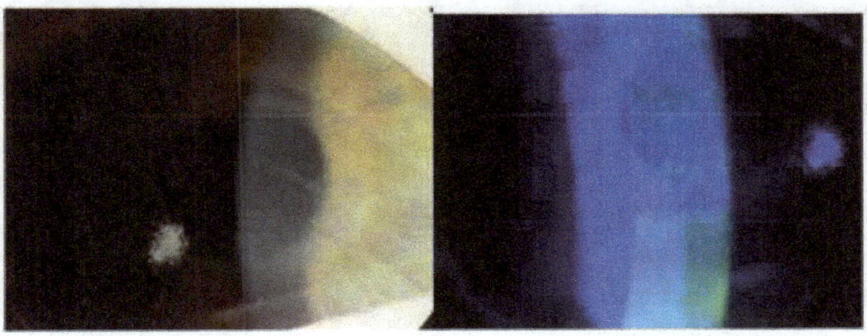

a)

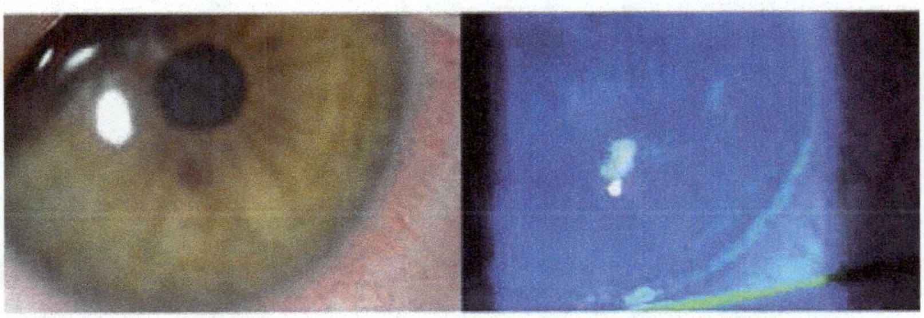

b)

Figure 6. a) Epithelial infiltrate with perineuritis in a patient with acanthamoeba keratitis. b) Diffuse stromal infiltrate in early acanthamoeba keratitis.

5.1.5. *Atypical*

This term is used to describe an infectious keratitis caused by atypical microorganisms like mycobacterium. The pattern of keratitis can be very confusing as it occurs usually in the context of postoperative, traumatic or previous corneal pathology situations. The course is always chronic, unresponsive to multiple previous treatments and the clinical picture varies between an epithelial and stromal form of keratitis with atypical features (Fig 7). Perhaps the most important aspect is the invariable presence of a significant risk factor like previous surgery, as this pathogen needs a significant break in the epithelial barrier to be able to invade and cause the condition due to its relative large size. The isolation of mycobacterium to confirm diagnosis depends on a high level of suspicion and the scrape or corneal biopsy culture that needs all the previously described media plus a Zhiel-Neelsen gram stain for identification of acid-fast bacteria and Lowenstein-Jensen agar for culture growth.

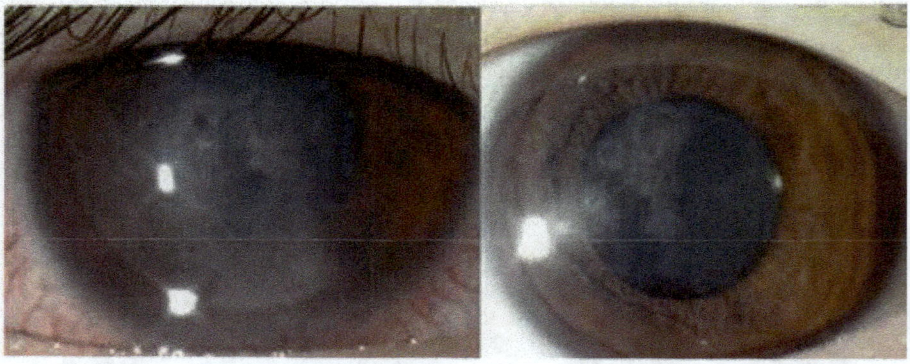

Figure 7. Atypical keratitis caused by mycobacterium abscessus after LASIK pre / post treatment.

5.2. Inflammatory — Autoimmune keratitis (Non suppurative keratitis)

Any condition that can induce an inflammatory response of the cornea can be classified in this group of causes of keratitis. There are autoimmune and no autoimmune related diseases.

5.2.1. Autoimmune

Like in any other autoimmune condition where the main target is the collagen in the body, the so-called autoimmune collagen or connective tissue diseases can be responsible for various forms of inflammatory keratitis, due to the high content of collagen seen in the corneal and scleral tissue. In some patients the cornea is the initial manifestation of the autoimmune process sometimes well in advance before the systemic condition manifests. The collagen diseases related to peripheral corneo-scleral ulceration or sclero-keratitis, include systemic lupus erythematosus, rheumatoid arthritis, Wegener's granullomatosis and polyarteritis nodosa. The form of keratitis seen in theses cases is epithelial with a significant stromal component mainly in the form of subtle infiltrate with severe stromal melting and associated episcleral or scleral vasculitis (Fig 8). In other circumstances the cornea is the only affected structure as it is seen in Mooren's or peripheral ulcerative keratitis, the characteristic clinical finding is corneal stromal melting associated to inflammation (Fig 9 a & b).

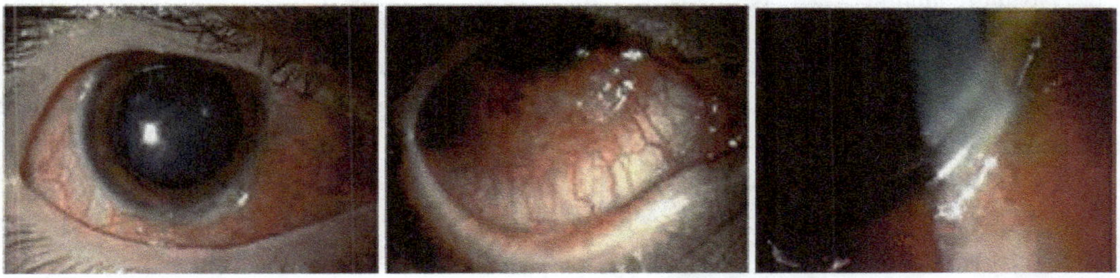

Figure 8. Sclerokeratitis in a patient with Wegener's granullomatosis.

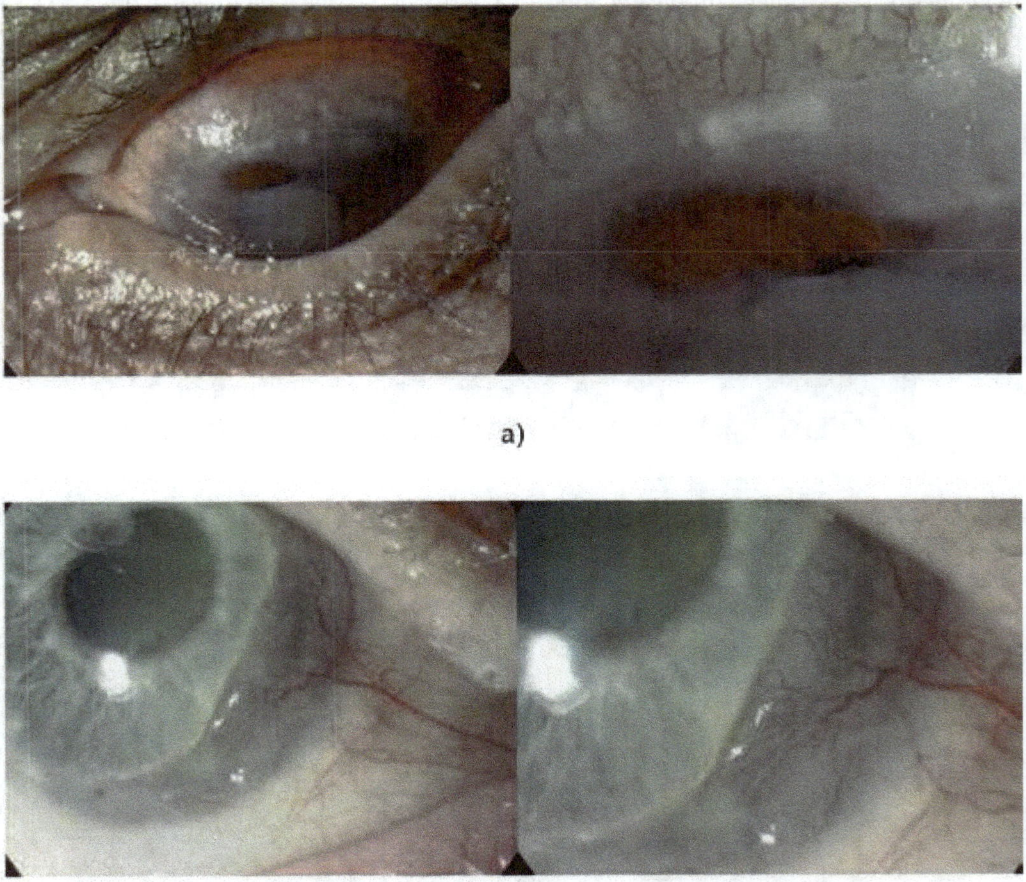

a)

b)

Figure 9. a) Peripheral ulcerative keratitis with associated scleritis and corneal stromal corneal infiltrate. b) Typical case of Mooren's keratitis.

5.2.2. Non autoimmune

In this group, we find conditions that can compromise the delicate functional triad between the cornea, the tear film and the lids. If any of these is affected it will indirectly affect the anatomy and function of the other, potentially causing an inflammatory keratitis. Lids conditions like blepharitis, rosacea, lagophthalmos, entropion, ectropion, tarsal calcareous concretions or tear film dysfunctions like the ones seen in Sjogren's or severe dry eye syndrome can directly or indirectly cause keratitis in the form of marginal keratitis (Fig 10), phlyctenular keratoconjunctivitis and sometimes diffuse punctate keratitis as seen in Thygeson's keratitis. Usually the clinical pattern in this form of keratitis is epithelial with isolated or multiple epithelial defects and sub-epithelial superficial mild infiltrates (Fig 11), filaments can also sometimes be seen. When chronically affected a peripheral corneal pannus can often be seen (Fig 12).

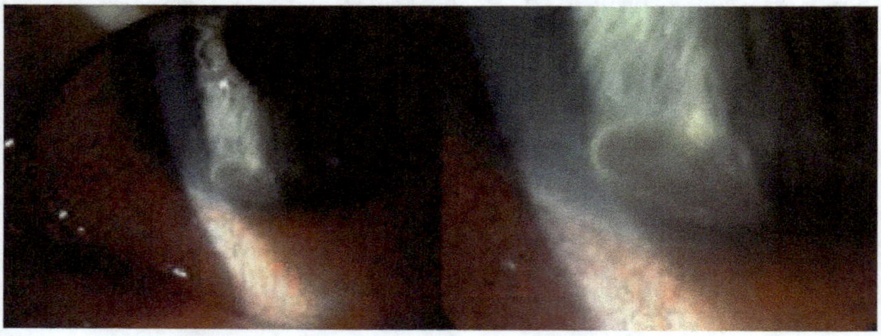

Figure 10. Typical marginal keratitis associated to rosacea.

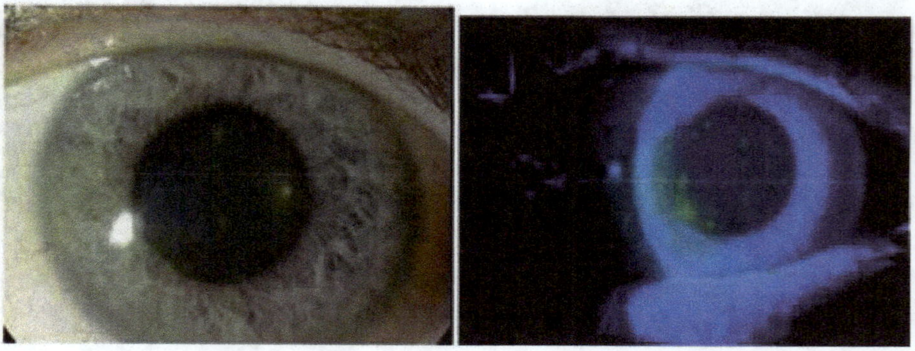

Figure 11. Superficial epithelial defects in dry eye syndrome.

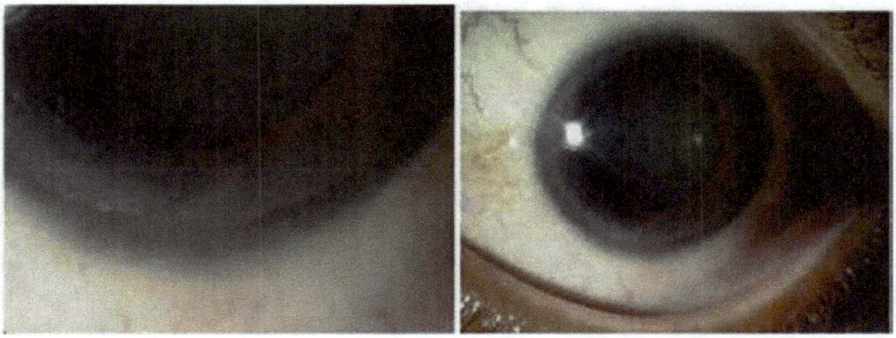

Figure 12. Peripheral pannus in chronic dry eye syndrome.

5.3. Neoplasia associated inflammatory corneal involvement

Any neoplastic process in the limbal region and surrounding conjunctiva can indirectly extend to the cornea and cause an inflammatory reaction, this is generally not considered in the differential diagnosis of keratitis and is perhaps the most rare and less suspected cause of corneal and limbal inflammation, however it is important to consider it in order to achieve an early diagnosis, as this type of conditions untreated can extend quickly with some mortality rate.

5.3.1. Conjunctival intraepithelial neoplasia and squamous carcinoma

Neoplasia of the conjunctival epithelial cells is more commonly seen in the elderly. There are different grades of penetration in the underlying tissue and the amount of cellular atypical cells defines also the degree of malignancy ranging from grade 1 to a carcinoma in situ. The more invasive the type of neoplasia, the more likely this will extend to the adjacent corneal tissue and regional lymphonodes; the corneal involvement always remains superficial (Fig 13, 14).

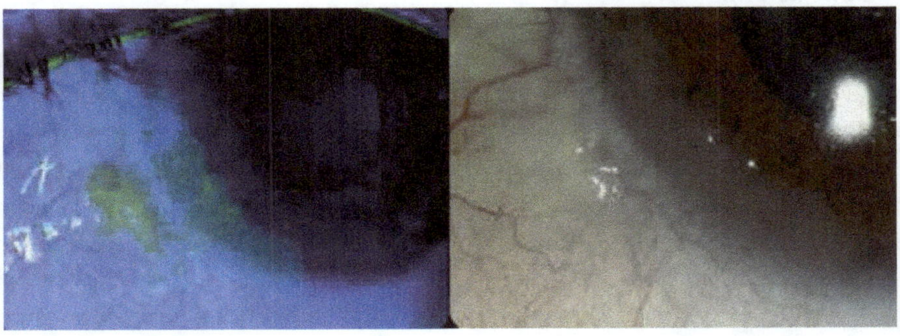

Figure 13. Conjunctival intraepithelial neoplasia (CIN) grade 3 with and without fluorescein staining.

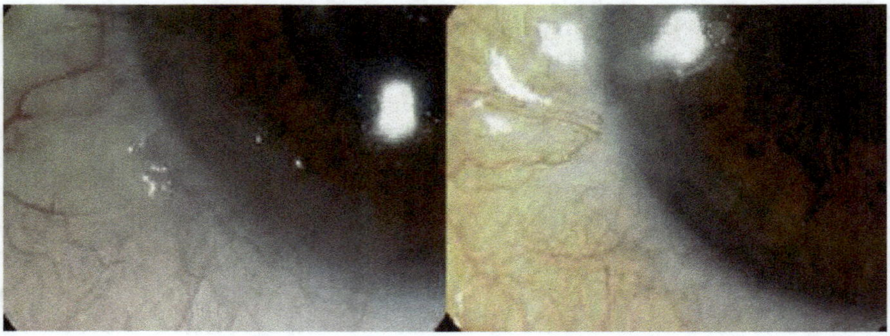

Figure 14. Conjunctival intraepithelial neoplasia (CIN) grade 3 treated with topical mytomicin C.

5.3.2. Conjunctival / limbal melanomas

They are rare but lethal. They can be very polymorphic with multiple types of different clinical presentation, pigmented (melanotic) or not pigmented (amelanotic), they are of rapid growth and can invade distant organs especially lungs and liver. The most likely origin is at the conjunctival epithelial cells when some pigmentation is associated. Isolated or multiple sentinel vessels are a pathognomonic feature (Fig. 15).

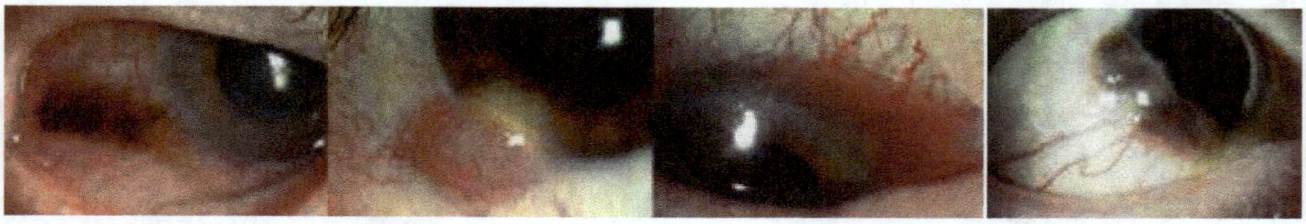

Figure 15. Four different conjunctival melanomas with corneal involvement, notice the polymorphism in clinical presentation.

5.4. Traumatic keratitis

In this group we can consider trauma by direct blunt injury with secondary corneal abrasion and corneal edema, or a surgical injury that damages the endothelial layer causing secondary corneal edema and endothelial failure with concurrent bullous keratopathy. The type of keratitis seen in these situations is mainly endothelial and stromal with multiple descemet folds, stromal collagen fibers disorganization, keratic precipitates and often associated anterior chamber reaction. At later stages if the endothelial layer does not recover from the insult, a severe corneal edema may lead to epithelial bullous formation and consequent epithelial keratitis. A clear history of trauma might not be obvious and the clinicians are encouraged to obtain it from the clinical history remembering that sometimes the traumatic event can precede the clinical manifestation for many years (i.e. previous cataract surgery, etc)

6. Keratitis: Treatment

The treatment of keratitis will depend on the direct cause; it is for this reason that an appropriate diagnosis is crucial at the moment of deciding the initial treatment.

6.1. Infectious causes

In viral herpetic keratitis cases, the drug of choice is acyclovir in topical or oral form depending on the extension of the keratitis within the corneal layers. A typical dose is ointment acyclovir 3% five times daily for one week or 400 mg orally five times a day for the same period. In severe cases both forms can be used to maximize effect. In children and the elderly the oral formulation is recommended due to difficulties in the application of the ointment. In resistant cases the alternative treatment will be topical trifluorthymidine 1% (F3T) or vidarabine 3% (Vira-A^{tm}). If high intraocular pressure (IOP) is detected this also need to be treated with lowering IOP agents. Other antiviral agents like topical ganciclovir 0.15% (Zirgan^{tm}) have started to be used more widely in recent years.

In bacterial suspected infections the initial treatment of choice is topical ciprofloxacin 0.3%, Ofloxacin 0.3% or levofloxacin 0.3% hourly, when significant anterior chamber reaction is found a cycloplegic/dilating drop to minimize pain and reduce the formation of posterior synechias is recommended and depending on the bacterial sensitivities results the treatment should be adjusted accordingly.

In acanthamoeba the treatment requires a combination of poly-hexyl-methyl-biguanide 0.02% (PHMB) and propamide isethionate 0.1% (Brolene^{tm}), alternatively preparations of chlorhexidine 0.02% can be used as well.

In atypical keratitis one can start treatment based on the suspicious on the most likely clinically apparent etyiological cause and adequate it based on the findings from the sampling.

6.2. Inflammatory / autoimmune

For autoimmune keratitis usually systemic therapy is needed, the important approach in the treatment is to identify corneal limbal ischemia and/or corneal melting as these are reasons not to use topical steroids due to the high risk of perforation. Severe cases will need high dose of oral steroids and immunosuppressant agents. No autoimmune cases, presenting with inflammatory features due to blepharitis and/or dry eyes with marginal infiltrates do benefit from topical steroids, however is also very important to treat the initial cause of corneal inflammation as this is usually secondary, i.e. removal of concretions and ectopic eyelashes, repair lagophthalmos or other lids malpositions, treat dry eyes with topical lubricants, etc.

6.3. Neoplasia associated

Surgical removal and biopsy is important as it is based on the histological diagnosis that further interventions like cryotherapy or radiotherapy might be indicated and planned. The excision of any suspicious lesion ideally has to have a margin of two centimeters of healthy tissue to prevent recurrences. In CIN cases concomitant cryotherapy is useful as well as topical mytomicin C or 5 – fluorouracil at different concentrations. In melanomas a systemic workup including chest CT scan and liver function tests at regular intervals to detect metastasis is important, concomitant local radiotherapy has been advocated as well at the time of removal of the lesion.

6.4. Traumatic

In cases of corneal abrasion the treatment of choice is to use topical antibiotic ointments to prevent infections and to pad the eye for 24 hours to allow epithelisation of the cornea, the use of preservative free cycloplegic drops initially to relief pain is recommended before padding. In blunt injuries the use of topical anti-inflammatory or steroid drops is useful depending on the severity of the inflammation. In cases of bullose keratopathy, endothelial corneal transplantation is highly successful, the use of highly osmotic drops like NACL 5% or bandage contact lenses can sometimes clear the corneal stroma and relief pain while waiting for a corneal donor.

7. Conclusion

A clear and simple approach to the differential diagnosis of keratitis has been presented. The methodological clinical diagnostic remains the cornerstone of medicine at anytime, the clinical history, examination of the patient and auxiliary diagnostic methods to confirm a suspected diagnosis are all crucial in achieving a clinical improvement of the clinical condition known as keratitis.

The simple classification based on clinical findings will help ophthalmologists, general practitioners to assess patients with this condition and start an adequate initial investigation and treatment

Keratitis remains one of the most frequent diagnoses in ophthalmology and a comprehensive review like the one here presented is useful for any levels of clinical practice.

Author details

Patricio A. Pacheco[1,2]

1 Moorfields Eye Hospital, London, UK

2 West Hertfordshire Hospitals, NHS trust, UK

References

[1] Chow, C.Y.; Foster, C.S. (1996). Mooren's ulcer. *International Ophthalmology clinics*, Vol. 36, (Winter 1996), pp. 1-13

[2] Donzis, P.B.; Mondino, B.J. (1987). Management of non infectious corneal ulcers. *Survey Ophthalmology*, Vol. 32, (January 1987), pp. 94-110

[3] Dua, H.S.; Faraj, L.A.; Said, D.G.; Gray, T.; Lowe, J. *Ophthalmology*, Vol. 120 (9), (September 2013), pp. 1778-1785

[4] Holland, E.J.; Schwartz, G.S. (1999). Classification of herpes simplex virus keratitis, *Cornea*, Vol. 18, (March 1999), pp. 144-154

[5] Kanski, J.; Pavesio C. & Tuft S. (2006). Ocular Inflammatory Disease, Mosby-Elsevier, ISBN 0-323-03737, 1st edition, Philadelphia, USA

[6] Ladas, J.G.; Mondino, B.J. (2000). Systemic disorders associated with peripheral corneal ulcération. *Current opinion Ophthalmology*, Vol. 11, (December 2000), pp. 468-471

[7] Radford, C.F.; Minassian, D.C. & Dart, J.K. (2002). Acanthamoeba keratitis in England and Wales: incidence, outcomes and risk factors. *British Journal Ophthalmology*, Vol. 86, (May 2002), pp. 536-542

[8] Rohatgi, J.; Dhaliwal, U. (2000). Phlyctenular eye disease. *Japanese Journal Ophthalmology*, Vol. 44, (March-April 2000), pp. 146-150

[9] Suchecki, J.K. ; Donshik, P. & Ehlers W.H. (2003). Contact lens complications. *Ophthalmology Clinics North America*, Vol. 16, (March 2003), pp. 471-484

[10] Solomon, A.; Karp, C.L. & Miller, D. (2001). Mycobacterium interface keratitis after laser in situ keratomileusis. *Ophthalmology*, Vol. 108, (December 2001), pp. 2201-2208

[11] Stern, M.; Gao, J & Siemasko, K. F. (2004). The rôle of the lacrimal functional unit in the pathophysiology of dry eye. *Experimental Eye Research*, Vol. 78, (March 2004), pp. 409-416

5

Structure and Function Relationship in Glaucoma-Historical Perspective to a Practical Approach

Elliot M. Kirstein

1. Introduction

Physicians, by nature, seem to strive for more precise means to diagnose, quantify and manage chronic disease. It seems intuitive that doing so will help us diagnose earlier, have an increased understanding for the relative severity of disease in individual patients and, ultimately, through more timely diagnosis, mitigate morbidities associated with that disease. In the example of diabetes, we can now look at glycosylated hemoglobin levels (HbA1c) and derive a reasonable understanding of risk level and relative treatment success for individual patients. While the HbA1c value is not flawless as a metric, it has become an extremely robust and accepted tool in diabetes management. Our efforts to coalesce ocular physical measurements with functional values seem to point to our desire to define glaucoma in one simple value. While the effort itself has already shed great benefits to our understanding of this complex disease, it ultimately seems unlikely that we will ever be able to adequately define glaucoma in terms of a singular value.

During the past century, the metrics used to diagnose and manage glaucoma have varied and evolved. In the 1950's, using Schiotz tonometry, Leydecker showed that approximately 2.5% of the population had intraocular pressures greater than 21mm Hg. It was also determined that a similar number of people in that study had glaucoma. From that point forward, 21mm Hg became the empirical metric for determining who was at risk. More than fifty years has passed since the publication of Leydecker's study and a cornucopia of compelling scientific literature has been presented which has shed light on the diversity and complexity of glaucoma and clearly diminishes its relevance as a stand-alone diagnostic feature. Ironically, the vast body of evidence which clearly discourages reliance of the old 21 mm red flag in glaucoma diagnosis seems not to have been sufficient to clear it from the minds and hearts of too many eye doctors in this century. It would appear that we have an inner need to strive for and adhere to simple answers to even the most complex problems.

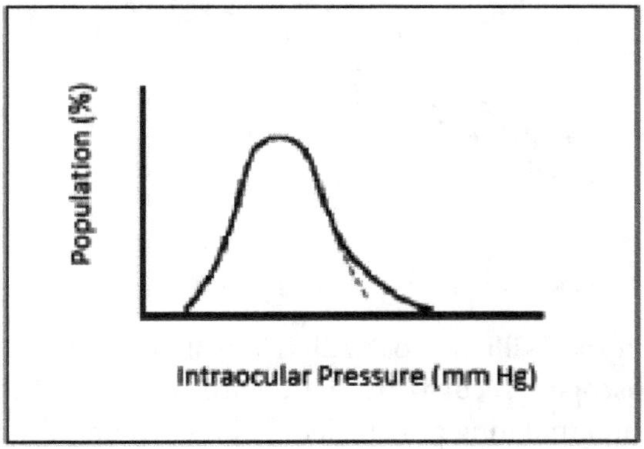

Figure 1. CURRENT SIGNIFICANCE OF 21 mmHg: The distribution of IOP in the general population as studied by Leydecker (normal IOP was statistically defined two standard deviations above and below mean, as 11-21 mmHg) is not Gaussian, but is slightly skewed towards higher IOP's [1]

Beyond the early observation that glaucomatous vision loss is generally accompanied with high intraocular pressure, scientists began to observe the physical changes within the eye that seemed to occur in concert with that loss. In 1885, Priestley Smith elegantly defined glaucoma, stating that "The excavation of the disc in glaucoma is not a purely mechanical result of exalted pressure; it is, in part at least, an atrophic condition which, though primarily due to pressure, includes vascular changes and impaired nutrition of the substance of the optic disc... which may possibly progress even though all excessive pressure be removed". Given this understanding, eye doctors started to look for tools to study the eye and its function in greater detail.

Today, eye doctors are challenged with a new puzzle. In current clinical practive we can obtain physical and psychometric data that was previously unimaginable. We are still attempting to determine which of the vast data has the greatest utility and specificity in regard to the diagnosis, quantification and management of glaucoma.

2. Observation and measurement of structure

2.1. Ophthalmoscopy

Understandably, long before doctors could document the eye's interior contents with imaging techniques, observation and evaluation of the nerve was performed by ophthalmoscopy. Observations were recorded with drawings. Though others produced earlier versions of the ophthalmoscope, in 1851, Hermann von Helmholtz reported its usefulness and, therein, revolutionized ophthalmology.

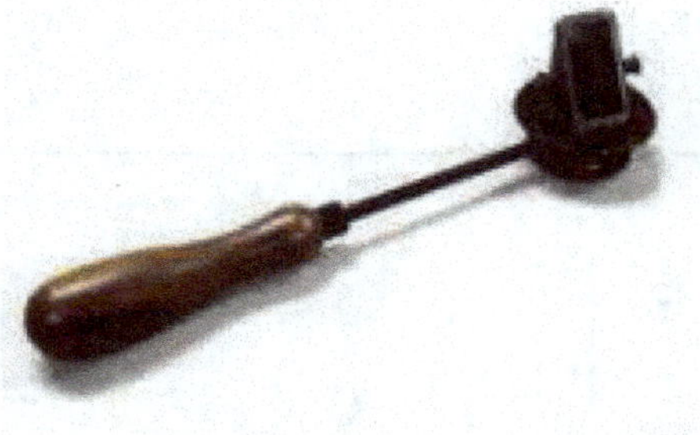

Figure 2. Early Welsh Allyn ophthalmoscope

In 1915, Francis A. Welch and William Noah Allyn invented the world's first hand-held direct illuminating ophthalmoscope, precursor to the device now used by clinicians around the world. This refinement and updating of von Helmholtz's invention enabled ophthalmoscopy to become one of the most ubiquitous medical screening techniques in the world today. The company started as a result of this invention is Welch Allyn. [2]

The need for stereopsis arose soon after the discovery of the ophthalmoscope. Given the limitations of a two dimensional view, the glaucomatous cup was, at first, mistaken for a swelling. At that time, Brewster's popular stereoscope was introduced, and its theory and method were then applied to ophthalmoscopy by Giraud-Teulon. His was the first binocular instrument, subsequently much improved by Zachariah Laurence. Binocular indirect ophthalmoscopy was abandoned toward the end of the 19th century in favor of direct monocular ophthalmoscopy, until it was revived in the 1950s by Schepens. More recently, hand held biomicroscopic lenses, which were popularized in the late 1980's by Volk Optical, Inc., are now a clinical standard for indirect three dimensional observations and evaluation of the nerve. [3]

3. Disc documentation

3.1. Drawings

Having the ability to view the nerve in vivo, proper scientific method deemed it necessary to document of these observations. For the better part of the twentieth century, manual drawing of the disc remained the clinical standard.

While disc drawing and careful direct observation of the nerve still have significant benefits, our scientific curiosity and our frank understanding of the likelihood of human variability and error with manual drawings, has driven us to develop methods of observation and recording which yield information down to the cellular level and render documentation which is relatively free of the obvious variability in individual observer skill and methodology.

Before the mid 1970's, eye doctors, in training, could not yet see photographs of the live human retina. Ophthalmic texts traditionally included drawings of normal and pathological eyes, which were rendered by professional medical artists.

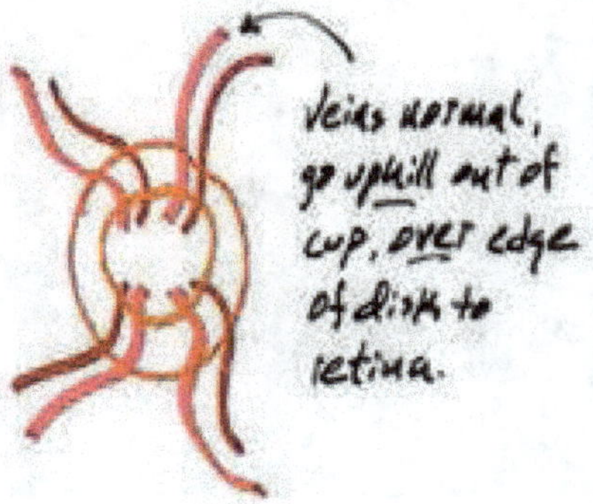

Figure 3. Typical clinician's disc drawing

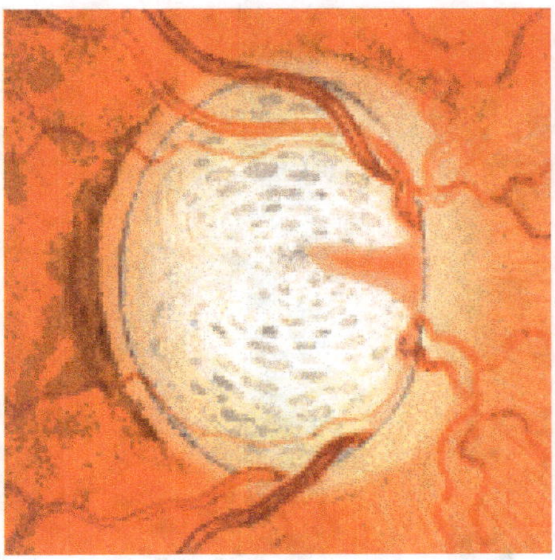

Figure 4. Medical artist's disc drawing of glaucomatous optic nerve

3.2. Photography

With fundus photography becoming commonplace by the early 1980's, stereo disc photography became possible and earned its place as the clinical gold standard in optic nerve documentation for the remainder of the twentieth century.

Recently, digital two and three dimensional photography have quickly outpaced conventional film photography of the nerve because of its obvious advantages in efficiency, economy and portability.

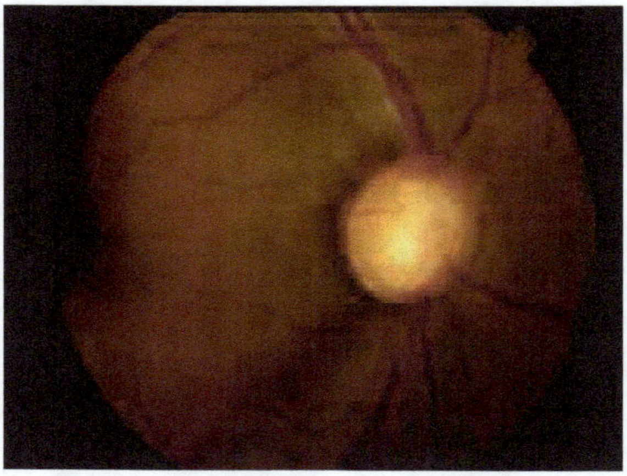

Figure 5. Optic nerve photograph

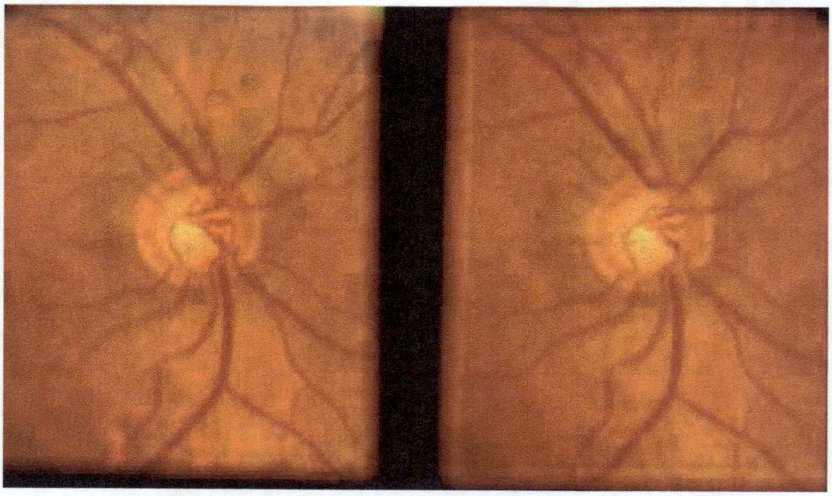

Figure 6. Simultaneous digital stereo disc photograph captured using the Nidek 3-DX system

3.3. Beyond photography

While photography had given us robust methodology for documentation of the appearance of the optic nerve head, it seemed natural to look for ways to numerically quantify various nerve attributes. An early attempt called the Glaucomascope, cast a series of infrared bars across the surface of the nerve. The variation in line contours signaled the instrument to make calculations regarding cup dimensions and, hopefully, track topographical change in concordance with glaucoma progression. The next generation of devices including the GDX (Carl Ziess) and the Heidelberg Retinal Tomograph (HRT) (Heidelberg Engineering), provided a more comprehensive perspective of nerve attributes and, with GDX, added new measurements of the nerve fiber layer surrounding the papilla. The HRT was the first to incorporate nerve progression analysis.

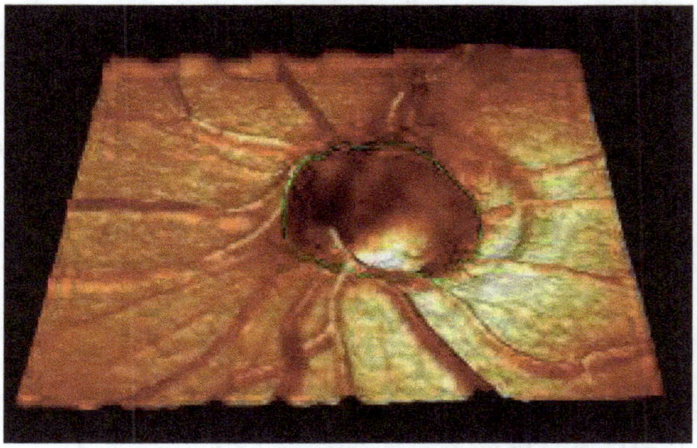

Figure 7. HRT 3-D image of the optic nerve and retinal nerve fiber layer (RNFL)

The Heidelberg Retina Tomograph (HRT) is a confocal scanning laser ophthalmoscope. A laser light scans the retina in 24 millisecond sequential scans, starting above the retinal surface, then capturing parallel images at increasing depths. The stacks of images can be combined to create a three-dimensional (3-D) topographic image of the retina. Images are aligned and compared using TruTrack™ software for both individual examinations and for detecting change between examinations.

When applying the technology to glaucoma, the HRT takes data from a 3-D stack of tomographic images of the optic nerve and retinal nerve fiber layer (RNFL), aligns the images and computes a 3-D topographic map of the surface of the retina. This 3-D topographic map is analyzed for signs of glaucomatous damage and the results are displayed on either a single eye examination report or on an OU examination report.

The GDx nerve fiber analyzers measures the retinal nerve fiber layer (RNFL) thickness with a scanning laser polarimeter based on the birefringent properties of the RNFL. Measurement is obtained from a band 1.75 disc diameters concentric to the disc.

The GDx projects a polarized beam of a light into the eye. As this light passes through the NFL tissue, it changes in speed. The detectors measure the change and convert it into thickness units that are graphically displayed. The GDx measures modulation around an ellipse just outside the optics disc and ratios of the thickest points either superiorly or inferiorly to the temporal or nasal regions.

The state of polarization of the light is change (retardation) as it passes through birefringent tissue (cornea and RNFL). Corneal birefringence is eliminated (in part) by a propriety 'corneal compensator'. The amount of retardation of light reflected from the fundus is converted to RNFL thickness.

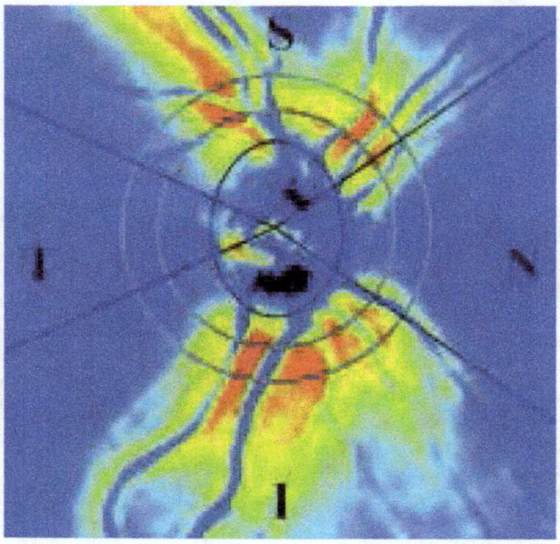

Figure 8. GDX ONH image

A Dutch study found that while there is a correlation between standard automated perimetry and GDx, variable corneal compensation (VCC) measurements in patients with glaucoma, suggesting that GDx VCC measurements relate well with functional loss in glaucoma. In healthy subjects, they found virtually no correlation between perimetry and GDx VCC measurements. This would cast doubt on its predictive value and suggests false positives. [4]

4. Ocular Coherence Tomography (OCT) – the new gold standard

Optical coherence tomography (OCT) has advanced considerably since it was first applied to the eye. It is an extension of a technique called low-coherence interferometry, which was initially applied to ophthalmology for in vivo measurements of eye axial length. OCT cross sections are used to evaluate the optic disc and retinal layers such as the retinal nerve fiber layer (RNFL). Scan patterns that enabled reproducible measurements were developed, and these eventually became incorporated into commercial systems. In 2000 Zangwill et al published a study comparing OCT nerve fiber thickness values against stereo photography and threshold visual field results showing that the OCT shows promise for providing quantitative measures of RNFL thickness for diagnosing and monitoring glaucoma. [5]

With these improvements in speed and sensitivity as seen in spectral domain OCT, it is now feasible to collect volumetric (three-dimensional; 3D) scans of tissue, whereas in the past, the amount of time required to do this would have been prohibitive. Broadband volumetric retinal imaging with SD-OCT have demonstrated speeds of up to 312,500. To date, most clinical systems operate at an acquisition rate of ~27,000 A-scans/s and an axial resolution of 5 to 6 μm.

The unprecedented speed and versatility of current forms of OCT have given us a new and vast data set, allowing us to seek out specific retinal measurements that are most highly specific for the diagnosis and observation of glaucomatous progression. Having the capacity to observe tissue at a cellular level, we now can more aptly compare between individuals and with specific individuals over time. The additional information at hand also allows us to emerge from cup/ disc ratio, the age old and weather beaten descriptive of the nerve in the context of glaucoma. It is now possible to look far deeper into retinal and nerve attributes and across a wider diameter of retina, to look for structural changes that are most highly pathognomonic of glaucoma and its progression. [6]

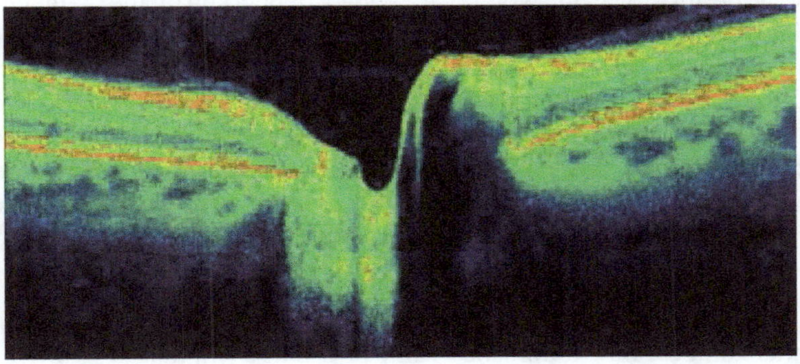

Figure 9. OCT crossectional view of the optic nerve

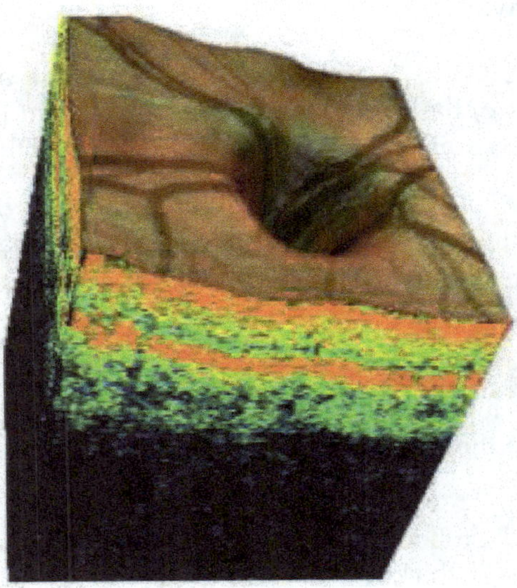

Figure 10. OCT three dimensional optic nerve scan

5. Measuring the nerve

5.1. Cup Disc Ratio (C/D)

In quantifying glaucoma risk and severity, the C/D ratio of the optic nerve has been the standard bearer during the past one hundred years. An eye with a low ratio was considered less apt to be glaucomatous and, if glaucoma was diagnosed, was known to be less advanced. High ratios implied high risk and or advanced disease. Some investigators noted that that the significance of a specific C/D value would vary widely depending on the diameter of the nerve itself. Investigators also began to note that nerve attributes such as rim thickness can be quite meaningful. For example, given two nerves with C/D=.50, one may have a well centered cup and no glaucomatous visual field loss, while another,.50 nerve, with loss if the inferior margin may show a severe superior nasal field defect. To further confuse the notion of C/D, more recent attention has been given to disc diameter and its implications on the significance of C/D in individual patients. Our current understanding is that nerve diameter plays a large role in the relative value of C/D. A C/D of.60 with a relatively small nerve is likely to have far greater implications with regard to glaucoma than the same C/D in a large nerve.

Given the additional perspective of the influence of cup position and nerve diameter, it should be easy to understand the now diminished value of C/D as a singular descriptive value of the state of disease. Reminiscent of the loss of relevance of the age old "21 mm Hg" standard, our current understanding of the scope of changes that occur within the nerve, surrounding the nerve and, more recently, those changes in the axonal bed and the peri papillary ganglion cell layer, further disenfranchises C/D and the meaningful descriptive of structural change in glaucoma.

5.2. Retinal nerve fiber layer

Technologies such as GDX and, more recently, OCT provide nerve fiber measurements outside of the boundaries of the disc and it has become evident that axonal changes in the area surrounding the nerve are important in understanding the nature and severity of glaucoma. [7, 8]

In a study performed by Bowd et al, clearly revealed that OCT revealed statistically significant quantitative differences in RNFL thickness between OHT and normal eyes within their study population. [9]

Additional studies such as those performed by Garas (2009), Sehi (2009) and Savini (2009) (table 1) have helped develop greater confidence in our ability to clinically determine RNFL thickness and to evaluate those findings in comparison to a reasonable field of normative data. [10-12]

Similar investigations in the following years helped give confidence that there was finally a method of determining RNFL thickness that was reliable enough so that meaningful comparisons could be made between normal and glaucomatous subjects. Beyond that general comparison, investigators could search for specific nerve and other retinal attributes which are more specific to the diagnosis and management of glaucoma. In 2010, Mansoori et al showed that SD-OCT identified differences in most parameters between eyes with glaucoma and normal eyes and also between eyes with glaucoma and OHT. It was important to note that they also observed that there was overlap of RNFL thickness between normal and OHT eyes, which somewhat limits the ability of this instrument to differentiate between normal and OHT subjects.[13]

	Garas			Sehi			Savini		
	Mean	Std. Dev.	95% Normal Range	Mean	Std.	95% Normal Range	Mean	Std. Dev.	95% Normal Range
Average RNFL	106.7	7.5	91.7 to 121.7	103.3	12.6	78.1 to 128.5	105.8	14.9	76.7 to 135.6
Superior	128.8	12.8	103.2 to 154.4	134.5	18.6	97.3 to 171.1	128.44	24.48	83.48 to 173.4
Inferior	136.6	12.7	111.2 to 162	129.7	16.9	95.9 to 163.5	137.15	21.99	93.17 to 181.13
S/I Ratio	0.943			1.037			0.936		

Table 1. Retinal nerve fiber layer thickness averages in normal patients. Garas et al 2009 (14 normals), Sehi et al (20 normals) and Savini et al (23 normals)

5.3. Ganglion cell layer

Most recently, the new abundant source of data rendered via spectral domain OCT measurements, allow us to document structural changes in the axonal bed as well as other retinal layers which were thought to, possibly, have close association with some types of glaucomatous progression. It seems intuitive that failing nerves might show changes at their endpoints before doing so in their mid-sections. Additionally, it seemed likely that axonal ganglia might show changes in concert with various types of axonal demise. Studies such as those conducted Desatnik et al and Ziemer et al in the 1990's helped point us to our new appreciation of the value of perimacular measurements. [14, 15]

Determining the extent of retinal ganglion cell loss may prove to be a superior method for identifying glaucomatous progression. The loss of these cells leads to functional deficits and structural changes in the retinal nerve fiber layer (RNFL). In their efforts to correlate structural and functional loss in glaucoma, Harwerth and associates showed that the number of retinal ganglion cells can be reliably estimated from either visual field sensitivity data or from OCT RNFL analysis. [16]

6. Functional measurement

6.1. Subjective testing

The first record of a visual field defect is found in Hippocrates description of a hemianopia from the late fifth century B.C. Ptolemy (150 B.C.) first attempted to quantify the visual field

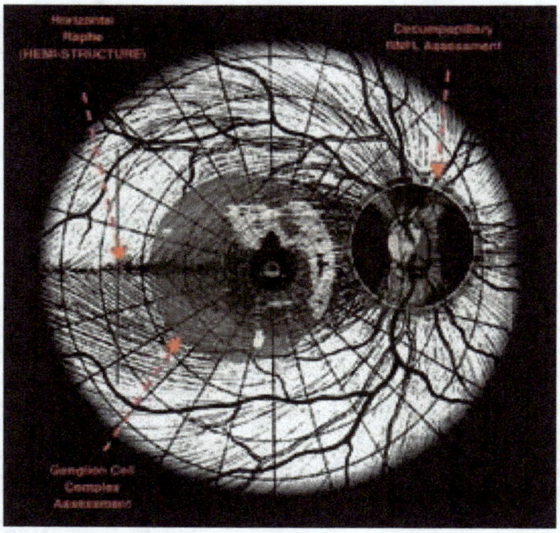

Figure 11. The RTVue scanning zones for assessment of the peripapillary retinal nerve fiber layer (RNFL) and the ganglion cell complex (GCC)

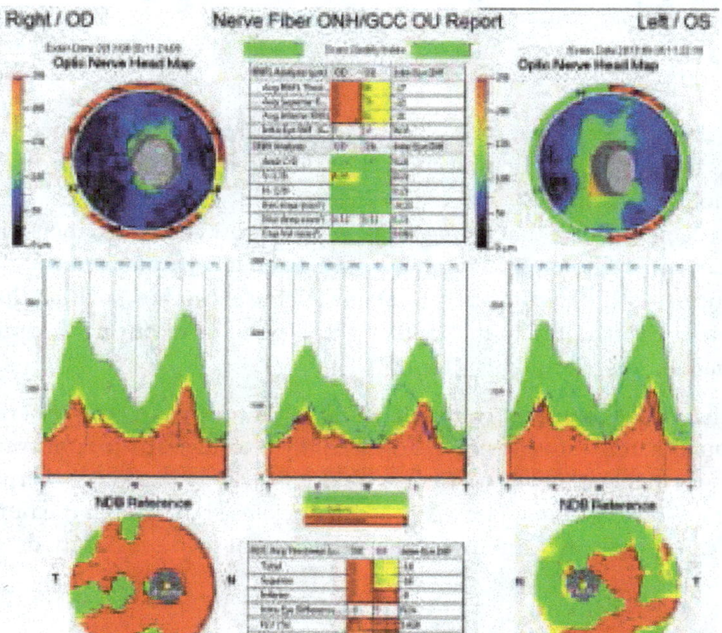

Figure 12. Optovue OCT report showing RNFL and GCC thickness. Colors green, yellow and red indicate normal, borderline and abnormal (low) findings.

and noted its circular form. According to Lloyd, Galen was the first physician "to record a recognition of Extramacular fields." He suggests the first illustration of the visual field was published in an article by Ulmus of Padua in 1602.

Early in the sixteenth century (about 1510) Leonardo da Vinci recognized that temporally the visual field reaches around more than 90 degrees from fixation. He said (Manuscript D. folio 8 verso), "the eye sees those objects behind it that are placed in lateral areas." He suggested that the cornea and the aqueous served to bend the light rays into the eye.

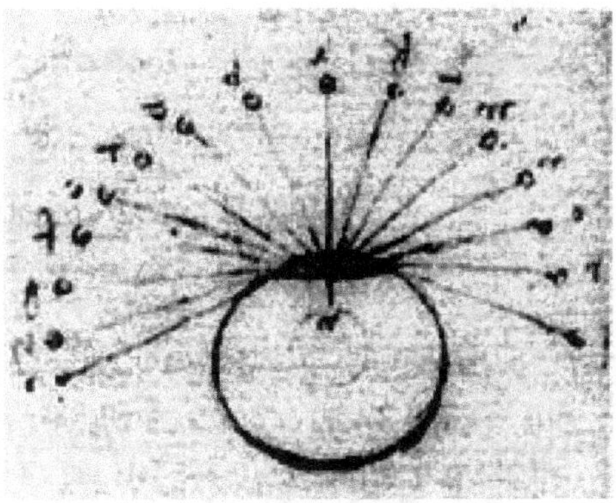

Figure 13. DaVinci's Illustration of rays approaching the cornea from different directions

Von Graefe (below) is credited with introducing perimetry into clinical medicine. In 1855, at the age of 28, he published "Examination of the Visual Functions in Amblyopic Affections." Von Graefe built on the work of Helmholtz. Helmholtz had recommended that, in order to keep one's bearing during the examination of the ocular fundus, a numbered grid be placed in front of the patient to direct the patient's eye into certain known directions of gaze. It was a piece of blackboard marked in this way that von Graefe used as a tangent screen. He worked at a distance of 18 inches and used as a test object a piece of white chalk, about 1 cm across, held in a wire. He made use of various symbols and dots as a fixation point so that the patient could recognize his deficits more easily. [17]

It was not until the late 1980's, when automated perimetry became widely available, that manual methods of visual field assessment were finally outpaced as the clinical standard. With the newfound ability to determine the relative depth of defect of a given point, clinicians had the ability to appreciate a three dimensional plot of one's visual status.

The introduction of computers and automation heralded a new era in perimetric testing. Static testing can be performed in an objective and standardized fashion with minimal perimetrist bias. A quantitative representation of the visual field can be obtained more rapidly than with manual testing. The computer allows stimuli to be presented in a pseudorandom, unpredictable fashion. Patients do not know where the next stimulus will appear, so fixation is improved, thereby increasing the reliability of the test. Random presentations also increase the speed with which perimetry can be performed by bypassing the problem of local retinal adaptation, which requires a 2-second interval between stimuli if adjacent locations are tested.

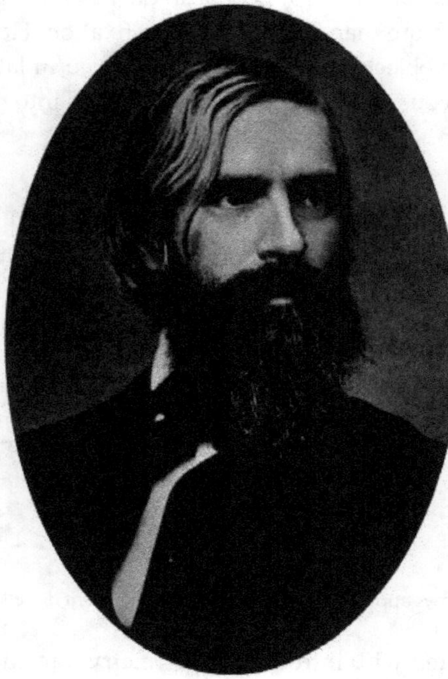

Figure 14. Albrecht von Graefe

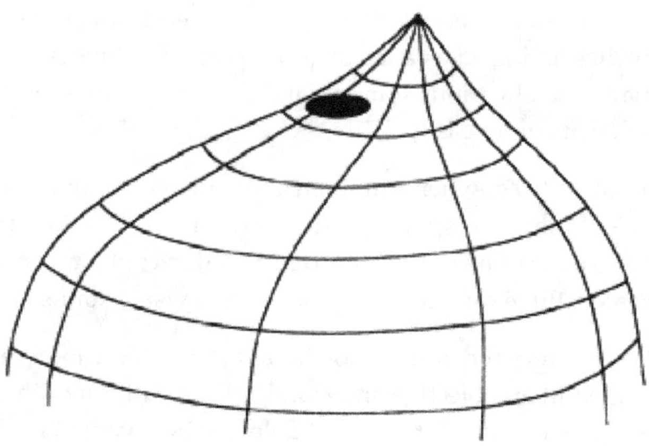

Figure 15. The normal island of vision. The hill is highest at fixation, where visual sensitivity is greatest. The height of the hill of vision declines toward the periphery as visual sensitivity diminishes.

Any clinically or statistically significant deviation from the normal shape of the hill of vision can be considered a visual field defect. In glaucoma, these defects are either diffuse depressions of the visual field or localized defects that conform to nerve fiber bundle patterns. [18]

6.2. Current choices in subjective functional testing

The addition of computerization to assessment of the eyes functional performance led the way to the development of several testing alternatives. Early white on white threshold testing strategies were followed with faster and more efficient programs such as Humphries Swedish Interactive Testing Algorithm (SITA) and the Haag-Streit Tendency Oriented Perimetry (TOP), Along with unenhanced test specificity, both strategies significantly reduce testing times by over 70%. The TOP strategy requires less than three minutes per eye per test.

A daunting point of frustration with the limits of threshold analysis came from the understanding that significant axonal loss had to have occurred before a repeatable threshold could be demonstrated. In 1982, Quigley reported that as much as 40% of optic nerve fibers may be lost before significant threshold visual field loss. [19]

Alternatives more recent methods in subjective field analysis, such as short wavelength (blue – yellow) and flicker strategies, were developed with the goal of reliably eliciting subject glaucomatous defects at an earlier point the progression of the disease. It is now shown that the flicker type tests such as Frequency Doubling Technology will have a role to play as a glaucoma screening tests, where as the the blue-yellow tests may not be as predictive as once throught. 20 Recently, there has been increased inteest in 10 degree white on white threshold fields because of its greater test point density and its apparent structure relationship to new OCT ganglion cell complex (GCC) imaging analyses. 14, 15

6.3. Objective testing

Objective methods such as Visual Evoked Potential (VEP), pattern electroretinography (pERG) (Diopsys, Inc.), and Relative Afferent Pupillary Defect (RAPDx) (Konan, USA) offer the potential of earlier and more specific functional testing but here continues to be a need to more reliably access functional loss at an earlier point in glaucomagenesis. While VEP and pERG measure the relative integrity of the electrical signal that passes through the nerve during the visual process,

RAPDx expands on the notion of diminished afferent pupillary reflex that may occur as nerve integrity is lost and glaucoma progresses.

With newer imaging methods such as OCT, we have made significant strides in earlier detection of structural loss, while our ability to detect functional loss earlier than what we achieve via white on white threshold field analysis remains a challenge. Given early evidence that VEP, pERG and RAPDx may offer some reliable evidence of early functional change, one can only hope that robust scientific evidence paired with more technical advancement of these types of tools may help us get a bit closer. [21-23]

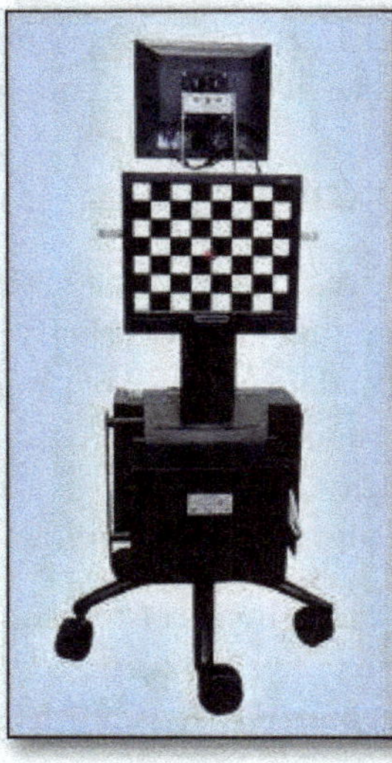

Figure 16. Visual Evoked Potential (VEP), pattern electroretinography (pERG) (Diopsys, Inc.)

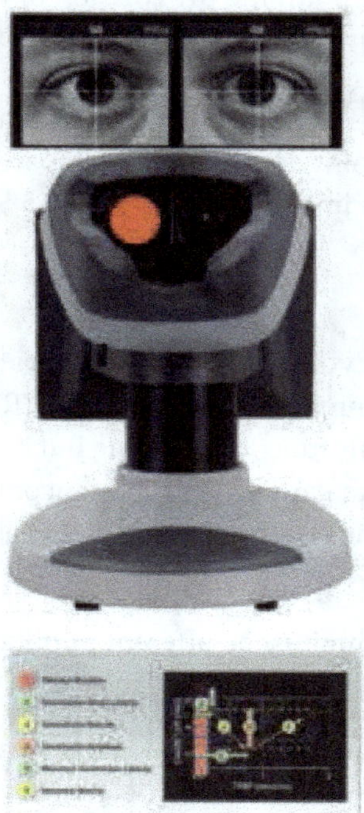

Figure 17. RAPDx (Konan, USA) measures Relative Afferent Pupillary Defect

7. Combining structural and functional data to optimize specificity in diagnosis

Along with our better understanding of the various limitations of either structural or functional analysis as a singular metric for glaucoma management, the obvious question has become can we, somehow, fortuitously coalesce both data sets? By combining the two, can we apprehend glaucoma earlier in its progression and develop better methods of dividing glaucoma into more meaningful subtypes? Will doing so allow us to treat more promptly, effectively and more specifically? Finally, is there a way to combine structural tests with functional tests to give us some type of unified glaucoma value?

Several investigators pioneered early structure function studies with the goal of establishing a better understanding of the relationships between various structural and functional values. In 1976, Stephen Drance described optic disc changes as they correlated to visual field defects in chronic open-angle glaucoma. Drance's studies were followed by Hoskins et al and Hitchings et al who also observed the nature of optic changes which occurred in concert with glaucomatous visual field changes (ref's). [24-26] These investigations were conducted with the goal of pairing specific anatomical changes commonly associated with glaucoma with associated functional (visual field) changes. Others tried to find a common more useful value in combining structural and functional data in different ways. [24-26]

Perhaps, the most renowned investigations which have established the foundations of our current understanding of the structure function relationship were performed by Quigley et al during the 1980's. Glaucomatous eyes were studied posthumously to determine how the number and distribution of human optic nerve axons compared with clinical measurements available the same eyes, including visual acuity, disc appearance, and visual field studies. Quigley reported that definite loss of axons occurs prior to reproducible visual field defects in some patients suspected of having glaucoma. In glaucoma, the superior and inferior poles of the nerve lose nerve fibers at a selectively greater rate, leading to an hourglass-shaped atrophy. He also reported that the pattern of atrophy in examples of toxic amblyopia, ischemic optic neuropathy and chronic papilledema differ from that of glaucoma, suggesting different mechanisms of damage in these conditions.

In later investigations, Harwerth et al described relationships between field loss and retinal ganglion cells. The data were analyzed by a model that predicted ganglion cell densities from standard clinical perimetry, which were then compared to histologic cell counts. Their work became part of the foundation for our current interest and understanding of functional loss in the context of retinal tissue changes beyond the losses previously described in retinal axons. [27-30]

In 2005, Gardiner et al produced a topographical map to demonstrate how sectors of the optic nerve head (ONH) are related to locations in the visual field, using empiric cross-sectional patient data. They observed one hundred nine subjects with healthy eyes and 166 subjects with diagnosed or suspected glaucoma (one test per patient) were evaluated using a Heidelberg Retina tomograph (HRT) and white-on-white standard automated perimetry (SAP). The

Tomograph ONH images were divided into 36 sectors; and the sector rim areas normalized to account for changes in the total rim area. These were then correlated with SAP thresholds. For each visual field location, a map was produced indicating the strength of correlation between the normalized sector rim areas and thresholds. Their efforts resulted in a map relating regions of the ONH to SAP test locations. This map may be useful in elucidating the structure-function relationship, particularly for cases of localized glaucomatous loss.

Their results also indicate that narrowing of the neuroretinal rim in some areas appeared to be more significant than in others, in terms of predicting functional loss; in particular in the polar areas of the ONH. This may account for some of the limitations of predictive power that has been shown of global HRT indices. [31]

In 2010, Harwerth et al attempted to build a model of these linking propositions using data from investigations of the relationships between losses of visual sensitivity and thinning of retinal nerve fiber layer over progressive stages of glaucoma severity. A foundation for the model was laid through the pointwise relationships between visual sensitivities (behavioral perimetry in monkeys with experimental glaucoma) and histological analyses of retinal ganglion cell densities in corresponding retinal locations. The subsequent blocks of the model were constructed from clinical studies of aging in normal human subjects and of clinical glaucoma in patients to provide a direct comparison of the results from standard clinical perimetry and optical coherence tomography. The final formulation is a nonlinear structure-function model that was evaluated by the accuracy and precision of translating visual sensitivities in a region of the visual field to produce a predicted thickness of the retinal nerve fiber layer in the peripapillary sector that corresponded to the region of reduced visual sensitivity. The model was tested on two independent patient populations, with results that confirmed the predictive relationship between the retinal nerve fiber layer thickness and visual sensitivities from clinical perimetry. Thus, the proposed model for linking structure and function in glaucoma has provided information that is important in understanding the results of standard clinical testing and the neuronal losses caused by glaucoma, which may have clinical application for inter-test comparisons of the stage of disease. The model was tested on two independent patient populations, with results that confirmed the predictive relationship between the retinal nerve fiber layer thickness and visual sensitivities from clinical perimetry. Thus, the proposed model for linking structure and function in glaucoma has provided information that is important in understanding the results of standard clinical testing and the neuronal losses caused by glaucoma, which may have clinical application for inter-test comparisons of the stage of disease. [16]

In 2012, Medeiros et al confirmed that an index combining structure and function performed better than isolated structural and functional measures for detection of perimetric and preperimetric glaucoma as well as for discriminating different stages of the disease. Observational study included 333 glaucomatous eyes (295 with perimetric glaucoma and 38 with preperimetric glaucoma) and 330 eyes of healthy subjects. All the eyes were tested with standard automated perimetry and spectral domain optical coherence tomography within 6 months. Estimates of the number of retinal ganglion cells (RGCs) were obtained from standard automated perimetry and spectral domain optical coherence tomography and a weighted averaging scheme was used to obtain a final estimate of the number of RGCs for each eye. The CSFI was calculated as the percent loss of RGCs obtained by subtracting estimated from expected RGC numbers. The performance of the CSFI for discriminating glaucoma from normal eyes and the different stages of disease was evaluated by receiver operating characteristic curves. [32, 33]

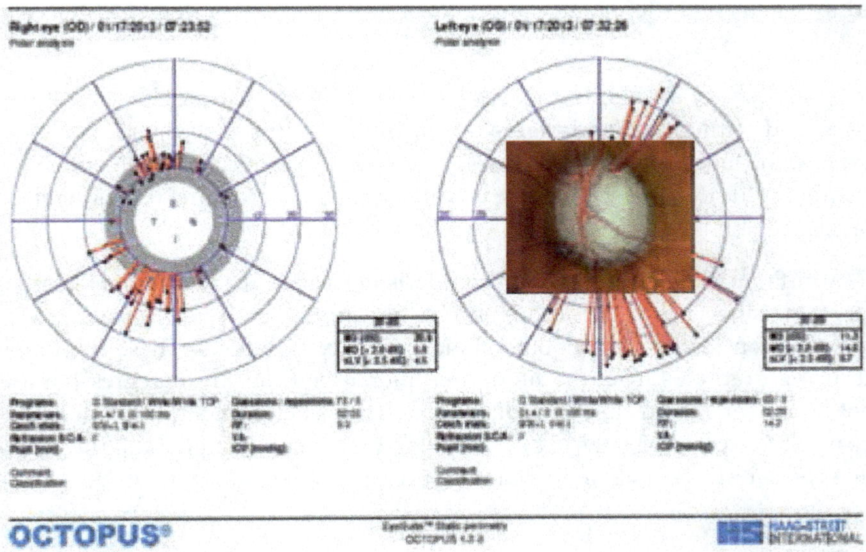

Figure 18. Polar analysis of a threshold visual field showing severity of the defect in concert with nerve anatomy. While traditional graphical reports of field analysis show projected (inverted) findings, the polar analysis is anatomically correct.

In 2013, Meira-Freitas et al demonstrated that baseline and longitudinal estimates of retinal ganglion cell counts based on combined structure and function tests may be helpful in predicting progression, and performed significantly better than conventional approaches for risk stratification of glaucoma suspects. The study included 288 glaucoma suspect eyes of 288 patients followed for an average of 3.8 ± 1.0 years. Estimates of RGC counts were obtained by combining data from SAP and OCT according to previously described method. Joint longitudinal survival models were used to evaluate the ability of baseline and rates of change in estimated RGC counts for predicting progression over time, adjusting for confounding variables. [34]

Also, in 2013, Le et al implemented fourier-domain optical coherence tomography (FD-OCT) system to map the macula and peripapillary regions of the retina in 56 eyes of 38 patients with perimetric glaucoma. The macular GCC and peripapillary NFL thicknesses were mapped and standard automated perimetry (SAP) was performed. Loss of GCC and NFL were correlated with the VF map on both a point-by-point and regional basis, showing that there are significant point-specific and regional correlations between GCC loss, NFL loss, and deficits on SAP. Their findings suggest that using these different data sources together may improve our understanding of glaucomatous damage and aid in the management of patients with glaucoma. [35]

In 2013, Hye-Young Shin et al Two hundred and thirteen eyes of 213 patients with glaucoma were observed to explore and compare the relationships between the visual field (VF) sensitivities assessed by standard automated perimetry (SAP) and the ganglion cell inner plexiform layer (GCIPL) and peripapillary retinal nerve fiber layer (pRNFL) thicknesses as measured by Cirrus high-definition optical coherence tomography (HD-OCT) in glaucomatous eyes.

The average and sectorial GCIPL thicknesses determined by Cirrus HD-OCT were significantly associated with global and regional VF sensitivity in patients with glaucoma. They concluded that the macular GCIPL thickness values may provide more valuable information than temporal profile thickness values for understanding the structure–function relationships of the macular region. [35]

In 2013, Marín-Franch et al reported their comparison structural and functional damage from glaucoma often using statistical methods such as linear regression, which was agreed to have limitations that can lead to inadequate clinical recommendations. These limitations were analyzed, using examples from the literature. Inferences from linear regression are model dependent. They concluded that tests of linear relations between structure and function in glaucoma may be improved by the use of Deming regression, although its application requires knowledge about test-retest variability of measures of glaucomatous damage. [37, 38]

8. Summary

It has been said that in Einstein's Grand Quest for a Unified Theory "He failed, of course, but he didn't exactly waste his time." Similarly, our search for a simplified common denominator to describe glaucoma in a simple way is likely to fail. Our methods of documenting the optic nerve and various ocular structures related to the genesis of glaucoma have evolved from direct observation paired with hand drawings to ocular corherance tomographic devices, which render elegant cross sectional views with as little as 5 microns of resolution. Quantification of the visual field has also evolved to sophisticated threshold subjective analyses and promising new objective strategies. In spite of this impressive technical evolution, we have yet to agree upon a practical combination of structural and functional data that can provide a single metric for risk of glaucoma and the level of its progression.

Perhaps, the solution to this conundrum can be derived from our acceptance that glaucoma does not appear to be one simple disease, but rather one that is the result of a litany of risk factors that commonly result in the untimely deterioration of the optic nerve. As investigators have and continue to examine the many structural and functional changes that may occur in the process of glaucoma, the field of clinical variables ironically seems to expand rather than contract. Physical changes may be observed at the neural retinal rim first, while in other patients changes in the peri macular ganglion cell layer may be the first signal of glaucomatous change. Some patients might show degradation in their peripheral visual fields while others seem to start with central changes. Recent investigators have even suggested that early changes, in glaucoma, may occur within the brain.

As with Einstein's Grand Quest, it can be argued that the efforts of researchers to find a "unified glaucoma value" have not been a waste of time. While there seems to be no simple solution to this puzzle in sight, we have been given a far better understanding of glaucoma's multivariate etiology which should enable more specific and prompt diagnosis and, ultimately, more specific and effective glaucoma therapies.

Author details

Elliot M. Kirstein*

Address all correspondence to: drkirstein@drkirstein.com

Harper's Point Eye Associates, Cincinnati, Ohio, USA

References

[1] The phasic variations in the ocular tension in primary glaucoma. Am J Ophthalmol. 1952 Jan;35(1):1–21.

[2] Ophthalmoscopes Part 1 http://www.college-optometrists.org/en/college/museyeum/online_exhibitions/optical_instruments/ophthalmoscopes/

[3] Mark HH, On the Evolution of Binocular Ophthalmoscopy. Ophthalmol. 2007;125(6): 830-833. doi:10.1001/archopht.125.6.830

[4] Reus NJ and Lemij HG. The Relationship between Standard Automated Perimetry and GDx VCC Measurements. Investigative Ophthalmology & Visual Science, March 2004, Vol. 45, No. 3

[5] Zangwill LM, Williams J, A comparison of optical coherence tomography and retinal nerve fiber layer photography for detection of nerve fiber layer damage in glaucoma. Ophthalmology Volume 113, Issue 9, Pages 1593-1602, September 2006

[6] Gabriele ML, Wollstein G, Ishikawa H, Kagemann L, Xu J, Folio L S and Schuman J S. Optical Coherence Tomography: History, Current Status, and Laboratory Work Investigative Ophthalmology & Visual Science, April 2011, Vol. 52, No. 5

[7] Bendschneider D, Tornow RP, Horn FK, Laemmer R, Roessler CW, Juenemann AG, Kruse FE, Mardin CY.Retinal nerve fiber layer thickness in normals measured by

spectral domain OCT.J Glaucoma. 2010 Sep;19(7):475-82. doi: 10.1097/IJG.0b013e3181c4b0c7

[8] Varma R, Skaf M, Barron E. Retinal nerve fiber layer thickness in normal human eyes. Ophthalmology. 1996 Dec;103(12):2114-9

[9] Bowd C, Weinreb RN; Williams JM, Zangwill LM. The Retinal Nerve Fiber Layer Thickness in Ocular Hypertensive, Normal, and Glaucomatous Eyes With Optical Coherence Tomography Arch Ophthalmol. 2000;118(1):22-26. doi:10.1001/archopht.118.1.22

[10] Garas A, Tóth M, Vargha P, Holló G. Comparison of repeatability of retinal nerve fiber layer thickness measurement made using the RTVue Fourier-domain optical coherence tomograph and the GDx scanning laser polarimeter with variable or enhanced corneal compensation. J Glaucoma. 2010 Aug;19(6):412-7. doi: 10.1097/IJG.0b013e3181bdb549

[11] Sehi M, Grewal DS, Sheets CW, Greenfield DS. Diagnostic ability of Fourier-domain vs time-domain optical coherence tomography for glaucoma detection. Am J Ophthalmol. 2009 Oct;148(4):597-605. doi: 10.1016/j.ajo.2009.05.030. Epub 2009 Jul 9.

[12] Savini G, Carbonelli M, Barboni P. Retinal nerve fiber layer thickness measurement by Fourier-domain optical coherence tomography: a comparison between cirrus-HD OCT and RTVue in healthy eyes. J Glaucoma. 2010 Aug;19(6):369-72. doi: 10.1097/IJG.0b013e3181bdb55d.

[13] Tarannum Mansoori, MS; Kalluri Viswanath, MS; Nagalla Balakrishna, PhD Quantification of Retinal Nerve Fiber Layer Thickness in Normal Eyes, Eyes With Ocular Hypertension, and Glaucomatous Eyes With SD-OCT Ophthalmic Surgery, Lasers & Imaging • Vol. 41, No. 6 (Suppl), 2010

[14] Desatnik H, Quigley HA, Glovinsky Y. Study of central retinal ganglion loss in experimental glaucoma in monkey eyes. J Glaucoma. 1996;5(1):46-53.

[15] Zeimer R, Asrani S, Zou S, et al. Quantitative detection of glaucomatous damage at the posterior pole by retinal thickness mapping: a pilot study. Ophthalmology. 1998;105(2):224-231.

[16] Harwerth RS, Wheat JL, Fredette MJ, Anderson DR. Linking structure and function in glaucoma. Prog Retin Eye Res. 2010 Jul;29(4):249-71. doi: 10.1016/j.preteyeres.2010.02.001. Epub 2010 Mar 11.

[17] Imaging and Perimetry Society History of the visual field before perimetry http://www.perimetry.org/PerimetryHistory/1-pre-perimetry.htm

[18] Piltz-Seymour J R, Heath Phillip O, Drance S M. Visual Fields in Glaucoma http://www.oculist.net/downaton502/prof/ebook/duanes/pages/v3/v3c049.html

[19] Quigley HA, Addicks EM, Green WR. Optic nerve damage in human glaucoma. III. Quantitative correlation of nerve fiber loss and visual field defect in glaucoma, ische-

mic neuropathy, papilledema, and toxic neuropathy. Arch Ophthalmol 1982 Jan; 100(1):135-46.

[20] Yoshiyama KK and Johnson CA. Which Method of Flicker Perimetry Is Most Effective for

[21] Detection of Glaucomatous Visual Field Loss? Investigative Ophthalmology & Visual Science, October 1997, Vol. 38, No. 11

[22] Pillai C, Ritch R, Derr P, Gonzalez A, Cox LK, Siegfried J, Liebmann JS and Tello C. Sensitivity and Specificity of Short-Duration Transient Visual Evolked Potentials in Discriminating Normal From Glaucomatous Eyes. Invest Ophthalmol Vis Sci. 2013 Apr 23;54(4):2847-52. doi: 10.1167/iovs.12-10097. f Short-Duration Transient Visual Evoked Potentials (SD-tVEP)

[23] Chang DS, Boland MV, Arora KS, Supakontanasan W, Chen BB, Friedman D. Wilmur Institute, Johns Hopkins August 2013 Symmetry of the Pupillary Light Reflex and its Relationship to Retinal Nerve Fiber Layer Thickness and Visual Field Defect Invest Ophthalmol Vis Sci. 2013 Aug 19;54(8):5596-601. doi: 10.1167/iovs.13-12142.

[24] Meira-Freitas D, Weinreb RN, Marvasti AH, Zangwill LM, and Madeiros FA. Estimation of retinal ganglion cell loss in glaucomatous eyes with a relative afferent pupillary defect. Ophthalmol. Vis. Sci. published 26 November 2013, 10.1167/iovs.13-12921

[25] Drance SM. Correlation between optic disc changes and visual field defects in chronic open-angle glaucoma. Trans Am Acad Ophthalmol Otolaryngol. 1976;81:224-226.

[26] Hoskins HD Jr, Gelber EC. Optic disk topography and visual field defects in patients with increased intraocular pressure. Am J Ophthalmol. 1975;80:284-290

[27] Hitchings RA, Spaeth GL. The optic disc in glaucoma II: Correlation of the appearance of the optic disc with the visual field. Br J Ophthalmol. 1977;61:107-113.

[28] Quigley HA, Addicks EM, Green WR. Optic nerve damage in human glaucoma. III. Quantitative correlation of nerve fiber loss and visual field defect in glaucoma, ischemic neuropathy, papilledema and toxic neuropathy. Arch Ophthalmol. 1982;100:135-146.

[29] Quigley HA, Dunkelberger GR, Green WR. Retinal ganglion cell atrophy correlated with automated perimetry in human eyes with glaucoma. Am J Ophthalmol. 1989;107:453-464.

[30] Harwerth RS, Carter-Dawson L, Smith EL 3rd, Crawford ML. Scaling the structure--function relationship for clinical perimetry. Acta Ophthalmol Scand. 2005;83:448-455.

[31] Harwerth RS, Quigley HA. Visual field defects and retinal ganglion cell losses in patients with glaucoma. Arch Ophthalmol. 2006;124:853-859.

[32] Gardiner SK, Johnson CA and Cioffi CA. Evaluation of the Structure-Function Relationship in Glaucoma. Copyright 2005 The Association for Research in Vision and Ophthalmology, Inc.

[33] Medeiros FA, Lisboa R, Weinreb RN, Girkin CA, Liebmann JM, Zangwill LM. A combined index of structure and function for staging glaucomatous damage. A combined index of structure and function for staging glaucomatous damage. Arch Ophthalmol. 2012 May;130(5):E1-10

[34] Medeiros FA, Zangwill LM, Anderson DR, Liebmann JM, Girkin CA, Harwerth RS, Fredette MJ, Weinreb RN. Estimating the rate of retinal ganglion cell loss in glaucoma. Am J Ophthalmol. 2012 Nov;154(5):814-824.e1. doi: 10.1016/j.ajo.2012.04.022. Epub 2012 Jul 27.

[35] Meira-Freitas D, Lisboa R, Tatham A, Zangwill LM, Weinreb RN, Girkin CA, Liebmann LM, and Medeiros FA. Predicting Progression in Glaucoma Suspects With Longitudinal Estimates of Retinal Ganglion Cell Counts Invest. Ophthalmol. Vis. Sci. 2013;54 4174-4183 7/2013 http://www.iovs.org/cgi/content/abstract/54/6/4174

[36] Phuc V. Le, Ou Tan, Vikas Chopra, Brian A. Francis, Omar Ragab, Rohit Varma, and David Huang. Regional Correlation Among Ganglion Cell Complex, Nerve Fiber Layer, and Visual Field Loss in GlaucomaInvest. Ophthalmol. Vis. Sci. 2013;54 4287-4295 http://www.iovs.org/cgi/content/abstract/54/6/4287

[37] Shin HY, Lopilly Park HY, Jung KI and Park CK. Comparative Study of Macular Ganglion Cell-Inner Plexiform Layer and Retinal Nerve Fiber Layer Measurement : Structure-Function Analysis IOVS IOVS-13-12667; published ahead of print October 15, 2013

[38] Marín-Franch I, Malik R, Crabb DP, and Swanson WH. Choice of Statistical Method Influences Apparent Association Between Structure and Function in Glaucoma Invest. Ophthalmol. Vis. Sci. 2013;54 4189-4196 7/2013 http://www.iovs.org/cgi/content/abstract/54/6/4189

[39] Mwanza JC, Warren JL, and BudenzInvest DL. Combining Spectral Domain Optical Coherence Tomography Structural Parameters for the Diagnosis of Glaucoma with Early Visual Field Loss Ophthalmol. Vis. Sci. published 26 November 2013, 10.1167/iovs.13-12749 http://www.iovs.org/cgi/content/abstract/iovs.13-12749v1

6

Disorders of Optic Nerve and Visual Pathways

Ipek Midi

1. Introduction

The evaluation of a patient with visual acuity and visual field defect depends on a detailed history, careful examination and knowledge of anatomic pathways. The structures which are responsible for these pathologies include the retina, optic nerve, optic chiasm, optic tract, optic radiation and visual cortex of the occipital lobe. These structures are called the afferent systems of visual pathways.

Multiple aetiologies can affect and cause different disorders. The history gives the information about the possible aetiologies of the optic neuropathy. There are simple and advanced investigation methods that can support the diagnosis of optic neuropathy. Visual field testing by either manual kinetic or automated static perimetry, cranial and orbital MR, visually evoked potentials and optic coherence tomography are the investigation methods that help in diagnosis. In this chapter optic nerve and visual pathway disorders will be discussed.

1.1. The anatomy of optic nerve and the visual pathways

The visual pathway begins from the globes and extends to the visual cortex in the occipital lobe [1]. The optic nerve (cranial nerve II) leaves the orbit; it reaches to the optic chiasm, which is located besides the pituitary gland. The optic nerve fibres originate from the nasal half of each retina decussate at the optic chiasm level and form an X-shaped structure; on the other hand the nerve fibres of the temporal retina continue their way without crossing [1-3]. From there, most of the axons of the nerve fibres terminate in the lateral geniculate nucleus of the thalamus which is called the **optic tract**, while the other axons terminate in the pretectal nucleus which is responsible for pupillary reflex movements. In its course from the lateral geniculate nucleus to the striate cortex, **optic radiation** fans out under the temporal and parietal lobes. Some of the optic radiation axons run out into the temporal lobe called Meyer's loop. Meyer's loop carries information from the superior portion of the contralateral visual field. More medial parts of the optic radiation, which pass under the cortex of the parietal lobe, carry information from the inferior portion of the contralateral visual field. Damage to parts of the temporal lobe results in a superior homonymous quadrantanopsia; damage to the optic radiation underlying the parietal cortex results in an inferior homonymous quadrantanopsia type in the visual field. Then the fibres from both the temporal and parietal lobe reach the visual cortex in the occipital lobe [1-3].

Signs of optic nerve dysfunction

1. Reduced visual acuity
2. Afferent pupillary defect
3. Dyschromatopsia (impairment of colour vision)
4. Diminished light brightness sensitivity
5. Diminished contrast sensitivity
6. Visual field defect

1.2. Examination of visual field

Confrontation technique is used to examine the central or peripheral visual dysfunction. The examiner asks the patient to cover one eye and the examiner also covers the opposite eye at the same time. The examiner moves a colourful object in his hand out of the patient's visual field and then brings it centrally. He has to tell the examiner when he notices the object. The same examination must be done for the opposite side [4].

1.3. Clinical features of visual field defect

Damage to the optic nerve causes permanent and severe loss of vision and pupillary reflex abnormalities. According to the localization of lesion, different type of visual field defect can occur. In general [1, 5]:

- If the optic nerve is damaged anterior to the optic chiasm, it causes loss of vision on the same side as the damage
- If the optic nerve is damaged in the optic chiasm level, it causes bitemporal hemianopia. This may occur in expanding pituitary adenoma (Figure 1).
- If optic nerve is damaged posterior to the optic chiasm (optic tract, optic radiation), it causes a visual field defect on the opposite side to the damage [5-7].

The main symptom is vision loss, frequently maximal within one or two days and varying from a small central or paracentral scotoma to complete blindness. Most patients complain of mild eye pain, which often feels worse with eye movements [3, 8].

Optic neuropathy describes abnormalities of the optic nerve [8].This may occur as a result of ischaemia, vascular and blood pressure abnormalities, toxins, compression, infiltrations and trauma [9,10]. Optic neuropathy is divided into anterior and posterior types: anterior optic

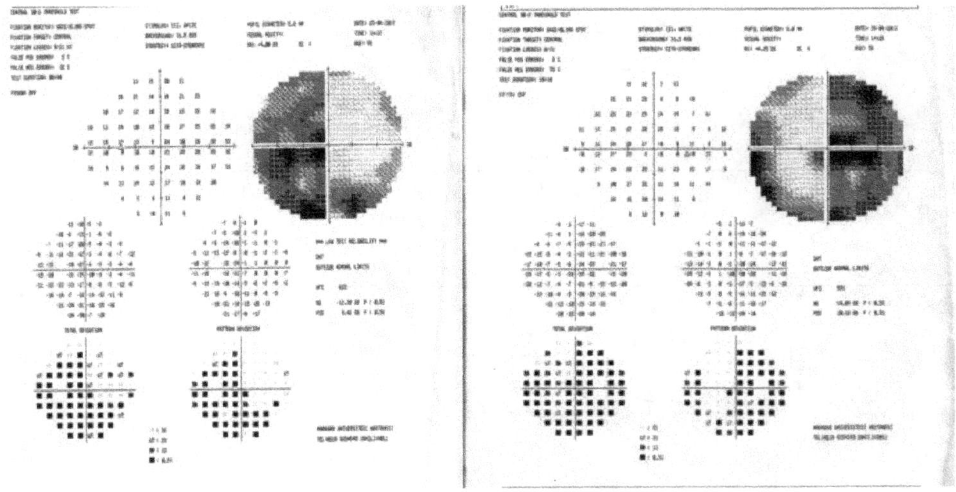

Figure 1. Visual field analysis shows bitemporal hemianophia in a patient with pituitary adenoma.

neuropathy, which causes a pale oedema of the optic disc; and posterior, in which the optic disc is not swollen and the abnormality occurs between the globe and the optic chiasm [3, 4, 8].

1.4. Optic disc oedema and papilloedema

Optic disc oedema is the swelling and elevation of the disc. It can be caused by a number of conditions. Papilloedema relates more specifically to optic nerve head swelling secondary to raised intracranial pressure (Table 1). Disc swelling is distinct from disc atrophy which refers to a loss of nerve fibres at the optic nerve head [2, 3, 11]. There are various signs visible during fundoscopic evaluation. These are: optic disc swelling, unclearness around the margin of the disc, optic disc hyperaemia, venous dilatation, peripapillary haemorrhages, disc exuda or exuda in peripapillar area and cotton wood spots [11].

The pathogenesis of optic disc oedema is mostly related to inhibition of axoplasmic flow. Although histopathological and ophthalmoscopic findings are similar, it is important for treatment approaches to find the causes of optic disc swelling. Often, the cause remains obscure despite undergoing a thorough evaluation [3-11].

Papilloedema is swelling of the optic nerve head, secondary to raised intracranial pressure. This may be due to obstruction of the ventricular system, space-occupying lesion, impairment of cerebro-spinal fluid (CSF) absorption, diffuse cerebral oedema or idiopathic (benign/essential) intracranial hypertension. The patient complains of headache (worse on waking and when coughing) and may have nausea/vomiting. There may be diplopia if there is a VI cranial nerve palsy [3].

In papilloedema, disc swelling is nearly always bilateral (it may be asymmetrical in the early phase) and may be hyperaemic; dilatation of veins and loss of spontaneous venous pulsation

Optic nerve lesions	Tumour (optic nerve sheath meningioma, glioma) Infiltrative lesions (leukaemia, lymphoma) Inflammatory lesions (sarcoidosis) Anterior ischemic optic neuropathy (hypertension, diabetes) Parainfectious and infectious optic neuropathy Trauma
Orbital lesions	Tumour Carotid-cavernous fistula Thyroid ophthalmopathy Trauma or surgery related
Intraocular events	Central retinal vein occlusion Uveitis Ocular hypotonia Papillophelibitis (optic disc vasculitis)
Systemic disease	Hypertension Anaemia Diabetes Mellitus
Leber's optic neuropathy	
Raised intracranial pressure: papilloedema	

Table 1. Causes of optic disc swelling

are the findings of fundoscopic examination. All other causes of disc oedema in the absence of raised intracranial pressure are referred to as disc swelling. But not all patients who have raised intracranial pressure will necessarily develop papilloedema [3]. Visual acuity (VA) is normal in the early stage and will be reduced in the late stage. Colour vision is impaired and there may have a relative afferent pupillary defect (RAPD). Transient obscurations are frequently seen. VI cranial nerve palsy and diplopia are the others clinical features of raised intracranial pressure. In some cases chronic papilloedema can progress to chronic atrophic papilloedema and in this situation visual loss develops [3, 8].

Papilloedema is a neurological emergency. The underlying cause needs to be investigated. After taking a detailed history and physical examination, Cranial CT or MRI has to be evaluated. If there is no space-occupying lesion on Cranial CT or MRI, lumbar puncture decreases the pressure.

2. Disorders of optic nerve (clinical symptoms/ diagnosis/ treatment/ imagings)

2.1. Arteritic ischemic optic neuropathy

Ischemic optic neuropathy is the most commonly seen neuropathy in elderly. Ischemic neuropathy is divided into two parts: 1) Anterior and 2) Posterior. (Both of them are also divided arteritic and non-arteritic forms.)

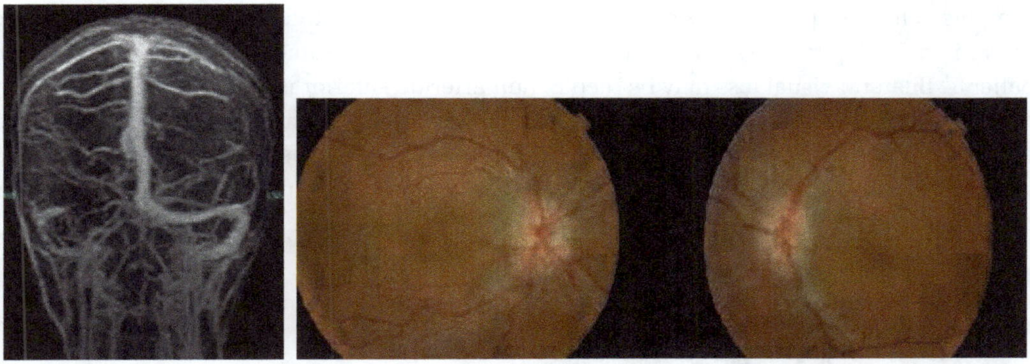

Figure 2. 37 year-old man with venous sinus thrombosis. Papilloedema in early phase is seen. The boundaries of the optic disc are not seen clearly. We do not observe vascular tortuousity (With the permission of Marmara University Dept. of Ophthalmology).

2.1.1. Non-Arteritic Anterior Ischemic Optic Neuropathy (NAAION)

Non-arteritic anterior ischemic optic neuropathy is the most common form of ischemic optic neuropathy. The underlying mechanism of **anterior ischemic optic neuropathy** is the interruption of the blood flow in the short posterior ciliary arteries that supply the optic nerve head. It generally occurs between the ages of 55 and 70 years old. The non-arteritic type involves mainly vascular occlusive disease or disorders that reduce the circulation of blood in the short posterior ciliary arteries. Predisposing systemic conditions include hypertension, diabetes mellitus, hypercholesterolaemia and collagen vascular disease (Table 2).

Visual loss may be sudden or occur over several days. Most of the patients complain of painless *monocular visual loss*. Visual acuity may be normal in about 30% of patients. Impairment of visual acuity in ischemic optic neuropathy may vary from moderate to severe with no light perception. Fundoscopic examination shows a pale, swollen optic disk, with peripapillary haemorrhages noticeable (Figure 3). Inferior altitudinal visual field defects are typical findings but other defects may also be seen. An afferent pupillary defect is present [3, 8, 12, 13].

Investigations: Fasting lipid profile and blood glucose, serological analysis, vasculitis markers, investigations of the carotid artery [3].

Treatment: There is no definite treatment to reverse the damage. Aspirin treatment is effective in reducing systemic vascular events but it does not appear to prevent the involvement of the other eye [3]. However, a recent large study has shown that if patients are treated with large doses of corticosteroid therapy during the early stages of NAION, there was visual acuity improvement in 70% of the treated group compared to 41% in the untreated group (odds ratio of improvement: 3.39; 95% CI:1.62, 7.11; $p < 0.001$) [14]. That study and a natural history study on NAION [15] showed that visual acuity can improve for up to six months.To minimize the risk of further visual loss in the other eye or the same eye, it is essential to reduce the risk factors.

Prognosis: In most patients, there is no further loss of vision but vision loss continues for six weeks in a small percentage of patients. Recurrence rate in the same eye occur is about 6% of patients. Bilateral visual loss may be seen in non-arteritic anterior ischemic optic neuropathy and it usually occurs sequentially instead of simultaneously [16].The second eye involvement occurs in about 10% of patients after two years and 15% after five years. When the second eye becomes involved, optic atrophy in one eye and disc oedema in the other eye gives the definition of "pseudo-Foster Kennedy Syndrome" [3].

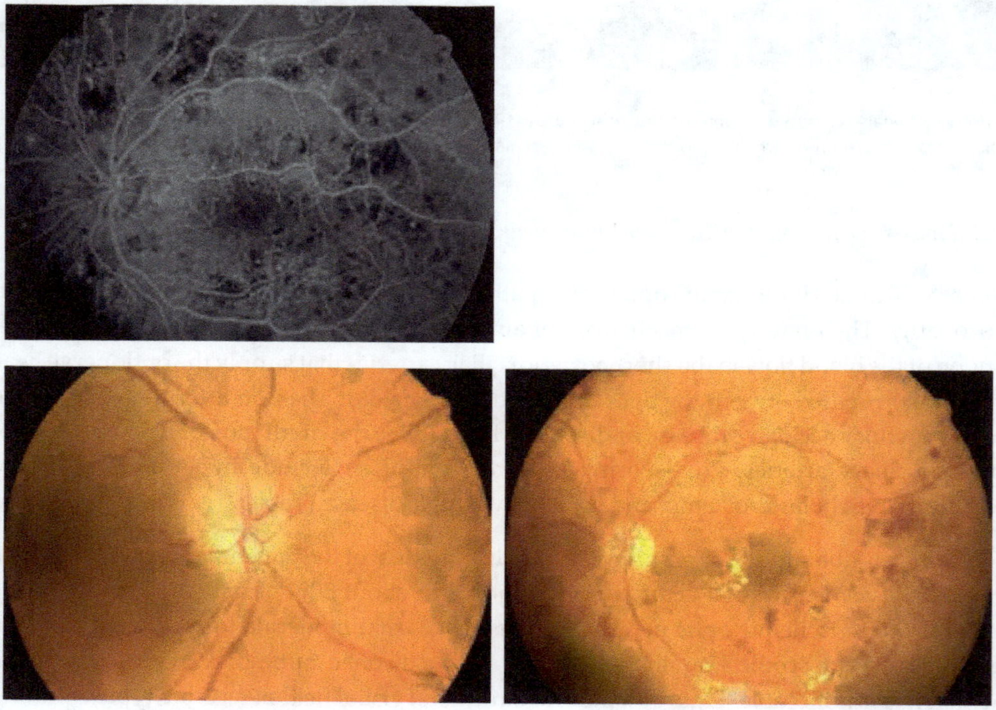

Figure 3. Non-arteritic anterior ischemic optic neuropathy: FFA shows hypofluorescence area caused by diffuse haemorrhage; diffuse microaneurysms, ischemic hypofluorescence area related to peripheric capillary blockages (right eye); crowded optic disc; oedema especially on the upper side; and boundaries on the nasal and temporal side show haemorrhages (left eye) diffuse haemorrhages, exudates and microvascular abnormalities in intraretinal segments (With the permission of Bezmialem University Dept. of Ophthalmology).

2.1.2. Arteritic Anterior Ischemic Optic Neuropathy (AAION)

The arteritic type is less common (25 %). Arteritic anterior ischemic optic neuropathy (AAION) is an acute ischaemia of the posterior ciliary arteries and/or ophthalmic artery due to inflammation. It is also known as giant cell arteritis. The ischaemia of the posterior ciliary arteries and/or the ophthalmic artery is caused by a granulomatous vasculitis of the vessel walls. Therapy is immediate intervention with systemic steroids, especially to protect against vision loss in the other eye [17-19].

The visual loss is sudden and unilateral, but if the treatment is delayed, bilateral visual loss may be seen. Patients with arteritic anterior ischemic optic neuropathy (AION) often have symptoms other than visual loss, such as malaise, weight loss, headache, scalp tenderness and loss of pulsation of one or both temporal arteries, jaw pain on mastication (jaw claudication), generalized muscle aches and swelling. [3, 20]

Investigations: ESR and CRP should be evaluated and they are usually raised. Temporal artery biopsy is the gold standard for diagnosis and should be performed within seven days of starting treatment. But the treatment should never be delayed while waiting for biopsy.

Treatment: Most patients' treatment continues for one or two years. a) Intravenous methyl-prednisolone: 1 gr/day for three days and oral prednisolone 80 mg/daily. The treatment regime continues by tapering the oral doses.

CRP is a sensitive marker in monitoring disease activity.

Prognosis: The course of the illness results in poor prognosis. Visual loss is generally permanent; partial visual recovery can be achieved by steroid therapy [3].

Posterior ischemic optic neuropathy is a rare type of neuropathy and diagnosis depends largely upon exclusion of other causes, such as stroke and brain tumour. Decreased visual acuity and altitudinal visual field defects are present. Decreased blood flow in the pial capillary plexus supplying the nerve, connective tissue disorders, diabetes mellitus, trauma and radiotherapy to the orbit have all been described as causes. It is also divided into two types; arteritic and non-arteritic [3, 12] (Table 2).

NON-ARTERITIC	ARTERITIC
Hypertension	Takayasu arteritis
Diabetes Mellitus	Romatoid arterid
Hypercholesterolaemia	Poliarteritis nodusa
Cardiac disease	Behçet's Disease
Anaemia, hypotension	Crohn's Disease
Cataract surgery	
Coagulopathies	
Collagen vascular disease	
Hyperhomocysteinaemia	
Antiphospholipid antibody synd.	
Sleep apnoea synd.	

Table 2. Anterior ischemic optic neuropathy

2.2. Inflammatory optic neuropathy

The dysfunction of the optic nerve due to inflammation is called optic neuritis. The acute demyelinating optic neuropathy is the most common type of inflammatory optic neuropathy. Systemic or local inflammations and infections can cause inflammatory optic neuropathy other than acute optic neurolopathy [21].

Symptoms are usually unilateral, with eye pain and partial or complete vision loss. Diagnosis is primarily clinical. Treatment is directed at the underlying condition; most cases resolve spontaneously [3, 8].

Optic neuritis: Optic neuritis is an inflammatory, demyelinating condition occurring in 50% of individuals at some point in the course of their illness [21]. Optic neuritis is highly associated with multiple sclerosis (MS), approximately 15-20% of MS patients attend hospital with optic neuritis and optic neuritis occurs in 50% of patients with established MS [3]. The ages of the patients are generally between 18 and 40 years. Symptoms develop over a few to several days, reaching maximum severity within two weeks. Fundoscopic examination shows that the appearance of optic disc is normal because the illness enhances the optic nerves of the retrobulber type. Ninety-five percent of patients demonstrate an optic nerve enhancement in Gadolinium-enhanced magnetic resonance imaging (MRI).

Patients typically present with subacute, monocular visual loss. The patients complain of pain in or around the eye which increases with ocular movement. Characteristic findings other than visual loss include a visual field deficit (usually central scotoma type), disturbed colour vision, an afferent pupillary defect, diminished light brightness and impairment contrast sensitivity. The Optic disc is normal in about two thirds of patients (inflammation is entirely retrobulbar).The rest show disc hyperaemia, oedema in or around the disk and vessel engorgement. A few exudates and haemorrhages may be present. Visual recovery is common and often complete; most patients achieve better vision over 6-12 months [3]. Despite the return of visual acuity, colour vision, contrast sensitivity and light brightness often remain abnormal [3]. Recurrent attacks may cause optic atrophy.

The Optic Neuritis Study Group published their findings in 2003 [22]. The aim of the study was to identify the factors associated with a high and low risk of developing multiple sclerosis after an initial episode of optic neuritis. Three hundred and eighty-eight patients who had acute optic neuritis were included the study and were followed up for the development of multiple sclerosis after an initial episode of acute optic neuritis for a 10 year risk. The 10-year risk of multiple sclerosis was 38% (95% confidence interval, 33%-43%). Patients (160) who had one or more typical lesions on baseline T2 weighted magnetic resonance imaging (MRI) scan of the brain had a 56% ; those with no lesions (191) had a 22% risk (P<.001, log rank test).

Diagnosis: Optic neuritis is suspected in patients with characteristic pain and vision loss. Gadolinium-enhanced orbital MRI may show an enlarged, enhanced optic nerve. Typical demyelinating lesions in a periventricular location in cranial MRI especially T2 or FLAIR weighed imaging may also help the diagnosis of multiple sclerosis (Figure 4).

Prognosis: Prognosis depends on the underlying condition. Most episodes resolve spontaneously, but > 25% have a recurrence in the same eye or in the other eye.

Treatment: Corticosteroids are an option, especially if multiple sclerosis is suspected. Treatment with methylprednisolone (1 gr /day) for five to seven days may speed recovery, but ultimate visual recovery is no different from those with observation alone.

Final visual outcomes are not influenced by treatment, but recovery can be reached quickly by intravenous methylprednisolone. Oral prednisone therapy alone is contraindicated because it is associated with a significantly higher recurrence rate. Patients at high risk for multiple sclerosis, assessed on the basis of MRI, may benefit from immunomodulatory therapy [3].

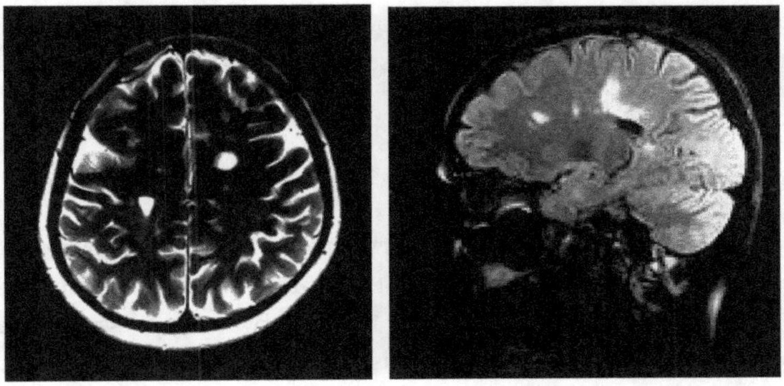

Figure 4. The hyperintense lesion on T2-and FLAIR weighted images. Corpus callosum involvement is noted on the sagittal T2WI.

2.3. Traumatic Optic Neuropathy (TON)

TON refers to the direct or indirect injury of the optic nerve secondary to trauma. The optic nerve runs in the optic canal and can be affected indirectly from blunt head trauma. The visual loss may be partial or complete and generally causes severe and permanent visual defects.

The incidence of traumatic optic neuropathy in a closed traumatic head injury ranges from 0.5-5%. The International Optic Nerve Trauma Study revealed that it was much more common in males (up to 85%) and that the average age of patients was 34 years old [23]. The most common causes were motor vehicle and bicycle accidents, followed by falls and assaults. Loss of consciousness can accompany 40-72% of cases. The diagnosis of TON is difficult and can be delayed when life-threatening systemic symptoms are present.

Direct optic nerve injury is generally rare because of the protecting effect of the orbital bones. It is caused by trauma to the head or orbit. In direct trauma, the anatomy and function of the optic nerve are disrupted. Penetrating injury to the orbit and bony fragments in the optic canal or orbit can result in optic nerve piercing. Orbital haemorrhage and optic nerve sheath haematoma can also cause TON by direct compression. The diagnosis of TON depends on the clinical signs. The cases of TON are generally of monocular involvement. Visual acuity is generally below 0.1. Visual defect is often seen in the acute phase. But delayed visual loss can develop in 10% of cases. The diagnosis of it is important because of the possibility of surgical intervention. Colour vision dysfunction, visual field defect and visual evoked potential are established.

Indirect injuries transmit force to the optic nerve without transgressing tissue planes. This type of injury is most common in the intracanalicular portion of the nerve. Direct optic nerve injuries crosses normal tissue planes and disrupts the anatomy and function of the optic nerve; e.g., a bullet or forceps that physically injures the optic nerve. Indirect injuries, like blunt trauma to the forehead during a motor vehicle accident, transmit force to the optic nerve without transgressing tissue planes. This type of force causes the optic nerve to absorb excess energy at the time of impact. The most common site of injury is the intracanalicular portion of the nerve. Optic neuropathy is most commonly seen in patients in an unconsciousness state associated with a fall [3, 8, 24, 25].

2.4. Compressive optic neuropathy (CON)

CON is the result of compression of the optic nerve. The optic nerve can be pressed in the orbit, the optic canal and the intracranial levels. But it is much more strongly related to orbital pathologies. The optic nerve is most vulnerable to injury by a compressive force in the orbital apex or optic canal [26]. The optic nerve is resistant to force in other parts of the orbita and intracranial level. The most common causes of compressive optic neuropathy in the orbit are inflammatory disease (thyroid orbitopathy, pseudotumour orbita, orbiata cellulitis), tumours and orbital traumas. A variety of tumours can produce optic nerve compression. Sellar and parasellar masses (craniopharyngioma, meningioma, or pituitary adenoma), optic nerve sheath meningiomas and metastatic lesions are included in the differential diagnosis. The other causes related to intracranial pathologies include hypophysis tumours, meningiomas, craniopharyngiomas and aneurisms [3, 8, 27].

Tumours can also infiltrate the optic nerve, particularly optic nerve gliomas (in neurofibromatosis), also lymphoma and other hematologic malignancies. These pathologies can also infiltrate rather than compress the optic nerve [28, 29].

Cranial computerized tomography is preferred as a means to detect orbital lesions and MRI is a useful technique to find out intracranial pathologies [3, 27].

Tumours and thyroid orbitopathy cause slowly progressive visual loss in the course of the disease [27, 30]. But in the situations like orbital trauma, hematoma and cellulitis cause acute vision loss. If compressive optic neuropathy cannot be treated, the results will be optic atrophy and blindness. Pain is variable in these cases.

2.5. Toxic and nutritional optic neuropathy

The causes of these disorders are various. A lot of drugs may cause toxic optic neuropathy; alcohol and tobacco have also a greater risk of causing toxic neuropathy [31-38].

2.6. Nutritional optic neuropathy

The predominant cause of nutritional optic neuropathy is thought to be a deficiency of B-complex vitamins while folic acid also seems to play a role. The toxic agents are summarized in Table 3.

Signs and symptoms: vision loss in toxic and nutritional optic neuropathy is bilateral, usually symmetric, painless, onset may be abrupt or gradual and progressive [3, 8, 32] (Figure 5).

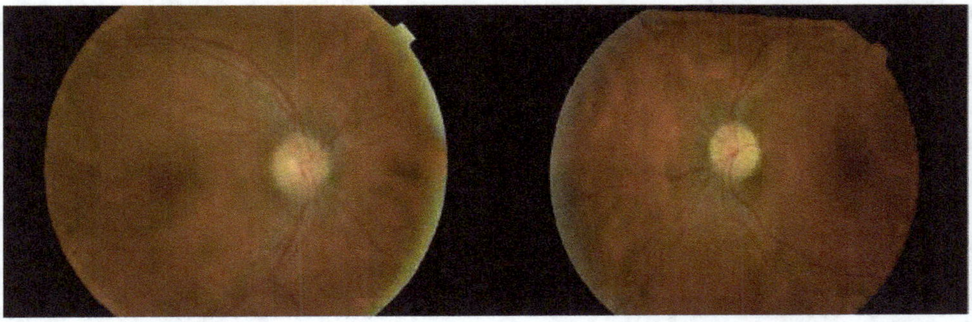

Figure 5. 56 year-old man who has a diagnosis of gastric cancer and is being treated with chemotherapy. Optic atrophy on the right eye and oedema of the optic nerve head on the left eye. The boundary of the optic disc is not seen clearly (With the permission of Marmara University Dept. of Ophthalmology).

DRUGS	Antibiotics: Chloramphenicol, linezolid, sulphonamides
	Antitubercular drugs: Ethambutol, isoniazid, streptomycin
	Antimalarials: Quinine, chloroquine
	Antiarrhytmic drugs: Amiodarone, digitals
	Anticancer drugs: Methotrexate, vincristine. 5FU, carboblastine
	Immune modulators and suppressants: Cyclosporine, tacrolimus, α interferon-2b
	Other: Sildenafil, cimetidine, infliximab, melatonin, sertraline hydrochloride (Zoloft)
ALCOHOLS	Alcohols derives: Methanol, ethylene glycol (antifreeze), toluen
METALS	Heavy metals: Lead, mercury, thallium
OTHERS	Carbon monoxide, tobacco, radiation (unshielded exposure to >3,000 rads)
NUTRITIONALS	Vitamin B1 (tiamin), vitamin B2 (riboflavin), vitamin B3 (niacin), vitamin B6 (pyridoxine), vitamin B12 (cyanocobalamin), folic acid

Table 3. Common causes of toxic and nutritional optic neuropathy

Management: The first step in the treatment of toxic optic neuropathy is to remove the offending agent. The prognosis is variable and dependent upon the affected individual, the nature of the agent, the total exposure duration and doses before the removal of agent and the degree of vision loss at diagnosis.

Patients with toxic/nutritional optic neuropathy should be observed initially every four to six weeks and then, depending on their recovery, every six to 12 months. The patient's visual acuity, pupils, optic nerves, colour vision and visual fields should be checked at each visit. Vision gradually recovers to normal over several weeks, though it may take months for full recovery. Some patients have a risk of permanent residual vision deficit. Visual acuity usually recovers before colour vision [30].

2.7. Hereditary optic neuropathy

Hereditary optic neuropathies are divided into two types. Primary hereditary optic neuropathy refers to cases in which optic nerve pathology is the only sign. On the other hand there are also other groups of hereditary diseases which include various neurological and systemic abnormalities other than optic nerve abnormalities. [(These include: autosomal recessive and maternal inheritance forms of optic atrophy with diabetes incipidus, diabetes mellitus and deafness (Wolfram syndrome, DIDMOAD); autosomal recessive bilateral optic atrophy with spastic paraparesia, chorea and cognitive impairment (Costeff syndrome)]. The most common of these disorders are autosomal dominant optic atrophy (Kjer's disease) and maternally-inherited Leber's hereditary optic neuropathy (Table 4) and these will be discussed in this chapter. However autosomal recessive and X-recessive pattern have been shown in very rare cases [3, 8, 39, 40].

Primary hereditary optic neuropathies
Autosomal Dominant Optic Atrophy (OPA1, Kjer's type)
Leber's Hereditary Optic Neuropathy (LHON)

Table 4. Primary hereditary optic neuropathies

With the remarkable advances in genetic science, the locus of the chromosome was defined and localized in optic neuropathies related to hereditary origin. Despite their genetic origin, these two hereditary optic neuropathies have a pathophysiology reflecting a common pathway in mitochondrial dysfunction. (LHON is a result of point mutations in the mitochondrial DNA and Dominant Optic Atrophy (DOA) is a consequence of mutations in nuclear chromosomes).

Kjer's type autosomal dominant optic atrophy: This is the most commonly seen hereditary optic neuropathy. The incidence of dominant optic atrophy has been estimated to be 1:50000 with a prevalence of 1:10000 in the Danish population. This entity primarily affects children in the first decade of life. But in some cases the beginning of the disease is delayed to 60-70 years of age. Bilateral visual acuity loss is commonly present and relatively symmetrical. Most patients cannot identify a precise onset and the illness usually shows mild, slow and gradual progression. More than 80% of patients maintain better than 20/200 vision, but interfamilial and intrafamilial variation in visual acuity can be seen [41]. There is pallor of the optic disc, cecocentral scotoma and colour vision loss also accompanies the visual acuity [42-43].

Kjer et al. have examined 62 patients from three large Danish families with autosomal dominant optic atrophy and followed up 30 patients retrospectively. They found great inter-

and intrafamiliar variation in visual acuity and visual decline. They analysed 175 chromosomal markers in 118 family members. All markers are located on chromosome 3q in the telomeric area. They found the most probable location for the OPA1 gene was D3S1601-OPA1-D3S1265. Using data from the Danish Family Register of Hereditary Eye Diseases, the minimum prevalence rate was estimated to be 1:12.301. With the results of this investigation, DOA has become the most common hereditary optic atrophy [44].

Leber's hereditary optic neuropathy (LHON): this is a rare disease when compared to Kjer's. Maternal inheritance is present. So this disorder affects young males predominantly (80 to 90% of patients) between the ages of 15 and 35 years. It is inherited through a mitochondrial DNA mutation. More than 90% of all cases have three mutations at positions 11778, 3460 and 14484 [45]. These genes are involved in the Complex I enzyme subunit in the mitochondrial respiratory chain [39].

The vision loss in patients with LHON is subacute and painless, severe, with sequential involvement of both eyes over a period of weeks to months. Fundoscopic examination usually shows circumpapillary telangiectasia, but up to 30% of patients can have normal disc appearance. Nerve fibre layer swelling around the disc can be seen; leakage from the disc or papillary area is not present in the fluorescein angiography [46]. Central vision is affected more severely. With the progression of the disease, telangiectasia vessels and pseudopapilloedema of the disc disappears and optic atrophy takes place. Optic nerve abnormality can be shown in MRI, but enhancement usually does not occur [47, 48]. LHON shows varying penetration and the prognosis for recovery depends on the mutation [45]. The 11778 mutation carries the worst prognosis.

Management: Therapies for mitochondrial disorders are very limited. Currently there is no effective therapy for dominant optic atrophy. Children of patients should be screened regularly for visual changes related to dominant optic atrophy. Nutritional supplements such as vitamin B12 and C, Coenzyme-Q10 and lutein have been suggested [49, 50].

2.8. Parainfectious optic neuritis

Optic neuropathy may be associated with postviral infections and occur as a post vaccination phenomenon [3, 8].Underlying mechanisms may be related to immune mediated process. Children are affected more frequently than adults and this may occur after immunizations [51].

Presentation: Severe acute visual loss, usually bilateral and occurs one to three weeks following a viral infection (e.g., measles, mumps, chickenpox, whooping cough, glandular fever). Other neurological features such as headache, seizure or ataxia may also be seen. There may also be a meningoencephalitis. Bilateral optic neuritis can also occur in Guillain-Barré syndrome [52, 53].

Ocular findings: The optic disc frequently shows bilateral papillitis or may be normal.

Treatment: Treatment is not necessary in the majority of patients. Spontaneous visual recovery is very good [3]. However when visual loss is severe and bilateral, intravenous steroids should be considered.

2.9. Infectious optic neuritis

Meningitis or encephalitis may cause optic neuritis, either as a direct effect of the infectious organism or from secondary vasculitis [51]. Signs and symptoms related to infection, MRI and CSF findings carry some information about causative agents [54-62]. When the meningitis is more indolent, as in some cases of tuberculosis and cryptococcus, optic nerve involvement may be a primary manifestation.

Sinus infections: Sinus related optic neuritis is a rare condition. It may occur following spheno-ethmoidal sinusitis. The underlying mechanisms include spread of infection directly, occlusive vasculitis and pressure by a mucocele. Patients complain of severe headaches and recurrent episodes of unilateral visual loss. Treatment with systemic antibiotics is necessary but surgical drainage of the sinus may also be needed.

Acute viral infections, as well as cat scratch disease and toxoplasmosis and others, can cause an isolated infection of the eye. Inflammation of the retina associated with the optic disc is called neuroretinitis. Neuroretinitis is another finding of ophthalmoscopic investigation. Fundoscopic examination usually reveals macular oedema, in addition to optic disc swelling. Corticosteroids and systemic antibiotics can be used for treatment. The West Nile virus in particular has been reported to produce optic neuritis in association with meningitis. Syphilitic optic neuritis may be monocular or binocular and is associated with vitreal inflammation; acute optic neuritis may occur both in the primary or secondary stages. Antibiotic therapy may improve the symptoms, but relapse may be seen. Lyme disease may cause acute retrobulbar optic neuritis and neuroretinitis. It may mimic multiple sclerosis symptoms. The treatment includes intravenous ceftriaxone [3].

Varicella-zoster virus: primary optic neuritis is uncommon unless the patient is immuno-compromised. Secondary optic neuritis arises from viruses spread from contiguous retinitis. Treatment is with intravenous (IV) antivirals. Cat-scratch fever: this self-limiting infection has a good prognosis with visual recovery. Treatment is with antimicrobial agents.

2.10. Infiltrative optic neuropathy

The optic nerve can be infiltrated by a variety of factors, including tumours, inflammation and infections [63].

The optic nerve has three parts as described by anatomic localization: intraocular, intraorbital and intracranial. The tumours which originate in these locations can expand to the optic nerve. Optic neuropathy related to tumours is generally of the compressive type, but the tumour cells can also infiltrate directly into the optic nerve, which cause infiltrative optic neuropathy. The difference between these two entities is important because removing the compression is the only solution in compressive neuropathy whereas in infiltrative neuropathy the eradication of tumour is the treatment. Tumours that infiltrate the optic nerve can be primary (optic gliomas, capillary haemangioma and cavernous haemangioma) or secondary (metastatic carcinoma, nasopharyngeal carcinoma, lymphoma and leukaemia). The underlying mechanism of paraneoplastic optic neuropathy is related to the development of autoantibodies (ex:anti-CV2) (Figure 6).

Infections, which include viruses, bacteria and opportunistic fungi, may also infiltrate the optic nerve. The appearance of the nerve on examination depends on the portion of the nerve that is affected. If the infiltration occurs in the proximal portion of the nerve, the optic nerve may be elevated. The optic nerve can be affected by a variety of systemic, auto-immune and infectious disorders such as sarcoidosis, systemic lupus erythematosus, Behçet's disease, inflammation, bowel disease, Sjogren's syndrome, Wegener's granulomatosis, syphilis, Lyme disease and cat-scratch disease. [8, 64, 65] (Figure 7).

Sarcoidosis is the most common inflammatory disorder that infiltrates the optic nerve. One to 5% of patients with neurosarcoid develop optic neuritis. Optic nerve head exhibits a characteristic lumpy appearance. Steroid treatment is effective and rapid, but some patients require long term low dose steroid therapy. In addition to steroids, some patients may also be given methotrexate treatment and methotrexate is an alternative to steroids for intolerant patients [3].

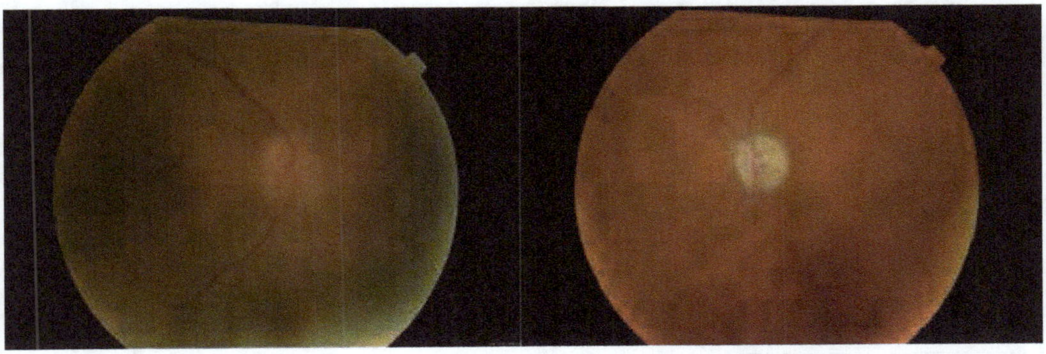

Figure 6. Optic neuropathy with underlying paraneoplastic aetiology (With the permission of Marmara University Dept. of Ophthalmology).

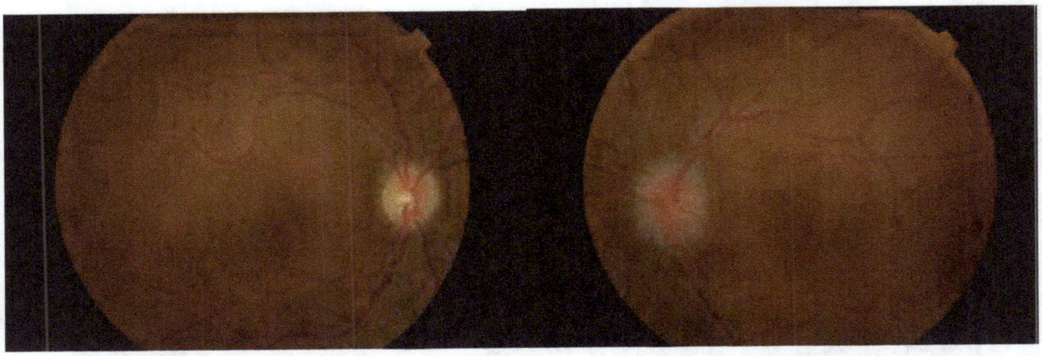

Figure 7. 43 year-old female patient using plaquenil (hydroxychloroquine) following diagnosis SLE. (With the permission of Marmara University Dept.Of Neurology)

2.11. Idiopathic intracranial hypertension *(pseudotumour cerebri, benign intracranial hypertension)*

Idiopathic intracranial hypertension (IIH) is known by raised intracranial pressure in the absence of a mass lesion or of hydrocephalus. It is mostly related to impaired cerebrospinal fluid (CSF) absorption from the subarachnoid space. It is common in obese woman of 20-40 years of age. The female to male ratio is between 3:1 and 8:1. Up to 90% of patients are overweight. IIH may result in permanent visual loss due to papilloedema (Figure 8). The clinical signs and symptoms are summarized in Table 5 (66). IIH may also be caused by drugs. Lumbar puncture (LP) is one of the treatment methods and is also useful for the diagnosis. If the opening pressure is >250 mm H2O and LP shows no inflammatory cells with normal CSF protein and glucose levels, the diagnosis will be achieved. Cranial MRI shows normal ventricles and often an empty sellar. Venous sinus thrombosis should be excluded by the cranial MR venography. Other secondary causes are summarized in Table 6. Regular perimetric examination is important to follow the progression of the disease [3].

Medical and lifestyle treatment: 1) weight loss, 2) Asetozolamide, 3) Furosemide, 4) Topiramate.

Surgical treatment: 1) repeated lumbar puncture, 2) optic nerve sheath decompressions, 3) ventriculoperitoneal shunt placements, 4) lumboperitoneal shunt placement [3]

Symptoms (68)	*Signs*
Headache (92%)	Papilloedema
Transient visual obscurations (72%)	Visual fields deficit
Pulsatil tinnitus (60%)	Contrast sensitivity loss
Photopsia (54%)	Decrease in visual acuity
Retrobulbar pain (44%)	Problems in colour vision
Diplopia (38%)	Relative afferent pupillary defect
Sustained visual loss (26%)	VI nerve paralysis (transient)

Table 5. Signs and symptoms in intracranial hypertension

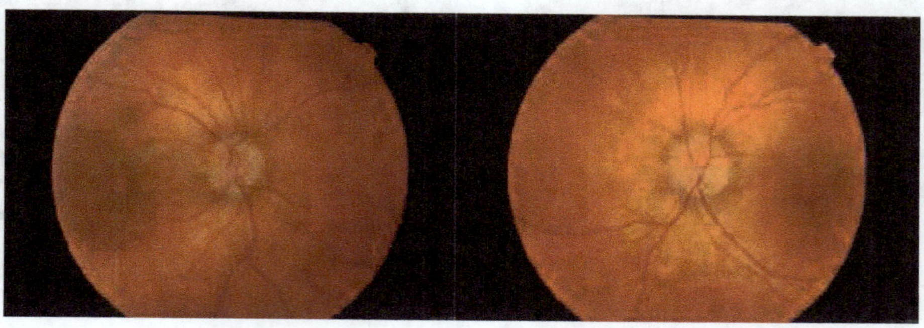

Figure 8. Early papilloedema (With the permission of Marmara University Dept. of Ophthalmology).

Endocrine	Addison disease, Cushing disease, puerpurium, polycystic ovarian syndrome, hyper and hypothyroidism, hypoparathyroidism
Venous hypertension	Venous sinus thrombosis
Metabolic disease	Renal insufficiency, Diabetes mellitus, iron deficiency, pernicious anaemia, hypercapnia, Addison disease, Cushing disease, puerpurium, polycystic over syndrome, hyper and hypothyroidism, hypoparathyroidism
Cranial trauma	
Parainfectious and immunological states	Behçet's disease, systemic lupus erithomatosus, sarcoidosis, HIV, Lyme
Meningial carsinomatosus	
Gliomatosus cerebri	
Medication and vitamin	cimetidine, corticosteroids, levothyroxine, lithium, minocycline, nalidixic acid, nitrofurantoin, tamoxifen, tetracycline, ciclosporin, oral contraceptive, recombinant and natural human growth hormone, Hypervitaminosis A
Obstructive sleep apnoea syndrome	

Table 6. Causes of secondary intracranial hypertension

2.12. Pseudopapilloedema (Drusen)

Hyaline-like calcific material on the optic nerve head is the characteristic feature of optic disc drusen. They are generally bilateral. In early childhood, its diagnosis is difficult because they lie deep. They may mimic papilloedema. Hyperaemia is absent and the surface vessels are not obscured. Disc is elevated without a physiological cup [3].

Ultrasound B-scan is the most reliable method and calcific deposits are detected easily. CT also shows the disc calcification but it is less sensitive than ophthalmic ultrasound [3] (Figure 9).

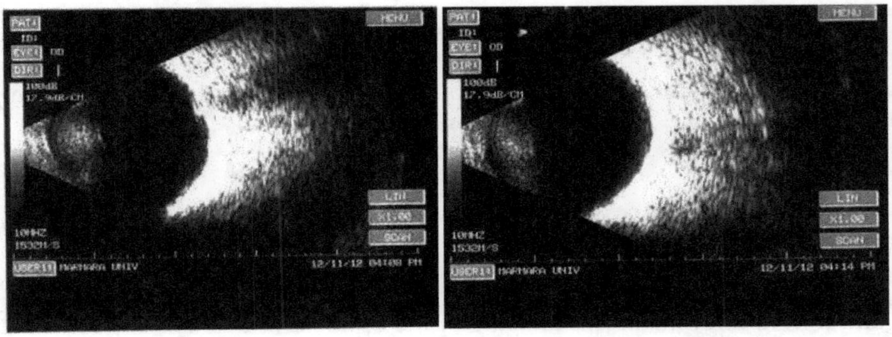

Figure 9. B-scan shows high acoustic reflectivity (With the permission of Marmara University Dept. of Ophthalmology).

In conclusion, disorders of the optic nerve may be related to congenital or acquired causes. There are many aetiologies that affect the optic nerve and according to the localization of lesion,

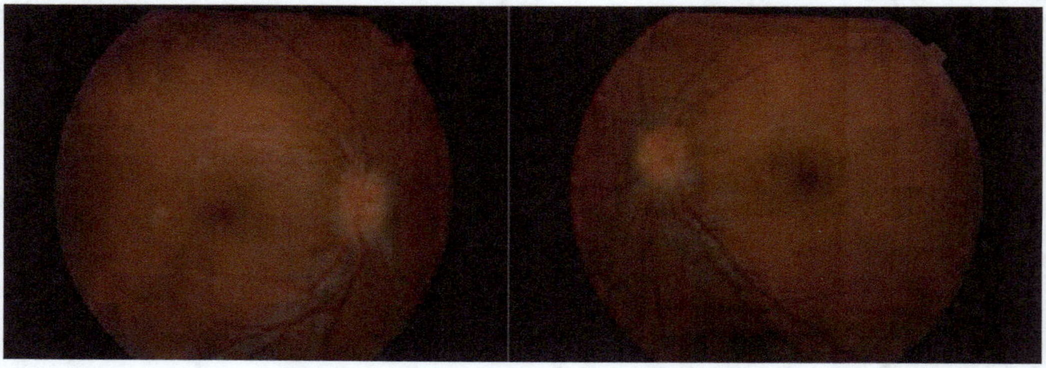

Figure 10. Optic disc drusen (With the permission of Marmara University Dept. of Ophthalmology).

different types of visual field defect can occur. The optic disc may show different abnormalities or may be of normal appearance on fundoscopic examination.

Acknowledgements

I greatly appreciate the Ophthalmology Department of Marmara University Hospital for supplying images for this chapter. I am very grateful to the following colleagues for their help Professor Dr. Ozlem Sahin, Assistant Dr. Umeyye Taka Aydin from Marmara University Dept. of Ophthalmology and Assistant Associate Professor Dr. Arif Koytak from Bezmialem University in the Dept. of Ophthalmology.

Author details

Ipek Midi*

Marmara University Pendik Research and Training Hospital, Department of Neurology, Istanbul, Turkey

References

[1] Smith MM, Strottmann JM. Imaging of the optic nerve and visual pathways. Semin Ultrasound CT MR. 2001; 22(6): 473-87.

[2] Anatomy and Physiology of the Retina and Optic Nerve. In Walsh & Hoyt's. Clinical Neuro-ophthalmology. 5th ed. The Essentials. Ed. NR Miller, NJ Newman. Williams & Wilkins. 1999: 59-86.

[3] Burton B. Chapter 21: Neuro-ophthalmology. In Clinical Ophthalmology A Systemic Approach. 6th ed. Ed. Kanski JJ. Butterworth Heinemann Elsevier 2007: 785-836.

[4] Kansu T. Chapter 2 (Section I): Afferent System (Examination and diagnosis) In Neuro-ophthalmology Handbook. 1st ed. Ed. O'Dwyer PA, Kansu T, Torun T. Güneş Medicine Publishing;2008: 9-17 (Turkish).

[5] Sadun AA. The afferent visual system: Anatomy and Physiology. In Ophthalmology, 2nd ed. Ed, Yanoff M, Duker JS. Mosby, St. Louis 2004: 186.

[6] Glaser JS. Topical diagnosis: Prechiasmal visual pathways. In Neuro-ophthalmology. Ed. Glaser JS. JB Lippincott, Philadelphia 1990: 83.

[7] Purves D, Augustine GJ, Fitzpatrick D, et al., Visual Field Deficits. In Neuroscience. 2nd ed. Ed. Sunderland (MA). Sinauer Associates; 2001.

[8] Osborne B, Balcer LJ. Optic Neuropathies. Section Ed: Brazis PW. Up to date 2013.

[9] Behbehani R. Clinical approach to optic neuropathies. Clin. Ophthalmol. 2007; 1(3): 233–46.

[10] Purvin VA. Optic neuropathies for the neurologist. Semin Neurol. 2000; 20(1): 97-110.

[11] Kadayifcilar S. Chapter 9 (Section II): Optic disc edema and papilloedema. In Neuro-ophthalmology Handbook. 1st ed. Ed. O'Dwyer PA, Kansu T, Torun T. Güneş Medicine Publishing;2008: 101-5. (Turkish).

[12] Bajin MS. Chapter 2 (Section II): Ischeic Optic Neuropathies. In Neuro-ophthalmology Handbook. 1st ed. Ed. O'Dwyer PA, Kansu T, Torun T. Güneş Medicine Publishing; 2008:51-8. (Turkish).

[13] Newman NJ, Scherer R, Langenberg P, Kelman S, Feldon S, Kaufman D, Dickersin K; Ischemic Optic Neuropathy Decompression Trial Research Group. "The fellow eye in NAION: report from the ischemic optic neuropathy decompression trial follow-up study." Am J Ophthalmol. 2002; 134(3): 317-28.

[14] Hayreh SS, Zimmerman MB. Non-arteritic anterior ischemic optic neuropathy: role of systemic corticosteroid therapy. Graefes Arch Clin Exp Ophthalmol. 2008; 246(7): 1029-46.

[15] Hayreh SS, Zimmerman MB. Non-arteritic anterior ischemic optic neuropathy: natural history of visual outcome. Ophthalmology 2008; 115:298–305.

[16] Anterior Ischemic Optic Neuropathy Author: Brian R Younge; Chief Editor: Hampton Roy Sr, et al. Medscape Jan 2012.

[17] Thorne JE, Jabs DA. Ocular manifestations of the rheumatic diseases. In: Duane's Clinical Ophthalmology. Ed. Tasman William. Vol. 5. Philadelphia: Lippincott Williams & Wilkins; 2005: 22–24.

[18] Hayreh SS, Zimmerman B, Kardon RH. Visual improvement with corticosteroid therapy in giant cell arteritis. Report of a large study and review of literature. Acta Ophthalmol Scand. 2002; 80:353–67.

[19] Foroozan R, Deramo VA, Buono LM, et al. Recovery of visual function in patients with biopsy-proven giant cell arteritis. Ophthalmology. 2003; 110: 539–42.

[20] Hayreh SS. Anterior ischaemic optic neuropathy, differentiation of arteritic from non-arteritic type and its management. Eye 1990; 4: 25–41;

[21] Acaroglu G. Chapter 1 (Section II): Inflammatory Optic Neuropathy. In Neuro-ophthalmology Handbook 1st ed. Ed. O'Dwyer PA, Kansu T, Torun T. Güneş Medicine Publishing;2008: 43-49 (Turkish)

[22] Beck RW, Trobe JD, Moke PS, GalRL, Xing D, BhattiMT, et al; Optic Neuritis Study Group. High-and low-risk profiles for the development of multiple sclerosis within 10 years after optic neuritis: experience of the optic neuritis treatment trial. Arch Ophthalmol.2003; 121(7): 944-9.

[23] Levin LA, et al., The treatment of traumatic optic neuropathy: the International Optic Nerve Trauma Study. Ophthalmology, 1999. 106(7): 1268-77.

[24] Steinsapir KD, Goldberg RA. Traumatic optic neuropathy: an evolving understanding. American Journal of Ophthalmology. 2011; 151: 928-933.

[25] Onder F. Chapter 3 (Section II): Afferent System (Examination and diagnosis). In Neuro-ophthalmology Handbook. 1st ed. Ed. O'Dwyer PA, Kansu T, Torun T. Güneş Medicine Publishing;2008: 59-64 (Turkish)

[26] Miller NR, Newman NJ, Biousse V. Walsh and Hoyt's Clinical Neuro-Ophthalmology. 6th ed. Lippincott, Williams & Wilkins; 2004.

[27] Yazici B. Chapter 4 (Section II): Compressive Optic Neuropathy. In Neuro-ophthalmology Handbook. 1st ed. Ed. O'Dwyer PA, Kansu T, Torun T. Güneş Medicine Publishing;2008: 65-71 (Turkish)

[28] Lee AG, Tang RA, Roberts D, et al. Primary central nervous system lymphoma involving the optic chiasm in AIDS. J Neuro-ophthalmol 2001; 21:95.

[29] Grimm SA, McCannel CA, Omuro AM, et al. Primary CNS lymphoma with intraocular involvement: International PCNSL Collaborative Group Report. Neurology 2008; 71:1355.

[30] Maheshwari R, Weis Ezekiel. Thyroid associated orbitopathy. Indian J Ophthalmol. 2012; 60(2): 87–93.

[31] Sharma P and Sharma R. Toxic optic neuropathy. Indian J Ophthalmol. 2011; 59(2): 137–141.

[32] Kargi SH. Chapter 6 (Section II): Toxic and Nutritional Optic Neuropathy. In Neuro-ophthalmology Handbook. 1st ed. Ed. O'Dwyer PA, Kansu T, Torun T. Güneş Medicine Publishing;2008: 81-88 (Turkish)

[33] Lim SA. Ethambutol-associated optic neuropathy. Ann Acad Med Singapore. 2006; 35(4): 274-8.

[34] Orssaud C, Roche O, Dufier JL. Nutritional optic neuropathies. J Neurol Sci. 2007; 262(1-2): 158-64.

[35] Murphy MA, Murphy JF. Amiodarone and optic neuropathy: the heart of the matter. J Neuroophthalmol. Sep 2005; 25(3): 232-6.

[36] Grzybowski A, Holder GE. Tobacco optic neuropathy (TON)-the historical and present concept of the disease. Acta Ophthalmol. 2011; 89(5): 495-9.

[37] Wilczynski M, Wilczynska O. Severe acute bilateral alcohol-induced toxic optic neuropathy-case report. Klin Oczna. 2012; 114(3): 208-12.

[38] Kerrison JB. Optic neuropathies caused by toxins and adverse drug reactions. Ophthalmol Clin North Am 2004: 17:481.

[39] Dogulu C. Chapter 7 (Section II): Hereditary Optic Neuropathy. In Neuro-ophthalmology Handbook. 1st ed. Ed. O'Dwyer PA, Kansu T, Torun T. Güneş Medicine Publishing;2008: 89-94 (Turkish).

[40] Newman NJ. Hereditary Optic Neuropathies: from the mitochondria to the optic nerve. Am J Ophthal. 2005; 140(3): 517-523.

[41] Votruba M, Fitzke FW, Holder CE, Carter A, Bhattacharya SS, Moore AT. Clinical features in affected individuals from 21 pedigrees with dominant optic atrophy. Arch Ophthalmol. 1998; 116(3): 353-358.

[42] Votruba M, Thiselton D, Bhattacharya SS.Optic disc morphology of patients with OPA1 autosomal dominant optic atrophy. Br J Ophthalmol 2003: 87:48.

[43] Alexander C, Votruba M, Pesch UE, et al. OPA1, encoding a dynamin-related GTPase, is mutated in autosomal dominant optic atrophy linked to chromosome 3q28. Nat Genet 2000: 26:211.

[44] Kjer B, Eiberg H, Kjer P, Rosenberg T. Dominant optic atrophy mapped to chromosome 3q region. II. Clinical and epidemiological aspects. Acta Ophthalmol Scand. 1996; 74(1): 3-7

[45] Howell N. LHON and other optic nerve atrophies: the mitochondrial connection. Dev Ophthalmol. 2003: 37:94.

[46] Smith JL, Hoyt WF, Susac JO. Ocular fundus in acute Leber optic neuropathy. Arch Ophthalmol 1973; 90:349.

[47] Kermode AG, Moseley IF, Kendall BE, et al. Magnetic resonance imaging in Leber's optic neuropathy. J Neurol Neurosurg Psychiatry 1989; 52:671.

[48] Lamirel C, Cassereau J, Cochereau I, et al. Papilloedema and MRI enhancement of the prechiasmal optic nerve at the acute stage of Leber hereditary optic neuropathy. J Neurol Neurosurg Psychiatry 2010; 81:578.

[49] Carelli V, La Morgia C, Sadun AA. Mitochondrial dysfunction in optic neuropathies: animal models and therapeutic options. Curr Opin Neurol. 2013; 26(1): 52-58.

[50] DiMauro S, Mancuso M. Mitochondrial diseases: therapeutic approaches. Biosci Rep. 2007; 27:125-3751-Golnik KC. Infectious optic neuropathy. Semin Ophthalmol 2002; 17:11.

[51] Ginestal RC, Plaza JF, Callejo JM, et al. Bilateral optic neuritis and Guillain-Barré syndrome following an acute Mycoplasma pneumoniae infection. J Neurol 2004; 251:767.

[52] Pfausler B, Engelhardt K, Kampfl A, et al. Post-infectious central and peripheral nervous system diseases complicating Mycoplasma pneumoniae infection. Report of three cases and review of the literature. Eur J Neurol 2002; 9:93.

[53] Venkatesh P, Garg SP, Verma L, et al. Combined optic neuropathy and central retinal artery occlusion in miliary tuberculosis. Retina 2001; 21:375.

[54] Rex JH, Larsen RA, Dismukes WE, et al. Catastrophic visual loss due to Cryptococcus neoformans meningitis. Medicine (Baltimore) 1993; 72:207.

[55] Fukushima A, Yasuoka M, Tsukahara M, Ueno H. A case of cat scratch disease neuroretinitis confirmed by polymerase chain reaction. Jpn J Ophthalmol 2003; 47:405.

[56] Gilden DH, Mahalingam R, Cohrs RJ, Tyler KL. Herpesvirus infections of the nervous system. Nat Clin Pract Neurol 2007; 3:82.

[57] Küçükerdönmez C, Akova YA, Yilmaz G. Ocular toxoplasmosis presenting as neuroretinitis: report of two cases. Ocul Immunol Inflamm 2002 10:229.

[58] Benz MS, Glaser JS, Davis JL. Progressive outer retinal necrosis in immunocompetent patients treated initially for optic neuropathy with systemic corticosteroids. Am J Ophthalmol 2003: 135:551.

[59] Ray S, Gragoudas E. Neuroretinitis. Int Ophthalmol Clin 2001: 41:83.

[60] Smith GT, Goldmeier D, Migdal C. Neurosyphilis with optic neuritis: an update. Postgrad Med J 2006: 82:36.

[61] Sibony P, Halperin J, Coyle PK, Patel K. Reactive Lyme serology in optic neuritis. J Neuroophthalmol 2005: 25:71.

[62] Tunc M. Chapter 5 (Section II): Inflammatory Optic Neuropathy. In Neuro-ophthalmology Handbooks. 1st ed. Ed. O'Dwyer PA, Kansu T, Torun T. Güneş Medicine Publishing;2008: 73-80 (Turkish)

[63] Jabs DA, Miller NR, Newman SA, et al. Optic neuropathy in systemic lupus erythematosus. Arch Ophthalmol 1986; 104:564.

[64] Kansu T, Kirkali P, Kansu E, Zileli T. Optic neuropathy in Behçet's disease. J Clin Neuroophthalmol 1989; 9:277.

[65] Wall M, George D. Idiopathic intracranial hypertension. A prospective study of 50 patients. Brain 1991; 114 (Pt 1A): 155.

7

Applications of Perceptual Learning to Ophthalmology

Jenni Deveau, Gary Lovcik and Aaron R. Seitz

1. Introduction

Our knowledge of the world is derived from our perceptions, and an individual's ability to navigate his/her surroundings or engage in activities of daily living such as walking, reading, watching TV, and driving, naturally relies on his/her ability to process sensory information. Thus deficits in visual abilities, due to disease, injury, stroke or aging, can have significant negative impacts on all aspects of an individual's life. Likewise, an enhancement of visual abilities can have substantial positive benefits to one's lifestyle. While a central concern of Ophthalmology is to address diseases of the eye (e.g. ocular impairments), an equally important component of vision is how the brain processes information that is received from the eye.

Vision is a synergistic effect of eye sensing and brain processing mechanisms. Vision can be compared to a satellite dish with the eye representing the dish or the sensor receiving aspect of the system. The eye/sensor captures light signals and transfers these signals to the brain, which is our visual processor. Through a series of brain processing stages, the image is processed by perceptual, higher order cognitive, and then motor systems resulting in decisions and responses. Thus, vision deficits can be due to eye mechanics, brain processing problems or both. Research of Perceptual Learning provides some answers and solutions for brain processing issues. This research demonstrates that the adult visual system is sufficiently plastic to ameliorate effects of low vision, including amblyopia [1], presbyopia [2], macular degeneration [3], stroke [4, 5], and late-life recovery of visual function [6]. Likewise, normal sighted individuals have the potential to further improve their vision through Perceptual Learning. These visual gains are related to brain function improvement (plasticity).

In this chapter we review the field of Perceptual Learning and its promise to achieve better outcomes in clinical practice. The significance of the development of effective, low-cost therapies to treat brain-based low vision can be life-altering for millions of people worldwide.

2. Perceptual Learning

Perceptual Learning (PL) refers to a long lasting improvement in perceptual abilities as a result of experience. Research of this topic has undergone tremendous development over the last 30 years. Plasticity in the sensory systems was previously thought to occur only in early development. This view has been substantiated by studies of a "critical period". The concept of a critical period states some processes develop early in life, and do not develop, or develop to a lesser degree, later in life. For example, classic experiments done in kittens demonstrate a critical period for ocular dominance where early patching enables inputs from the open eye to take over much of primary visual cortex, however, in adult cats patching has little impact on connectivity [7, 8]. This data was used to support the hypothesis that the low-level sensory stages need to consistently process primitive sensory features; such as in vision, orientation, spatial frequency, and local motion. However, studies of perceptual learning show that even in adults, perceptual abilities can be sharpened with repeated exposure or training. For example, perceptual abilities, including elementary processes (e.g., contrast sensitivity [9] and visual acuity [1, 2, 10, 11]) can be strengthened through appropriate training approaches.

Perceptual Learning is exemplified by long-lasting improvement on simple but difficult perceptual tasks. The effects of perceptual learning have been shown to last months, even years [12-14]. The field of perceptual learning is one of growing interest largely due to the fact training on visual perception can be highly specific to the trained visual features and can give clues into the stages of processing at which learning occurs. For example, a series of studies conducted by Schoups and colleagues [15, 16] showed that training subjects (human and monkey) on an orientation discrimination task around a particular reference orientation yielded learning effects that failed to transfer to other stimulus orientations at the trained location or that same orientation at a different retinotopic location. They postulated that these learning effects were consistent with plasticity in neurons residing in primary visual cortex, which show a high degree of both retinotopic and orientation specificity. Physiological studies by this group confirmed these predictions with the demonstration of plasticity of orientation tuning across early visual cortex [15, 17]. Consistent with this, numerous behavioral studies show perceptual learning can be highly specific to a wide range of trained stimulus features including retinotopic location [18, 19], visual orientation [15, 20] and direction [12, 19], among others. Likewise, many neuroscientific studies provide evidence of sensory plasticity in all stages of visual processing through single-unit recording in monkeys [15, 21-23] and fMRI signal changes in humans [24-26].

An important caveat is that psychophysical studies of perceptual learning are only a rough tool for making inferences of the underlying neural structures. Accordingly, physiological studies demonstrating low-level perceptual learning typically fail to explain the magnitude of the behavioral changes [27] and some models of perceptual learning demonstrate that channel reweighting in the readout of sensory areas can account for some aspects of perceptual learning specificity without requiring plasticity in primary sensory areas [28-31]. Other studies have found plasticity in higher-level visual areas that were originally hypothesized to be lower level features [14, 32-34]. For instance, Law and Gold [33] failed to find plasticity in monkey area middle temporal cortex (MT), but found learning effects in a later area (lateral intraparietal cortex; LIP) that largely explained behavioral changes after training in a visual motion task. Likewise, learning in visual area V4 has been found to be more robust than that in V1 [17, 22, 32, 35, 36]. Also, some aspects of learning could be taking place in other brain regions, an interesting case was recently found in which the superior colliculus [37, 38] and frontal brain areas [39] develop tuning to motion directions after extensive training. While the exact locus of visual plasticity in a given study is often an issue of significant controversy, as a whole these studies give indication that plasticity is likely occurring at all stages of visual processing; although with a distribution that varies across tasks and training paradigms.

3. Perceptual Learning as a method to improve vision

Software programs integrating perceptual learning are being utilized more frequently to optimize outcomes in specific visual conditions, both in research/clinical studies and commercially. Using computer generated visual stimuli presented in repetitive patterns, users interact with visual stimuli and the training process induces neurological visual system plasticity and patient benefits. The observed benefits can include increased neuro-adaptation to new visual environments, improved contrast sensitivity and increases in spatial or visual acuity. Recent research provides examples of perceptual learning techniques that result in visual improvements for a variety of visual conditions.

4. Amblyopia

Amblyopia results in a lack of stereovision and poor vision in the amblyopic eye (even after the optics of the eye, and misalignment between the eyes, are corrected). Amblyopia impacts 2-3% of the population and is conventionally considered untreatable in adults. The gold standard for treating amblyopia is to restore stereovision. To accomplish this, (1) cortical processing of the amblyopic eye needs to be strengthened, (2) suppression from the non-amblyopic eye needs to be lessened, and (3) binocular integration needs to process correctly in the visual system. Amblyopia is typically treated only children, where traditional approaches focusing on patching or the use of atropine in the non-amblyopic eye, with no treatment attempted in adults due to a believed lack of plasticity.

However, recently perceptual learning paradigms have been found to be effective in improving acuity and stereopsis in adults, and in children where traditional patching was unsuccessful [40-42]. More recently there has been focus on binocular interactions in amblyopia with push-pull trainings that put the eyes in competition successfully lessening suppression in the amblyopic eye [43, 44], or binocular integration, which trains the two eyes to work better together [45]. Perceptual learning techniques, or more recently commercial video games [46], have also been found to reduce crowding [47], and improve spatial frequency and contrast discrimination, which also transferred to untrained spatial frequencies in adults with amblyopia [48]. Together these approaches have led to numerous examples which demonstrate substantial benefits in vision in the amblyopic eye and provide great promise for future perceptual learning based treatment approaches.

5. Age-related Macular Degeneration (AMD)

Age-related Macular Degeneration (AMD) is the leading cause of central low vision in adults. The prevalence of AMD increases after age 50, and is expected to affect nearly three million Americans by 2020 (*The Eye Diseases Prevalence Research Group, 2004*). AMD patients suffer a retinal disorder in which photoreceptors are damaged or displaced, resulting in visual field loss, spatial distortions to the visual field, and impairments of acuity and contrast sensitivity. Despite a range of treatments to arrest the progress of AMD, damage to the retina cannot be reversed, resulting in a need for effective visual training therapies. There are a number of studies that show both functional learning in the development of preferred looking points [49-51] and cortical reorganization in foveal responses to peripheral stimuli [3, 52]. Difficulty reading is a common complaint in AMD patients due to the central vision loss. Recently, Chung [53] demonstrated that perceptual learning could improve reading speed in these patients after training. Additionally, Liu et al [54] trained profoundly visually impaired individuals (including AMD, glaucoma, retinitis pigmentosa, and other conditions) on a visual search task. Search speed and accuracy improved after training, effects that remained for at least one month.

While, there are limited perceptual-learning studies in AMD patients and it is unclear the extent to which normally occurring reorganizations are driven through use-dependent mechanisms [55], there is significant potential benefit to applications of perceptual learning in AMD.

6. Age related visual decline

It is well documented that vision declines with age [56]. Deficits are seen in many aspects of vision including eye optics, luminance, contrast, orientation, motion processing, form, scene and depth perception, and optical flow. Recent research has found perceptual learning can improve visual performance in older individuals. For example, after training on a visual discrimination task older participants improved up to the same performance level of untrained college age participants, with improvements lasting at least 3 months after training [57]. Additionally, older individuals improved on a motion detection task (either drifting sine wave gratings or random dot motion), and learning transferred to the untrained motion type [58].

The most common age related visual deficit is presbyopia. Presbyopia is a progressive normal aging process where the elasticity of the lens of the eye is reduced [59]. Although the decrease in elasticity of lens starts at birth, this condition, noticed by most people in their early 40's, manifests as a reduced ability to focus on nearby stimuli and a reduction of contrast sensitivity

[2]. There is no cure for presbyopia. Typical treatments are reading glasses or multifocal lenses, contact lenses or more recently, surgery like the Laser-Assisted in Situ Keratomileusis (LASIK). While treatments do exist, their use can be inconvenient for some as many treatments are not ideal for all daily activities, or can represent a significant challenge to others. All treatment options of presbyopia induce further reduction in optical contrast [60, 61]. Additionally, the use of multifocal lenses (common form of therapy) introduces unnatural viewing conditions where the point of focus depends upon gaze angle and optical aberration in transition regions. Of note, encouraging research from Polat and colleagues [62] suggest perceptual learning can ameliorate the effects of presbyopia, and in some cases, enable mild presbyopes to read without glasses. After training on a contrast detection task using Gabor patches of a range of spatial frequencies participants improved near vision acuity, reading speed, contrast detection and discrimination without changing the optics of the eye.

In general, perceptual learning also shows great promise for conditions for which there are no standard treatments. These include the conditions mentioned above as well as other low-vision conditions such as glaucoma, night vision deficits, retinitis pigmentosa, low myopia, diabetes, etc., as well as a complement to medical technologies such as LASIK, intraocular lens implantations, retinal implants, and other treatments that yield improvements in vision but for which suboptimal cortical processing leaves patients without the full potential benefit of the optical improvements that they've gained.

7. Applying Perceptual Learning in ophthalmology practice

As eyecare technology advances, so do patient expectations. Optimizing outcomes and managing expectations is a consistent challenge in clinical practice. Eye practitioners agree that good vision promotes healthier lifestyles [63], aids educational processes [64] and visual impairment is detrimental to life itself [65, 66]. An international online survey sponsored by Bausch and Lomb called NSIGHT (Needs, Symptoms, Incidence, Global Eye Health Trends) found that "seeing better" was the most important consideration for choosing vision products. Patients prefer vision related products that emphasize vision improvement, therefore therapy goals need to involve products and methods to improve vision to a maximum. Clinicians pay tremendous attention to the "eye side" of the visual system but emerging research shows that we need to pay more attention to the neurological or brain processing aspect of vision which lies outside of conventional treatments.

Vision training is not a new phenomenon in Ophthalmology, eye exercises have been used for hundreds of years. The most common vision training procedures, currently and traditionally, focus on exercising the optics of the eye (e.g. flippers, prisms, and alternating fixation between distances). However these techniques lack reliable evidence of success [67]. Alternatively, recent perceptual learning based software intervention programs for eye related disorders have shown great promise and there is increasing evidence of their efficacy. Historically reserved for database and assessment tool functions, eyecare software is expanding rapidly into therapeutic interventions and treatment. Computer software is now finding real world use in the visual world of binocular disorders, amblyopia, neuro-rehabilitation and visual enhancement. Researchers and software developers are encouraged by research showing that specific software use actualizes the potential of the visual system and translates into real life gains. Therefore, the science of improving brain processing is not only relevant but utilizing these tools to treat these disorders can prove life changing. With that said, not all computer programs produce positive visual benefits and the results derived from training can vary from individual to individual. In other words, a simple software program may create entertainment but does not necessarily create real world vision improvement.

Here, we highlight a few perceptual training products currently on the market that doctors are using to help patients.

GlassesOff is an iOS app that enhances contrast sensitivity. Studies have found that contrast sensitivity decreases in disease states but also diminishes with age [68, 69]. Therefore, presbyopia is a combination of both decreased accommodation but also decreased contrast sensitivity. GlassesOff reports several studies on their website related to their product. A recent study found acuity and contrast sensitivity improved in presbyopes after using GlassesOff for approximately 3 months [62]. A perceptual learning technique called "collinear facilitation" is utilized to strengthen neural connections and reduce visual noise. The reduction of visual noise then increases visual clarity. It claims a 90% success rate for dismissing glasses for reading. For more information see glassesoff.com.

Nova Vision is a home computer training program used to reduce visual field deficits and provide visual benefits to patients suffering from the effects of stroke and traumatic brain injury. Nova studies show that visual field can be expanded an additional 5% over time [70]. According to another study, 75% of the trainees reported improved mobility after training [71]. Ideal training consists of using the technology twice daily for 30 minutes a session for approximately 6 months. One can find more information at Novavision.com.

RevitalVision/NeuroVision was developed to aid doctors in the treatment of amblyopia, presbyopia and cataract surgery. RevitalVision has also been used to enhance the vision of sports athletes. Depending on the visual condition, the program requires 40 training sessions for the treatment of amblyopia and 20 sessions for other conditions. Three sessions are recommended weekly and each session lasts up to 30 minutes. Stated benefits include increased contrast sensitivity, enhanced visual acuity, reduction in haloes and improved sense of night vision [72]. The program is used at home on a Windows PC. Some doctors are prescribing the technology to patients to accelerate adaptation to altered visual states due to cataract or LASIK surgery. For more information see Revitalvision.com

ULTIMEYES is a recent application that works on a home computer (Windows PC, Apple Mac) or iOS or Android to train vision. Implementing recent neuroscience advances, ULTIMEYES training combines paired visual and auditory stimuli and was designed in a video-game like way, to make the training more enjoyable for the patient. Benefits include improved contrast sensitivity, enhanced visual acuity, increased night vision and a reduction of haloes. Training time requires 4 weekly sessions for a total of 30 sessions, and each training session takes approximately 25 minutes to complete. A recent study found improved acuity and contrast sensitivity in normal sighted individuals after 2 months of ULTIMEYES training [10]. ULTIMEYES has also been used in the treatment of low vision conditions including presbyopia, amblyopia, post-LASIK rehabilitation, and post-cataract surgery rehabilitation (especially effective for multifocal patients), and with athletes for improved sports performance [11]. For more information see Ultimeyesvision.com.

This is not an exhaustive list of available technologies but gives the reader an idea of commercially available products using software technology to tune brain processing and create better visual performance.

8. Principles of Perceptual Learning

An important question in evaluating studies of PL, is how do we know *what* to learn? In other words, how does a neural system know which information is behaviorally relevant and which is not? Given that plasticity can occur in adult sensory systems, there must be some mechanism that gates what is learned (i.e. to control what aspects are allowed and what aspects are restricted). In the following sections, we review different mechanisms and approaches that help guide perceptual learning.

8.1. Attention

Attention refers to a set of fundamental mental process that selectively modulates the processing of relevant information over irrelevant information; it informs decisions, guides memory processes, and our executive control to direct resources to act upon the world. A common belief is that perceptual learning cannot occur without persistent and intensive attention to the feature to be learned [73]. Profound learning effects are often present for task-relevant features but are typically absent or very limited for the task-irrelevant and unattended features. For example, Ahissar and Hochstein [74] found no or little transfer of learning effects between two tasks that involved judgments on different stimulus attributes (either orientation of local elements or global shape) of the same stimuli. It was also reported that the ability of subjects to discriminate the orientation of a line did not improve when the brightness rather than orientation of the line was attended [75]. Additionally, a single-unit recording study in monkeys found neuronal plasticity manifested as a change in the orientation tuning curves of V1 cells with receptive fields overlapping the spatial location of the training task. No plasticity was found for cells with receptive fields overlapping the location of task-irrelevant stimuli presented at a different location from those relevant to the task [15]. While in the next section we'll discuss how attention to stimuli is not actually required to achieve on those stimuli, nonetheless attention plays an important role in selecting what we do (and do not) learn.

8.2. Reinforcement

Theories of reinforcement learning show that rewards and punishment sculpt when and what we learn. At these times reinforcement signals are released to better learn aspects of the environment (even those for which the organism is not consciously aware) that are predictive or co-vary with the event. For example, in a natural environment a target (e.g., a predator) to which one needs to direct attention is usually presented in the same or similar context. Thus, gaining higher sensitivity to features in such a context may lead one to more easily notice that he/she is in the environment in which a target tends to appear and to better recognize the target [e.g. 76].

Recent research demonstrates the fundamental importance of reinforcement processes in guiding perceptual learning. For example, the research paradigm of "task-irrelevant perceptual learning" shows that sensory plasticity occurs without attention being directed to the learned stimuli, and even for those that participants are not aware [19, 77-88]. Seitz and Watanabe [84] found that a sensitivity enhancement occurred as the result of temporal-pairing between the presentation of a subliminal, task-irrelevant, motion stimulus and a task-target. In this experiment, four different directions of motion were presented an equal number of times during the exposure stage, but a single direction of interest was consistently paired (temporally preceded and then overlapped) with the task-targets. Learning was found only for the motion-direction that was temporally-paired with the task-targets, not for the other motion-directions. Similar results were obtained when the luminance contrast of the dots (100% coherence) was made so low that the subjects did not notice the presentation of the motion stimuli [81]. These results suggest that task-irrelevant perceptual learning does not occur as a result of purely passive exposure, but that the irrelevant feature must be related to task performance. These results have led to the idea that plasticity is gated by confluence between a spatially diffusive task-related signal and a task-irrelevant feature signal [79]. Later research confirmed this idea by demonstrating that task-irrelevant perceptual learning can arise through pairing a stimulus with a liquid reward [80].

Seitz and Watanabe [79] suggested a model of perceptual learning where learning results from interactions between spatially diffusive task-driven signals and bottom-up stimulus signals. Namely, that learning is gated by behaviorally relevant events (rewards, punishment, novelty, etc). At these times reinforcement signals are released to better learn aspects of the environment (even those for which the organism is not consciously aware) that are predictive or co-vary with the event. By now, task-irrelevant perceptual learning has been shown to be a robust learning phenomenon that generalizes to a wide range of stimulus features, for example, motion processing [19], orientation processing [89], critical flicker fusion thresholds [82, 83], contour integration [90], auditory formant processing [91], and phonetic processing [92]. Importantly, task-irrelevant perceptual learning produces learning effects that are often as strong, and sometimes stronger, than learning effects produced through direct training [91, 93]. While the phenomenon of task-irrelevant perceptual learning has been studied in most detail in the case of low-level perceptual learning, recent research has identified a high-level, fast form, of task-irrelevant perceptual learning (fast-task-irrelevant perceptual learning) [94-101]. In this fast-task-irrelevant perceptual learning paradigm, participants conducted target detection tasks (looking for a target, letter, color, or word among a series of distractors), while also memorizing other stimuli (images, pictures) that were consistently paired with the stimuli of the target-detection task. Similar to task-irrelevant perceptual learning for low-level perceptual learning, visual memory was enhanced for stimuli that were paired with the targets of the target-detection task. Thus task-irrelevant perceptual learning is arguably a basic mechanism of learning in the brain that spans multiple levels of processing and sensory modalities.

While we have discussed attention and reinforcement as separate processes, this distinction may be overly simplistic (e.g. [79, 86]). For example, the orienting of attention, in the direction of the target-arrow, has been linked with the acetylcholine neuromodulatory system [102]. The same neuromodulatory system has been suggested to have an important role in learning: some studies indicate that a reduction of the cholinergic input reduces cortical plasticity [103] and impairs learning [104-106]. However, other neuromodulatory systems, such as dopamine and norepinephrine have also been linked to both attention [107, 108] and to learning [109, 110]. Indeed, these three neuromodulators (acetylcholine, norepinephrine, and dopamine) have been linked to the three attentional systems described by Posner and Petersen (1990): the alerting network that involves temporal cueing and the maintenance of an alert state (norepinephrine; [111-113]; the orienting network that spatially selects information from sensory input (acetylcholine; [102]; and the executive control network that resolves conflict among responses (dopamine; [114]). These studies indicate that attention and reinforcement are deeply interrelated and that a good training approach should aim to direct both attention and reinforcement in a manner to promote learning.

8.3. Applying rules of synaptic plasticity

At the cellular level, it is widely accepted that the process of synaptic plasticity underlies learning and memory. Synaptic plasticity is the ability of the strength of the connections between synapses to change, strengthening or weakening the connections of existing neurons to modulate the effectiveness of their communication. Bliss and Lomo discovered a method to experimentally induce a persistent synaptic plasticity termed long-term potentiation (LTP) [115]. By inducing brief high frequency electrical stimulation in the perforant pathway of anaesthetized rabbits and recording in the dentate gyrus they discovered an increase of excitatory post-synaptic potentials (EPSPs) over baseline response that lasted up to 10 hours. Conversely, long-term depression (LTD) is induced by persistent low frequency electrical stimulation, resulting in weakened synaptic connections.

Recent research has established that non-invasive exposure-based stimulation protocols can be applied to the sensory systems and result in plasticity of the corresponding sensory cortices. Passive high frequency stimulation (HFS) (20 Hz) of the fingertip resulted in the behavioral improvement of a 2-point discrimination task, and low frequency stimulation (LFS) (1 Hz) decreased performance on this task [116]. Additionally, improvements on the behavioral task after HFS was correlated with cortical reorganization as assessed by mapping somatosensory evoked potentials. This effect was abolished by oral application of an NMDA receptor antagonist, indicating this effect shares similar requirements to cellular LTP and long-term memory formation as identified in the animal model [117]. Using a visual stimulation protocol Beste and colleagues [118] demonstrated behavioral changes on a change-detection task. Here, two bars were presented where a change could occur in the luminance of one bar, the orientation of one bar, the luminance and orientation of the same bar, or the luminance of one bar and the orientation of the other bar. The participants had to report a change in luminance, and ignore a change in orientation. The orientation change in the last condition was highly distracting, and made the luminance detection more difficult. A visual stimulation protocol consisted of alternating black and white bars flashing at either a high (20 Hz) or low (1 Hz) frequency with the goal of increasing or decreasing luminance saliency. The authors found a high frequency visual stimulation protocol improved the behavioral outcome on the detection task tested up to 10 days after induction. Conversely, a low frequency LTD-like protocol impaired performance. These studies of exposure-based learning provide a clear connection between the animal model and the human system, and suggest that approaches based upon knowledge of synaptic plasticity can be applied to improved perception in humans.

8.4. Multisensory facilitation

The human brain has evolved to learn and operate optimally in natural environments in which behavior is guided by information integrated across multiple sensory modalities. Crossmodal interactions are ubiquitous in the nervous system and occur even at early stages of perceptual processing [119-123]. Until recently, however, all studies of perceptual learning focused on training with one sensory modality. This unisensory training fails to tap into natural learning mechanisms that have evolved to optimize behavior in a multisensory environment. Recent research shows that subjects trained with auditory-visual stimuli exhibit a faster rate of learning and a higher degree of improvement than found in subjects trained in silence [124, 125]. Critically, these benefits of multisensory training are even found for perceptual tests *without* auditory signals. In other words, *multisensory training facilitates unisensory learning*. While, to date, most vision training procedures either don't include sounds as part of the task (other than as feedback) or include sounds that are not coordinated with visual stimuli, the advantage of multisensory training over visual-alone training is substantial; reducing the number of sessions required to reach asymptote by ~60%, while also raising the maximum performance [126]. We suggest that having complementary information about the target objects come from different sensory modalities allows the senses to work together to facilitate learning.

8.5. Promoting transfer of learning

Classically, a translational barrier to perceptual learning has been its high degree of specificity to trained stimulus features [127]; such as orientation [20], retinal location [128] or even the eye of training [80, 129]. For example training with a single visual stimulus at a single screen location can result in learning that is specific to that situation. While such studies have been informative regarding the mechanisms of learning, specificity limits therapeutic benefits.

Recent research suggests methods of how this "curse of specificity" can be overcome. Approaches that depart from the most simple training approaches, such as those using multi-stimulus training [130, 131] and off-the-shelf video games [132, 133] show a greater generalization of learning. For example, the recently developed technique of 'double training' found that the specific learning effects found in their paradigms can show broad transfer when more than one stimulus attribute is trained at a time. Xiao, Zhang [131] trained participants on the Vernier discrimination task at a specific orientation at a specific location in the visual field, which normally yields location and orientation specific learning effects [129]. But when they subsequently trained a second orientation at a different spatial location, they found that the training induced changes for the second orientation transferred to the first location. Such findings of broad location transfer undermine the argument that this learning is due to plasticity in retinotopic visual areas.

There exist a growing number of studies that address how specificity, or its opposite, transfer, is controlled by different factors. In a discrimination task, Jeter, Dosher, Petrov and Lu [134] showed that transfer was observed in low-precision transfer tasks while specificity was observed in high-precision transfer tasks. Then, Jeter, Dosher, Liu and Lu [135] showed that specificity was the result of an extensive training, confirming more classical results [20, 128, 136], while a substantial transfer was observed at early in the training. Interestingly, another study, reported by Aberg, Tartaglia and Herzog [137] presented a series of experiments showing, in one hand, that the number of trials per session influenced the overall improvement of the participant's performance, and in another hand, the transfer depended on the number of trials presented during each session, not the total number of trials. Zhang *et al.*, [138] showed a peripheral orientation discrimination task transferred to new locations only after a pre-test was given to participants. These studies add to the double-training studies that show transfer after training multiple features or at multiple locations [130, 131]. Together these studies show that many factors (extent of training, blocking of trials, precision of training stimuli, diversity of training set, etc), influence the transfer of learning.

9. Conclusion

While extant applications of perceptual learning to Ophthalmology show great promise, a limitation of modern perceptual learning research is that learning is studied in very specific ways, focusing on one particular stimulus or factor. This narrow focus has limited understanding of the multiple learning factors that are present in natural settings and how these factors interact to determine the speed and nature of learning. We suggest a new paradigm of integrating perceptual learning methodologies into a coordinated approach that achieves a more comprehensive form of perceptual learning than typically studied in the lab. For example the approach used in the ULTIMEYES program combines many factors that are known to promote neural plasticity and generalization of learning [10, 11]. Furthermore, findings that playing off-the-shelf video games can improve vision [132, 133, 139] suggests another avenue of research where principles derived from video games should be combined with those from the field of perceptual learning to create an enriching user experience that encourages compliance with treatment while effectively optimizing how the brain process its ocular inputs.

Author details

Jenni Deveau[1], Gary Lovcik[2] and Aaron R. Seitz[1]

*Address all correspondence to: aseitz@ucr.edu

1 Department of Psychology, University of California – Riverside, Riverside, CA, USA

2 Anaheim Hills Optometric Center, Anaheim, CA, USA

References

[1] Levi, D.M. and R.W. Li, *Perceptual learning as a potential treatment for amblyopia: a mini-review.* Vision Res, 2009. 49(21): p. 2535-49.

[2] Polat, U., *Making perceptual learning practical to improve visual functions.* Vision Res, 2009. 49(21): p. 2566-73.

[3] Baker, C.I., et al., *Reorganization of visual processing in macular degeneration.* J Neurosci, 2005. 25(3): p. 614-8.

[4] Huxlin, K.R., et al., *Perceptual relearning of complex visual motion after V1 damage in humans.* J Neurosci, 2009. 29(13): p. 3981-91.

[5] Vaina, L.M. and C.G. Gross, *Perceptual deficits in patients with impaired recognition of biological motion after temporal lobe lesions.* Proc Natl Acad Sci U S A, 2004. 101(48): p. 16947-51.

[6] Ostrovsky, Y., A. Andalman, and P. Sinha, *Vision following extended congenital blindness.* Psychol Sci, 2006. 17(12): p. 1009-14.

[7] Hubel, D.H. and T.N. Wiesel, *Effects of Monocular Deprivation in Kittens.* Naunyn Schmiedebergs Arch Pharmacol, 1964. 248: p. 492-7.

[8] Hubel, D.H. and T.N. Wiesel, *Binocular interaction in striate cortex of kittens reared with artificial squint.* J Neurophysiol, 1965. 28(6): p. 1041-59.

[9] Adini, Y., D. Sagi, and M. Tsodyks, *Context-enabled learning in the human visual system.* Nature, 2002. 415(6873): p. 790-3.

[10] Deveau, J., G. Lovcik, and A.R. Seitz, *Broad-based visual benefits from training with an integrated perceptual-learning video game.* Vision Res, 2014.

[11] Deveau, J., D.J. Ozer, and A.R. Seitz, *Improved vision and on field performance in baseball through perceptual learning.* Curr Biol, 2014. 24(4).

[12] Ball, K. and R. Sekuler, *Adaptive processing of visual motion.* J Exp Psychol Hum Percept Perform, 1981. 7(4): p. 780-94.

[13] Sagi, D. and D. Tanne, *Perceptual learning: learning to see.* Curr Opin Neurobiol, 1994. 4(2): p. 195-9.

[14] Crist, R.E., W. Li, and C.D. Gilbert, *Learning to see: experience and attention in primary visual cortex.* Nat Neurosci, 2001. 4(5): p. 519-25.

[15] Schoups, A., et al., *Practising orientation identification improves orientation coding in V1 neurons.PG-549-53.* Nature, 2001. 412(6846).

[16] Schoups, A.A., R. Vogels, and G.A. Orban, *Human perceptual learning in identifying the oblique orientation: retinotopy, orientation specificity and monocularity.* J Physiol, 1995. 483 (Pt 3): p. 797-810.

[17] Raiguel, S., et al., *Learning to see the difference specifically alters the most informative V4 neurons.* J Neurosci, 2006. 26(24): p. 6589-602.

[18] Crist, R.E., et al., *Perceptual learning of spatial localization: specificity for orientation, position, and context.* J Neurophysiol, 1997. 78(6): p. 2889-94.

[19] Watanabe, T., et al., *Greater plasticity in lower-level than higher-level visual motion processing in a passive perceptual learning task.* Nat Neurosci, 2002. 5(10): p. 1003-9.

[20] Fiorentini, A. and N. Berardi, *Perceptual learning specific for orientation and spatial frequency.* Nature, 1980. 287(5777): p. 43-4.

[21] Li, C.S., C. Padoa-Schioppa, and E. Bizzi, *Neuronal correlates of motor performance and motor learning in the primary motor cortex of monkeys adapting to an external force field.* Neuron, 2001. 30(2): p. 593-607.

[22] Yang, T. and J.H. Maunsell, *The effect of perceptual learning on neuronal responses in monkey visual area V4.* J Neurosci, 2004. 24(7): p. 1617-26.

[23] Zohary, E., et al., *Neuronal plasticity that underlies improvement in perceptual performance.* Science, 1994. 263(5151): p. 1289-92.

[24] Furmanski, C.S., D. Schluppeck, and S.A. Engel, *Learning strengthens the response of primary visual cortex to simple patterns.* Curr Biol, 2004. 14(7): p. 573-8.

[25] Schwartz, S., P. Maquet, and C. Frith, *Neural correlates of perceptual learning: a functional MRI study of visual texture discrimination.* Proc Natl Acad Sci U S A, 2002. 99(26): p. 17137-42.

[26] Vaina, L.M., et al., *Neural systems underlying learning and representation of global motion.* Proc Natl Acad Sci U S A, 1998. 95(21): p. 12657-62.

[27] Roelfsema, P.R. and A. van Ooyen, *Attention-gated reinforcement learning of internal representations for classification.* Neural Comput, 2005. 17(10): p. 2176-214.

[28] Dosher, B.A. and Z.L. Lu, *Perceptual learning reflects external noise filtering and internal noise reduction through channel reweighting.* Proc Natl Acad Sci U S A, 1998. 95(23): p. 13988-93.

[29] Sotiropoulos, G., A.R. Seitz, and P. Series, *Perceptual learning in visual hyperacuity: A reweighting model.* Vision Res, 2011. 51(6): p. 585-99.

[30] Dosher, B.A. and Z.L. Lu, *Mechanisms of perceptual learning.* Vision Res, 1999. 39(19): p. 3197-221.

[31] Petrov, A., A. Dosher, and Z. Lu, *Perceptual learning without feedback in non-stationary contexts: data and model.* Vision Res, 2006. in press.

[32] Ghose, G.M., T. Yang, and J.H. Maunsell, *Physiological correlates of perceptual learning in monkey V1 and V2.* J Neurophysiol, 2002. 87(4): p. 1867-88.

[33] Law, C.T. and J.I. Gold, *Neural correlates of perceptual learning in a sensory-motor, but not a sensory, cortical area.* Nat Neurosci, 2008. 11(4): p. 505-13.

[34] Gu, Y., et al., *Perceptual learning reduces interneuronal correlations in macaque visual cortex.* Neuron, 2011. 71(4): p. 750-61.

[35] Rainer, G., H. Lee, and N.K. Logothetis, *The effect of learning on the function of monkey extrastriate visual cortex.* PLoS Biol, 2004. 2(2): p. E44.

[36] Ghose, G.M., *Learning in mammalian sensory cortex.* Curr Opin Neurobiol, 2004. 14(4): p. 513-8.

[37] Horwitz, G.D., A.P. Batista, and W.T. Newsome, *Direction-selective visual responses in macaque superior colliculus induced by behavioral training.* Neurosci Lett, 2004. 366(3): p. 315-9.

[38] Horwitz, G.D., A.P. Batista, and W.T. Newsome, *Representation of an abstract perceptual decision in macaque superior colliculus.* J Neurophysiol, 2004. 91(5): p. 2281-96.

[39] Zaksas, D. and T. Pasternak, *Directional signals in the prefrontal cortex and in area MT during a working memory for visual motion task.* J Neurosci, 2006. 26(45): p. 11726-42.

[40] Huang, C.B., Y. Zhou, and Z.L. Lu, *Broad bandwidth of perceptual learning in the visual system of adults with anisometropic amblyopia.* Proc Natl Acad Sci U S A, 2008. 105(10): p. 4068-73.

[41] Polat, U., et al., *Improving vision in adult amblyopia by perceptual learning.* Proc Natl Acad Sci U S A, 2004. 101(17): p. 6692-7.

[42] Polat, U., T. Ma-Naim, and A. Spierer, *Treatment of children with amblyopia by perceptual learning.* Vision Res, 2009. 49(21): p. 2599-603.

[43] Ooi, T.L., et al., *A push-pull treatment for strengthening the 'lazy eye' in amblyopia.* Curr Biol, 2013. 23(8): p. R309-10.

[44] Xu, J.P., Z.J. He, and T.L. Ooi, *Effectively reducing sensory eye dominance with a push-pull perceptual learning protocol.* Curr Biol, 2010. 20(20): p. 1864-8.

[45] Li, J., et al., *Dichoptic training enables the adult amblyopic brain to learn.* Curr Biol, 2013. 23(8): p. R308-9.

[46] Li, R.W., et al., *Video-game play induces plasticity in the visual system of adults with amblyopia.* PLoS Biol, 2011. 9(8): p. e1001135.

[47] Hussain, Z., et al., *Perceptual learning reduces crowding in amblyopia and in the normal periphery.* J Neurosci, 2012. 32(2): p. 474-80.

[48] Astle, A.T., B.S. Webb, and P.V. McGraw, *Spatial frequency discrimination learning in normal and developmentally impaired human vision.* Vision Res, 2010. 50(23): p. 2445-54.

[49] Fletcher, D.C. and R.A. Schuchard, *Preferred retinal loci relationship to macular scotomas in a low-vision population.* Ophthalmology, 1997. 104(4): p. 632-8.

[50] Kwon, M., A.S. Nandy, and B.S. Tjan, *Rapid and persistent adaptability of human oculomotor control in response to simulated central vision loss.* Curr Biol, 2013. 23(17): p. 1663-9.

[51] Kwon, M., et al., *Contour enhancement benefits older adults with simulated central field loss.* Optom Vis Sci, 2012. 89(9): p. 1374-84.

[52] Baker, C.I., et al., *Reorganization of visual processing in macular degeneration: replication and clues about the role of foveal loss.* Vision Res, 2008. 48(18): p. 1910-9.

[53] Chung, S.T., *Improving reading speed for people with central vision loss through perceptual learning.* Invest Ophthalmol Vis Sci, 2011. 52(2): p. 1164-70.

[54] Liu, L., T. Kuyk, and P. Fuhr, *Visual search training in subjects with severe to profound low vision.* Vision Res, 2007. 47(20): p. 2627-36.

[55] Dilks, D.D., et al., *Reorganization of visual processing in macular degeneration is not specific to the "preferred retinal locus".* J Neurosci, 2009. 29(9): p. 2768-73.

[56] Andersen, G.J., *Aging and Vision: Changes in Function and Performance from Optics to Perception.* Wiley Interdiscip Rev Cogn Sci, 2012. 3(3): p. 403-410.

[57] Andersen, G.J., et al., *Perceptual learning, aging, and improved visual performance in early stages of visual processing.* J Vis, 2010. 10(13): p. 4.

[58] Lu, Z.L. and B.A. Dosher, *Characterizing observers using external noise and observer models: assessing internal representations with external noise.* Psychol Rev, 2008. 115(1): p. 44-82.

[59] Koretz, J.F., et al., *Accommodation and presbyopia in the human eye--aging of the anterior segment.* Vision Res, 1989. 29(12): p. 1685-92.

[60] Llorente-Guillemot, A., et al., *Visual performance with simultaneous vision multifocal contact lenses.* Clin Exp Optom, 2012. 95(1): p. 54-9.

[61] Alarcon, A., et al., *Visual quality after monovision correction by laser in situ keratomileusis in presbyopic patients.* J Cataract Refract Surg, 2011. 37(9): p. 1629-35.

[62] Polat, U., et al., *Training the brain to overcome the effect of aging on the human eye.* Sci Rep, 2012. 2: p. 278.

[63] Fong, C.S., et al., *Correction of visual impairment by cataract surgery and improved survival in older persons: the Blue Mountains Eye Study cohort.* Ophthalmology, 2013. 120(9): p. 1720-7.

[64] Basch, C.E., *Healthier students are better learners: a missing link in school reforms to close the achievement gap.* J Sch Health, 2011. 81(10): p. 593-8.

[65] De Leo, D., et al., *Blindness, fear of sight loss, and suicide.* Psychosomatics, 1999. 40(4): p. 339-44.

[66] CDC. *The State of Vision, Aging, and Public Health in America.* 2013; Available from: cdc.gov/visionhealth/pdf/vision.pdf.

[67] Helveston, E.M., *Visual training: current status in ophthalmology.* Am J Ophthalmol, 2005. 140(5): p. 903-10.

[68] McKendrick, A.M., et al., *Contrast sensitivity changes due to glaucoma and normal aging: Low-spatial-frequency losses in both magnocellular and parvocellular pathways.* Investigative Ophthalmology & Visual Science, 2007. 48(5): p. 2115-2122.

[69] Ross, J.E., D.D. Clarke, and A.J. Bron, *Effect of age on contrast sensitivity function: uniocular and binocular findings.* Br J Ophthalmol, 1985. 69(1): p. 51-6.

[70] Kasten, E., et al., *Computer-based training for the treatment of partial blindness.* Nat Med, 1998. 4(9): p. 1083-7.

[71] Mueller, I.P., D.A.; Kenkel, S.; Kasten, E. and Sabel, B.A., *Vision Restoration Therapy after brain damage; subjective improvements of activities of daily life and their relationship to visual field enlargements.* Vision Impairment Research, 2003(5): p. 157-178.

[72] Revitalvision.com. *Amblyopia Effectiveness* 2013; Available from: Revitalvision.com/amblyopia/effectiveness.

[73] Ahissar, M. and S. Hochstein, *Attentional control of early perceptual learning.* Proc Natl Acad Sci U S A, 1993. 90(12): p. 5718-22.

[74] Ahissar, M. and S. Hochstein, *Task difficulty and the specificity of perceptual learning.* Nature, 1997. 387(6631): p. 401-6.

[75] Shiu, L.P. and H. Pashler, *Improvement in line orientation discrimination is retinally local but dependent on cognitive set.* Percept Psychophys, 1992. 52(5): p. 582-8.

[76] Chun, M.M., *Contextual cueing of visual attention.* Trends Cogn Sci, 2000. 4(5): p. 170-178.

[77] Nishina, S., et al. *The spatial spread of task-irrelevant perceptual learning*. in *Society for Neuroscience 35th Annual Meeting*. 2005. Washington, D.C.

[78] Seitz, A., et al., *Requirement for high-level processing in subliminal learning.* Curr Biol, 2005. 15(18): p. R753-5.

[79] Seitz, A. and T. Watanabe, *A unified model for perceptual learning.* Trends Cogn Sci, 2005. 9(7): p. 329-34.

[80] Seitz, A.R., D. Kim, and T. Watanabe, *Rewards evoke learning of unconsciously processed visual stimuli in adult humans.* Neuron, 2009. 61(5): p. 700-7.

[81] Seitz, A.R., et al., *Seeing what is not there shows the costs of perceptual learning.* Proc Natl Acad Sci U S A, 2005. 102(25): p. 9080-5.

[82] Seitz, A.R., et al., *Visual experience can substantially alter critical flicker fusion thresholds.* Hum Psychopharmacol, 2005. 20(1): p. 55-60.

[83] Seitz, A.R., et al., *Perceptual learning of motion leads to faster flicker perception.* PLoS ONE, 2006. 1: p. e28.

[84] Seitz, A.R. and T. Watanabe, *Psychophysics: Is subliminal learning really passive?* Nature, 2003. 422(6927): p. 36.

[85] Seitz, A.R. and T. Watanabe, *Is task-irrelevant learning really task-irrelevant?* PLoS ONE, 2008. 3(11): p. e3792.

[86] Seitz, A.R. and T. Watanabe, *The phenomenon of task-irrelevant perceptual learning.* Vision Res, 2009. 49(21): p. 2604-10.

[87] Tsushima, Y., A.R. Seitz, and T. Watanabe, *Task-irrelevant learning occurs only when the irrelevant feature is weak.* Curr Biol, 2008. 18(12): p. R516-7.

[88] Watanabe, T., J.E. Nanez, and Y. Sasaki, *Perceptual learning without perception.* Nature, 2001. 413(6858): p. 844-8.

[89] Nishina, S., et al., *Effect of spatial distance to the task stimulus on task-irrelevant perceptual learning of static Gabors.* Journal of Vision, 2007. 7(13): p. 1-10.

[90] Rosenthal, O. and G.W. Humphreys, *Perceptual organization without perception: the subliminal learning of global contour.* Psychol Sci, 2010. 21(12): p. 1751-8.

[91] Seitz, A.R., et al., *Unattended exposure to components of speech sounds yields same benefits as explicit auditory training.* Cognition, 2010. 115(3): p. 435-43.

[92] Vlahou, E., A.R. Seitz, and A. Protopapas. *Implicit learning of non-native speech stimuli.* in *Acoustical Society of America*. 2009. Portland, OR.

[93] Vlahou, E.L., A. Protopapas, and A.R. Seitz, *Implicit training of nonnative speech stimuli.* J Exp Psychol Gen, 2012. 141(2): p. 363-81.

[94] Swallow, K.M. and Y.V. Jiang, *The Attentional Boost Effect: Transient increases in attention to one task enhance performance in a second task.* Cognition, 2010. 115(1): p. 118-32.

[95] Swallow, K.M. and Y.V. Jiang, *The role of timing in the attentional boost effect.* Atten Percept Psychophys, 2011. 73(2): p. 389-404.

[96] Lin, J.Y., et al., *Enhanced memory for scenes presented at behaviorally relevant points in time.* PLoS Biol, 2010. 8(3): p. e1000337.

[97] Leclercq, V. and A.R. Seitz, *Enhancement from targets and suppression from cues in fast task-irrelevant perceptual learning.* Acta Psychol (Amst), 2012. 141(1): p. 31-8.

[98] Leclercq, V. and A.R. Seitz, *Fast-TIPL occurs for salient images without a memorization requirement in men but not in women.* PLoS ONE, 2012. 7(4): p. e36228.

[99] Leclercq, V. and A.R. Seitz, *The impact of orienting attention in fast task-irrelevant perceptual learning.* Atten Percept Psychophys, 2012. 74(4): p. 648-60.

[100] Leclercq, V. and A.R. Seitz, *Fast task-irrelevant perceptual learning is disrupted by sudden onset of central task elements.* Vision Res, 2012. 61: p. 70-6.

[101] Leclercq, V., C.C. Le Dantec, and A.R. Seitz, *Encoding of episodic information through fast task-irrelevant perceptual learning.* Vision Res, 2013.

[102] Davidson, M.C. and R.T. Marrocco, *Local infusion of scopolamine into intraparietal cortex slows covert orienting in rhesus monkeys.* J Neurophysiol, 2000. 83(3): p. 1536-49.

[103] Juliano, S.L., W. Ma, and D. Eslin, *Cholinergic depletion prevents expansion of topographic maps in somatosensory cortex.* Proc Natl Acad Sci U S A, 1991. 88(3): p. 780-4.

[104] Easton, A., et al., *Unilateral lesions of the cholinergic basal forebrain and fornix in one hemisphere and inferior temporal cortex in the opposite hemisphere produce severe learning impairments in rhesus monkeys.* Cereb Cortex, 2002. 12(7): p. 729-36.

[105] Winkler, J., et al., *Essential role of neocortical acetylcholine in spatial memory.* Nature, 1995. 375(6531): p. 484-7.

[106] Warburton, E.C., et al., *Cholinergic neurotransmission is essential for perirhinal cortical plasticity and recognition memory.* Neuron, 2003. 38(6): p. 987-96.

[107] Fan, J., et al., *Mapping the genetic variation of executive attention onto brain activity.* Proc Natl Acad Sci U S A, 2003. 100(12): p. 7406-11.

[108] Posner, M.I. and S.E. Petersen, *The attention system of the human brain.* Annu Rev Neurosci, 1990. 13: p. 25-42.

[109] Dalley, J.W., et al., *Distinct changes in cortical acetylcholine and noradrenaline efflux during contingent and noncontingent performance of a visual attentional task.* J Neurosci, 2001. 21(13): p. 4908-14.

[110] Bao, S., V.T. Chan, and M.M. Merzenich, *Cortical remodelling induced by activity of ventral tegmental dopamine neurons.* Nature, 2001. 412(6842): p. 79-83.

[111] Witte, E.A. and R.T. Marrocco, *Alteration of brain noradrenergic activity in rhesus monkeys affects the alerting component of covert orienting.* Psychopharmacology (Berl), 1997. 132(4): p. 315-23.

[112] Coull, J.T., et al., *A fronto-parietal network for rapid visual information processing: a PET study of sustained attention and working memory.* Neuropsychologia, 1996. 34(11): p. 1085-95.

[113] Marrocco, R.T., E.A. Witte, and M.C. Davidson, *Arousal systems.* Curr Opin Neurobiol, 1994. 4(2): p. 166-70.

[114] Fossella, J., et al., *Assessing the molecular genetics of attention networks.* BMC Neurosci, 2002. 3(1): p. 14.

[115] Bliss, T.V. and T. Lomo, *Long-lasting potentiation of synaptic transmission in the dentate area of the anaesthetized rabbit following stimulation of the perforant path.* J Physiol, 1973. 232(2): p. 331-56.

[116] Ragert, P., et al., *Differential effects of tactile high-and low-frequency stimulation on tactile discrimination in human subjects.* BMC Neurosci, 2008. 9: p. 9.

[117] Dinse, H.R., et al., *Pharmacological modulation of perceptual learning and associated cortical reorganization.* Science, 2003. 301(5629): p. 91-4.

[118] Beste, C., et al., *Improvement and impairment of visually guided behavior through LTP-and LTD-like exposure-based visual learning.* Curr Biol, 2011. 21(10): p. 876-82.

[119] Calvert, G., C. Spence, and B.E. Stein, *The handbook of multisensory processes.* 2004: The MIT Press.

[120] Driver, J. and T. Noesselt, *Multisensory interplay reveals crossmodal influences on 'sensory-specific' brain regions, neural responses, and judgments.* Neuron, 2008. 57: p. 11-23.

[121] Ghazanfar, A. and C.E. Schroeder, *Is neocortex essentially multisensory?* Trends Cogn Sci, 2006. 10(6): p. 278-285.

[122] Shimojo, S. and L. Shams, *Sensory modalities are not separate modalities: plasticity and interactions.* Current Opinion in Neurobiology, 2001. 11: p. 505-509.

[123] Schroeder, C.E. and J. Foxe, *Multisensory contributions to low-level, 'unisensory' processing.* Current Opinion in Neurobiology, 2005. 15: p. 454-458.

[124] Kim, R.S., A.R. Seitz, and L. Shams, *Benefits of stimulus congruency for multisensory facilitation of visual learning.* PLoS ONE, 2008. 3(1): p. e1532.

[125] Seitz, A.R., R. Kim, and L. Shams, *Sound facilitates visual learning.* Current Biology, 2006. 16: p. 1422-1427.

[126] Seitz, A.R., R. Kim, and L. Shams, *Sound facilitates visual learning.* Curr Biol, 2006. 16(14): p. 1422-7.

[127] Fahle, M., *Perceptual learning: specificity versus generalization.* Curr Opin Neurobiol, 2005. 15(2): p. 154-60.

[128] Karni, A. and D. Sagi, *Where practice makes perfect in texture discrimination: evidence for primary visual cortex plasticity.* Proc Natl Acad Sci U S A, 1991. 88(11): p. 4966-70.

[129] Poggio, T., M. Fahle, and S. Edelman, *Fast perceptual learning in visual hyperacuity.* Science, 1992. 256(5059): p. 1018-21.

[130] Yu, C., et al., *Rule-Based Learning Explains Visual Perceptual Learning and Its Specificity and Transfer.* Journal of Neuroscience, 2010. 30(37): p. 12323-12328.

[131] Xiao, L.Q., et al., *Complete Transfer of Perceptual Learning across Retinal Locations Enabled by Double Training.* Curr Biol, 2008. 18(24): p. 1922-6.

[132] Green, C.S. and D. Bavelier, *Action video game modifies visual selective attention.* Nature, 2003. 423(6939): p. 534-537.

[133] Li, R., et al., *Enhancing the contrast sensitivity function through action video game training.* Nat Neurosci, 2009. 12(5): p. 549-51.

[134] Jeter, P.E., et al., *Task precision at transfer determines specificity of perceptual learning.* J Vis, 2009. 9(3): p. 1 1-13.

[135] Jeter, P.E., et al., *Specificity of perceptual learning increases with increased training.* Vision Res, 2010. 50(19): p. 1928-40.

[136] Ball, K. and R. Sekuler, *A specific and enduring improvement in visual motion discrimination.* Science, 1982. 218(4573): p. 697-8.

[137] Aberg, K.C., E.M. Tartaglia, and M.H. Herzog, *Perceptual learning with Chevrons requires a minimal number of trials, transfers to untrained directions, but does not require sleep.* Vision Res, 2009. 49(16): p. 2087-94.

[138] Zhang, T., et al., Decoupling location specificity from perceptual learning of orientation discrimination. Vision Res, 2010. 50(4): p. 368-74.

[139] Green, C.S. and D. Bavelier, Action-video-game experience alters the spatial resolution of vision. Psychol Sci, 2007. 18(1): p. 88-94.

8

Ibopamine – A New Alpha-Adrenergic and D1-Dopaminergic Drug

Italo Giuffré

1. Introduction

Ibopamine (3,4 di-isobutyrrylester of N-methyldopamine) at 2% concentration, when instilled in the conjunctival sac, stimulates ocular D1-dopaminergic and α-adrenergic receptors [1,2]. It is a pro-drug of epinine (N-methyldopamine) (Figure 1). It has positive inotropic effects: it improves cardiac function and it is effective in the treatment of congestive heart failure. The pharmacological ocular characteristics of ibopamine are as follows:

- It increases aqueous humor production following D1-dopaminergic stimulation;
- It is a provocative test for evaluating the function of aqueous humor outflow structures;
- It can be used to treat ocular hypotension;
- It induces a noncycloplegic mydriasis (α-adrenergic action);
- It is very useful, apart from genetic testing, to detect a predisposition to ocular hypertension and even glaucoma in relatives of glaucoma patients.

In the conjunctival sac, ibopamine is fastly hydrolysed to epinine by the esterases of the aqueous humor and ocular tissues. This hydrolysis suggests that epinine is the active component of the molecule. The half-life of ibopamine in the aqueous humor is short (about 2 minutes) and epinine formation precedes the mydriatic effect [3,4] (Figure 1). It has been proved that after the instillation of ibopamine, only epinine can be found in the aqueous humor [3].

When hydrolysed to epinine, ibopamine stimulates the α-adrenergic and D1 dopaminergic receptors. The mydriatic effect of ibopamine is due to the stimulation of the α-adrenergic receptors of the dilating muscle of the pupil. Since ibopamine has no effect on the ciliary muscle, the mydriasis is not accompanied by cycloplegia. Mydriasis can be antagonized and

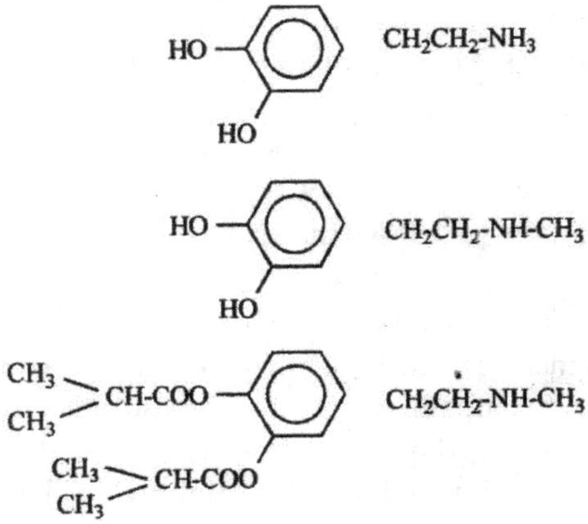

Figure 1. Dopamine → Epinine → Ibopamine (3,4 dyisobutyrrilester of N-methyldopamine).

reversed by pre-treatment by α-blocking agents (such as thymoxamine and dapiprazole). Some Randomized Clinical Trials (RCTs) show that the D1 dopaminergic activity of the drug increases aqueous humor production and intraocular pressure (IOP) in open-angle glaucoma (POAG) patients [5].

Ibopamine has low toxicity both at systemic and local levels. LD_{50} is 2056 mg/Kg, 4930 mg/Kg and 1786 mg/Kg in mice, rats and guinea pigs respectively. Ibopamine is well tolerated without any significant change to the haematological and behavioural parameters. 2% ibopamine eye drops show that ibopamine is well tolerated at local level, without systemic side-effects and tachyphylaxis phenomena. One drop of 2% ibopamine contains 1 mg of the compound, while the oral dosage is higher than 400 mg/day. Electrophysiological assessment showed that ibopamine is not retinotoxic at all [6].

2. Clinical use

2.1. Non-cycloplegic mydriatic activity

In binocular indirect examination of fundus oculi with scleral indentation, fluorescein and indocyanine angiography, and in the laser treatment of retinal lesions, ibopamine can induce a fast, short-lasting (2-3 hours) maximal mydriasis without cycloplegic effects or local a/or systemic side-effects [7]. The mydriatic effect of ibopamine can be prolonged if repeatedly administered (every 30 minutes). Ibopamine-induced mydriasis can be reversed by local application of α-blockers such as thymoxamine and dapiprazole. Ibopamine can substitute phenylephrine in association with tropicamide a/or cyclopentolate to avoid the typical discomfort of cycloplegia mostly in adults [7]. Ibopamine eye drops is effective in inducing pre-operative mydriasis, without effects on the cardiovascular system [7]. In the post-operative period ibopamine can induce a fast and short-lasting mydriasis to induce pupil dilatation.

2.2. Pathophysiology of IOP

2% ibopamine eye drops increases IOP only in patients suffering from POAG. Ibopamine is useful in different ways:

- Physiological studies on IOP;
- Evaluation of trabecular outflow pathways (pressure-dependent outflow);
- Treatment of ocular hypotony.

The instillation of ibopamine increases the IOP only in about 96% of eyes with POAG [8,9,10] (Figures 2, 3). In normal eyes, 2% ibopamine does not significantly affect IOP, with a possible mild hypotensive effect (1-2 mmHg) (Figure 4). The IOP, in POAG patients, increases by a maximum value of 10-11 mmHg within 45 minutes from the instillation and lasts about 180 minutes [7,8,9,10,11,12,13,14]. To observe this effect, 2 drops of 2% ibopamine have been instilled 5 minutes apart, and IOP was measured 45 minutes after the first instillation. The ibopamine provocative test shows a significant correlation with the highest intraocular pressure in the diurnal tension curve in glaucoma patients [15]. Indeed, in glaucoma patients with early visual field defect, the ibopamine provocative test has shown better sensitivity/ specificity than the water drinking test [16]. Ibopamine test does not modify the results of visual field tests in normal individuals [17].

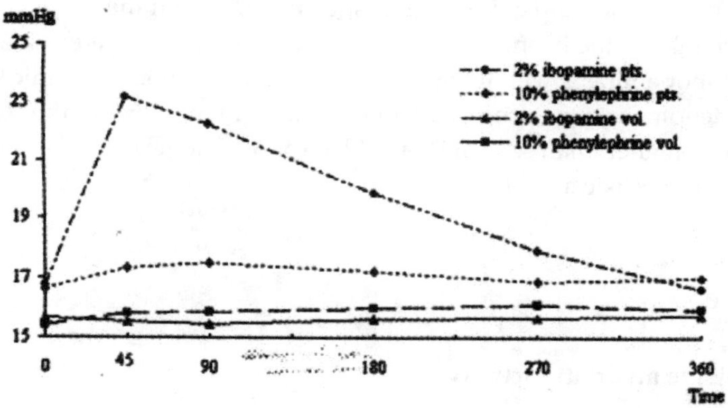

	Maximum increase	Area under the curve
Ibo pts. vs. Ibo vol.	p = 0.0001	p = 0.0001
Ibo pts. vs. Phn pts.	p = 0.0001	p = 0.0001
Ibo vol. vs. Phn vol.	p = n.s.	p = 0.01
Phn pts. vs. Phn vol.	p = n.s.	p = n.s.

Figure 2. Effect on the intraocular pressure of 2% ibopamine and 10% phenylephrine in glaucomatous patients and in normal volunteers.

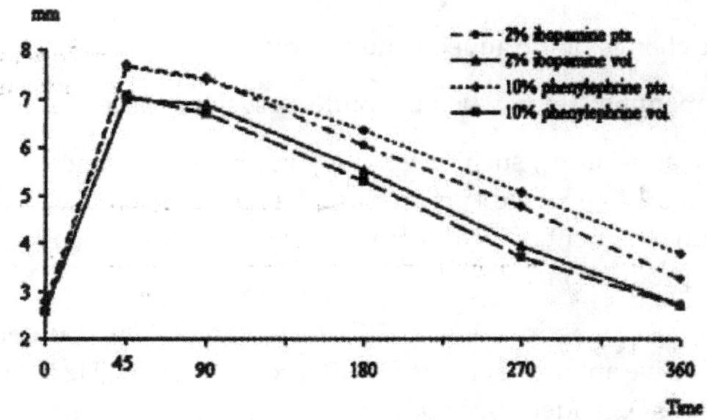

	Maximum increase	Area Under the Curve
Ibo pts. vs. Ibo vol.	p = n.s.	p = n.s.
Ibo pts. vs. Phn pts.	p = n.s.	$p < 0.05$
Ibo vol. vs. Phn vol.	p = n.s.	p = n.s.
Phn pts. vs. Phn vol.	p = n.s.	p = 0.0002

Figure 3. Effect on the pupillary diameter of 2% ibopamine and 10% phenylephrine in glaucomatous patients and in normal volunteers.

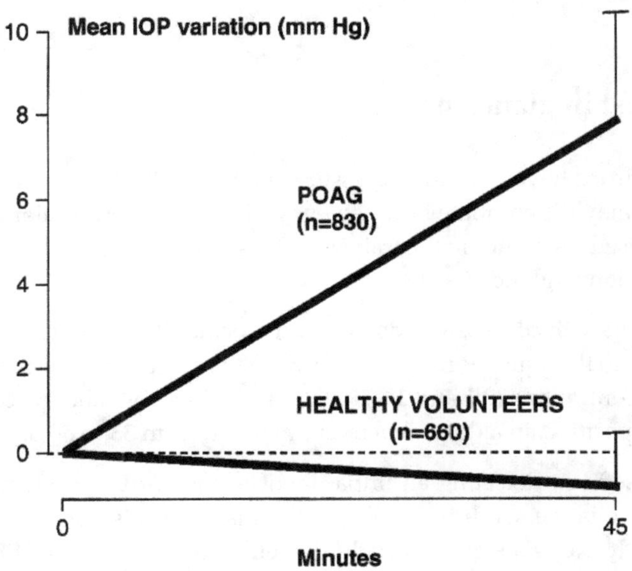

Figure 4. ibopamine induces a transient ocular hypertensive effect (mean, 8.31±2.14 mmHg) in 96% of eyes of patients affected by POAG, whereas in healthy eyes there is a reduction of intraocular pressure (IOP) by 1 to 2 mmHg.

Several studies have been performed to assess the following issues:

- Identification of the responsible receptor (agonist and antagonist);
- Evaluation of the change of the aqueous humor dynamics;
- Evaluation of ibopamine effects when the outflow system was experimentally impaired.

Only the D1 agonist substances, such as fenoldopam, have the same effect as ibopamine on IOP in POAG patients. D1 agonist drugs increase the IOP only in POAG, but never in healthy eyes, stressing the involvement of D1 dopaminergic receptors on the mechanism stimulating the aqueous humor production.

The hypertensive effect of ibopamine in POAG is completely counteracted by the pre-treatment with a selective antagonist of the D1 receptors such as SCH23390. A clear receptorial antagonism for IOP has been identified. Ocular anti-hypertensive drug, such as β-blockers and α-agonists do not antagonize the hypertensive effects of ibopamine in POAG [14]. The partial antagonism performed by glycerol is due to an osmotic reduction of the vitreous mass.

When there is a marked increase of aqueous humor production, due to the D1 dopaminergic effect of ibopamine, the healthy eye increases its outflow mantaining the homeostasis. Instead, in glaucomatous eyes, the impaired trabecular outflow fails to maintain the hydrodynamic equilibrium and IOP increases. Fluorophotometry proves that the D1 dopaminergic stimulation, induced by 2% ibopamine, undoubtedly increases the aqueous humor production.

Ibopamine, when instilled, prior to the Laminaria, into the healthy rabbit eyes does not significantly affect the IOP, while in the eyes treated with Laminaria digitata induces ocular hypertension.

3. Provocative test in glaucoma

Ibopamine 2% eye drops have a positive pressure effect in 50% of suspected normal-tension glaucoma eyes and may differentiate between eyes with normal trabecular outflow capacity and eyes with increased resistance in the trabecular meshwork that are ready to have pressure peaks and deterioration to glaucoma [18].

A long-term treatment with corticosteroids can induce ocular hypertension. They increase the IOP by interfering with the aqueous humor outflow system. By administering dexamethasone at two different concentrations (0.1 and 1%) in eyes suffering from allergic conjunctivitis, the ibopamine test was positive, in a dose-dependent manner, from 33 to 50%.

Ibopamine test is useful in detecting an impairment of the outflow system also in patients affected by psudoexfoliative syndrome (PEX) [19]. This test is also positive when PEX syndrome is unilateral. It exerts a significant additive effect on mydriasis of PEX eyes induced with 10% phenylephrine-0.5% tropicamide with only minimal increase in IOP [20].

The ibopamine test is positive in 44.33% of offspring of one glaucoma parent without glaucomatous damage. It signifies an impaired function of the outflow structures and, therefore, a predisposition to intraocular hypertension and possible glaucoma in some years [21,22].

Ocular hypotony is a pathological condition of the IOP when it decreases to values below 6-7 mmHg. IOP values below 4 mmHg usually cause progressive damage to the eye [23]. Ocular hypotony can be caused by a damage to ciliary body from trauma or inflammation. In the treatment of ocular hypotony, ibopamine can be administerd every 3 hours or 3-4 times daily, associated to corticosteroid therapy [24,25].

4. Conclusion

In conclusion, 2% ibopamine eye drops test is a useful pharmacological tool allowing us to study the pathophysiology of hydrodynamic disorders and in evaluating the outflow impairment. It is useful as a therapeutic drug in ocular hypotony secondary to filtering surgery, vitreo-retinal surgery or long-lasting uveitis. That's why its use is adviced in all the Ophthalmological Department in EU and USA.

Author details

Italo Giuffré*

Address all correspondence to: italogiuffre@libero.it

Department of Ophthalmology – Medical School – Catholic University of Roma, Italy

References

[1] Virno M., Taverniti L., Motolese E. et al. Ibopamina: nuovo midriatico non cicloplegico (nota preliminare). Boll. Ocul. 1986; 65: 11-2.

[2] Virno M., Taverniti L., De Gregorio F et al. Increase in aqueous humor production following D1 receptors activation by means of ibopamine. Int. Ophthalmol. 1997; 20: 141-6.

[3] Soldati L., Gianesello V., Galbiati I. et al. Ocular pharmacokinetics and pharmacodynamics in rabbits of ibopamine, a new mydriatic agent. Exp. Eye Res. 1993; 56: 247-54.

[4] Ugahary L.C., Ganteris E., Veckeneer M. et al. Topical ibopamine in the treatment of chronic ocular hypotony attributable to vitreoretinal surgery, uveitis, or penetrating trauma. Am. J. Ophthalmol. 2006; 141: 571-3.

[5] De Gregorio F., Pecori-Giraldi J, Pannarale L. et al. Ibopamine in glaucoma diagnostics: a new pharmacological provocative test. Int. Ophthalmol. 1997; 20: 151-5.

[6] Giuffre' I., Falsini B., Gari M.A., Balestrazzi E. Pattern-electroretinogram assessment during ibopamine test in ocular hypertension. Eur. J. Ophthalmol. 2013 Jun 24; 23 (6): 819-22.

[7] Giuffre' I., Taverniti L., Di Staso S. The effects of 2% ibopamine eye drops on the intraocular pressure and pupil motility of patients with open-angle glaucoma. Eur. J. Ophthalmol. 2004; 14; 6:508-13.

[8] Giuffre' I. Ibopamine stimulates α-adrenergic receptors and D1 dopaminergic receptors in the eye. Curr. Drug Therapy 2007, 2: 1-7.

[9] Magacho L., Costa M.L., Dessimoni A., de Avila M.P. Comparison between the 1% and 2% ibopamine provocative test in primary open-angle glaucoma patients: sensitivity, specificity and tolerability. Arq. Bras Oftalmol. 2006 Sep-Oct; 69 (5): 695-9.

[10] Ullrich K., Craig J.E., Landers J. The ibopamine challenge test can be used to differentiate glaucoma suspects from glaucoma patients. Clin. Experiment. Ophthalmol. 2013 Sep. 3.

[11] Marchini G., Babighian S., Tosi R. et al. Comparative study of the effects of 2% ibopamine, 10% phenylephrine, and 1% tropicamide on the anterior segment. Invest. Ophthalmol. Vis. Sci. 2003; 44: 281-9.

[12] Boles Carenini B., Brogliatti B., Boles Carenini A. et al. Ibopamine: a new drug and its use as provocative test for the diagnosis of glaucoma. New Trends Ophthalmol. 1992; 7: 3.

[13] Nuti A., Ciappetta R., Diadori A., Frezzotti R. Ibopamine provocative test in the diagnosis of hydrodynamic disorders. Exp. Eye Res. 1992; 55 (suppl.): S185.

[14] Virno M., Pecori-Giraldi J., Taverniti L. et al. Indagini sul meccanismo d'azione dell'aumento tensionale di ibopamina nell'iperteso oculare. Boll. Ocul. 1989; 68 (suppl. 2): 379-84.

[15] Pecori-Giraldi J., De Gregorio F., Carbone F. et al. Curva tonometrica e positivita' al test della ibopamina nella prima diagnosi di glaucoma. Boll. Ocul. 1994; 73 (suppl. 2): 319-23.

[16] Magacho L., Reis R., Pigini M.A., Avila M.P. 2% ibopamine vs. water-drinking test as a provocative test for glaucoma. Arq. Bras. Oftalmol. 2008 Jul-Aug; 71 (4): 499-503.

[17] Pigini M.A., Avila M.P., Magacho L. Effects of 2% ibopamine eye drops on the results of computerized visual field. Arq. Bras. Oftalmol. 2009 May-Jun; 72 (3): 365-9.

[18] Kniestedt C., Romppainen T., Gloor B.P., Sturmer J. Positive ibopamine provocative test in normal-tension glaucoma suspects. Klin. Monbl. Augenheilkd 2007 Apr; 224 (4): 255-9.

[19] Di Staso S., D'Andrea D., Giuffre' I. et al. Test dell'ibopamina nella sindrome da pseudoesfoliazione. Boll. Ocul. 1994; 73 (suppl. 2): 325-30.

[20] Scuderi G.L., Regine F., Perdicchi A. et al. Efficacy of 2% ibopamine on the dilation of patients with pseudoexfoliation syndrome. Eur. J. Ophthalmol. 2010 Jan-Feb; 20 (1): 120-3.

[21] Pecori-Giraldi J., Damiano A., Gabrielli A. et al. Ocular hypertension induced by ibopamine early discloses glaucoma suspects among relatives of glaucomatous patients. Boll. Ocul. 2002; 81: 91.

[22] Virno M., Sanpaolesi R., Pecori-Giraldi J. et al. Ibopamine: D1-dopaminergic agonist in the diagnosis of glaucoma. J. Glaucoma 2013; 22: 5-9.

[23] Pivetti Pezzi P., Da Dalt S., La Cava M. et al. Ibopamine treatment in chronic hypotony secondary to long-lasting uveitis. A case report. Eur. J. Ophthalmol. 2000; 10: 332-4.

[24] Ganteris-Gerritsen E., Ugahary L.C., Jansen J. et al. Six months treatment with ibopamine in patients with hypotony after vitreoretinal surgery for retinal detachment, uveitis or penetrating trauma. Retina 2012 Apr; 32 (4): 742-7.

[25] Virno M., De Gregorio F., Pannarale L., Arrico L. Topical ibopamine and corticosteroids in the treatment of post-surgery ocular hypotony. Int. Ophthalmol. 1997; 20:147-50.

9

Clinical Research Progress of Glaucomatocyclitic Crisis

He-Zheng Zhou, Wen-Shan Jiang, Han-Guang Jie, Chang Feng, Wen-Qiang Zhang, Qian Ye, Jian-Guo Wu, Yan-Ping Song and Qin Ding

1. Introduction

1.1.Definition

Glaucomatocyclitic crisis was initially described in detail by Posner and Schlossman in 1948, so it was also called Posner – Schlossman syndrome (PSS). PSS is a special form of anterior uveitis with glaucoma, mainly seen in young adults, characterized by non-granulomatousiri-docyclitis with significant elevation of intraocular pressure. In most cases, the disease takes an acute form of recurrent and monocular onset.

1.2. Morbidity

This disease is often seen in people aged from 20 to 50, and rarely in people above 60 years old. Five percent or less of PSS cases were reported in people above 60 years old [3]. The disease is rare in Western countries, it was reported that 19 in one million people have suffered from PSS in Finland [4]. As PSS is a kind of disease attacks intermittently, it is difficult to diagnose PSS in intermittent period for the lack of diagnostic signs and investigate the morbidity with epidemiology methods. We used the full text VIP Chinese literature retrieval system and Medeline retrieval system to find PSS reports from 1975 to 2011 in both English and Chinese literature and divided into review, case, experimental study and clinical report four categories, then analyzed the regional distribution of the authors and cases (Chinese reports were divided into the Yangtze river and the other, English reports were divided into Asia and the other).

The report which contained the most number of cases was chosen if there were more than two from a same author statistical results shows that 1262 cases were reported by 33 Chinese clinical reports in which 991 cases were reported by 20 reports from the area near the Yangtze river, and 271 cases were reported by 13 reports from the other area. The other 211 cases were reported by 16 English clinical reports in which 144 cases were reported by 7 reports from the Asia area and 67 cases reported by 9 reports from the other area. The results above suggest that there are much more literature and cases related to PSS in the area near the Yangtze river and infer that the prevalence of PSS in that area may be higher.

Literature types	Region	Review	Case	Experimental research	Clinical report	Aggregate
Chinese	Near the Yangtze river basin	0	11	1	20	32
	Other areas	2	11	0	13	26
English	Asia	2	0	2	7	11
	Other areas	3	12	0	9	24
Aggregate		7	34	3	49	93(total)

Table 1. The regional distribution of the authors

1.3. Possible etiology

1. Many factors were considered to be related to the onset of PSS, such as allergy, fatigue, mental fatigue, mental stress, decreased body resistance, infection, hypothalamic disorders, autonomic dysfunction, abnormal reactions of ciliary vascular and nervous system and abnormal development in angle of anterior chamber.[1]
2. Recent research had confirmed that concentration of prostaglandins (PGs) in the anterior chamber aqueous increased obviously in the PSS cases, especially that of PGE. [5]
3. Infection by herpes virus.

The conclusion that PSS was caused by herpes simplex virus (HKS) was reported by Yainamotos in 1995, and was confirmed by many following researches. A recent report showed that antiviral treatment reduced the frequency of the outbreak of the disease. [6-7]

It was reported that aqueous humor of a binocular PSS case was collected after suffering from herpes viral keratitis for five months with anterior chamber paracentesis, then DNA of cytomegalovirus (CMV) and HKS were measured by means of quantitative polymerase chain reaction(PCR), the results showed CMV was positive but HKS was negative. It was speculated that CMV which belongs to herpes virus genera would also lead to PSS. It was considered that PSS is not a separate disease, but a kind of anterior uveitis relating to infections of herpes virus.

A study from Singapore showed that the CMV DNA of aqueous humor was positive for 24 of 104 anterior uveitis cases with monocular high IOP, in which 18 cases were PSS, 5 cases were Fuchs heterochromic iridocyclitis (FHI). [8]Another study showed CMV DNA was positive in 35 of 67 PSS cases (52.2%) and in 15 of 35 FHI cases (41.7%). Although the keratic precipitates (KP) in CMV DNA positive anterior uveitis cases was consider to be accompanied with an endothelial halo, clinical difference was not so significant between CMV DNA positive and negative cases as less aqueous humor in sample and weak sensitivity of detection method. In 2008, aqueous analysis for CMV by PCR was performed in 103 eyes of 102 patients with presumed PSS or FHI at the Singapore National Eye Centre. Their records were reviewed for clinical features and human immunodeficiency virus (HIV) status of the CMV-positive patients. The main parameters were age, gender, maximum intraocular pressure, endothelial cell count, endothelial changes, PCR results, and presence of uveitic cataract and/or glaucoma. It was found that there was no clinically detectable differences between CMV-positive and negative presumed PSS eyes. CMV-positive presumed FHI patients are more likely to be male, older at diagnosis or have nodular endothelial lesions. [9]

4. Helicobacter pylori infection.

It was reported in South Korean that there was a significant difference of the positive rate of helicobacter pylori serum antibody between cases with PSS (80%) and cases without PSS (56.2%). In another prospective study, 40 cases with PSS and 73 cases without PSS received serologic analysis for the presence of H. pylori infection by an enzyme-linked immunosorbent assay. The positive rate of serum anti-H. pylori IgG was compared between the two groups. It was proved that H. pylori infection occurred significantly more often in PSS patients. This study suggests that exposure to H. pylori infection is associated with PSS in Korea. [10]

1.4. Clinical features of typical cases [1, 2, 3, 11, 12, 13]

1. In most cases, the disease always attacks the identical eye repeatedly, binocularly affected cases is not common; PSS results in paroxysmal increase of IOP repeatedly, which reaches as high as 40 to 60 mmHg, and lasts for 1 to 14 days generally, 1 month occasionally, 2 months rarely; interval of onset is from months to 2 years;
2. Symptoms are not obvious, just mild discomfort for most cases;
3. Eyesight is normal generally, blurred vision when suffers from corneal edema at onset;
4. Pupil becomes slightly bigger with normal reaction to light, and never adheres to lens;
5. The KP of PSS appeared in a few days after or before the elevation of IOP with number of 1 to 25, took a form of hoar and suet-shaped and disappeared days to 1 month after the IOP returned normal, distributed mainly in the inferior part of the cornea or concealed in the trabecular meshwork. There were no or at most a few planktonic cells in aqueous while the flare was negative.There is no inflammatory cell in vitreous body (See Figure 1);
6. The anterior chamber angle is open, no matter IOP is normal or elevated; visual field and fundus of most cases are normal generally, but a reversible expanding of vascular shadow may occur during an acute onset.
7. Coefficient of outflow facility (C value) descends in episodes and recovers in intermission; various stimulation tests for glaucoma are negative in intermission;
8. The forms of onset of PSS could be divided into three kinds: KP, high IOP and intermediate type, according to relationship between KP and IOP.

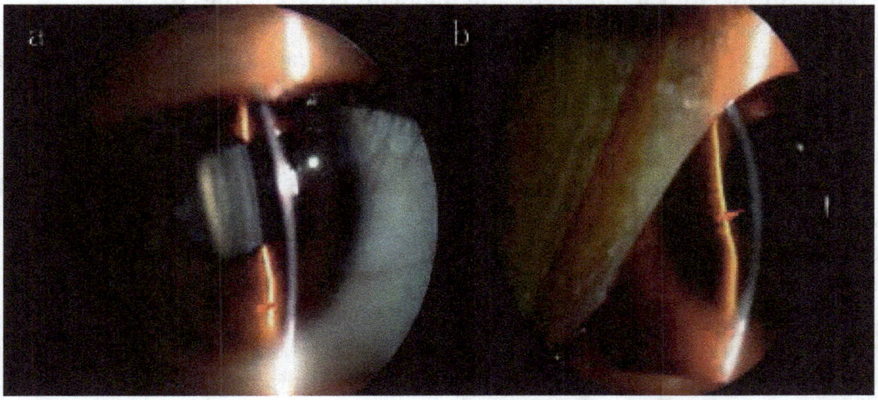

Figure 1. Anterior segment of a case with PSS in episodes. Arrows indicate the typital hoar and suet-shaped KP.

Typical case

A patient complained of her blurred vision two months ago, examination in other hospital showed: conjunctiva of her left eye wasn't congestive and the cornea was edematous mildly, IOP: 34/ 18(R/L) mmHg; there were some round lipid-like KP in the left cornea, aqueous flare(-). She came to our hospital on June 7, 2012, ophthalmologic examination: vision was 0.5/ 1.5(R/L), best corrected vision of left eye was 1.2(-1.25DS), IOP: 18/ 13 (R/L) mmHg. Her right eye was normal, conjunctiva of her left eye wasn't congestive and there were five rounds lipid-like KP in the left cornea, binocular C/D was 0.4. Her KP faded away after the treatment of chloromethyl and pranopulin (three times a day) for three weeks. Examination of FFA, ICGA and Virus screening were normal on July 10.The measurement of her 24 hours IOP performed two weeks after she ceased the drugs was 20-14mmHg(R), 15-12 mmHg (L). The result of her visual field and the OCT for glaucoma was normal. She was diagnosed as PSS in left eye and suggested to be observed and treated timely.

1.5. Treatment of typical cases in episodes

1. Anti-inflammation: Corticosteroid drugs is needed in most cases, but it should not be used too long at a time, so as not to cause the corticosteroid glaucoma.

2. It is a better select in some cases to apply non-steroidal anti-inflammatory drugs (NSAIDs) such as eye drops of pranoprofen, indomethacin and flufenamic acid.

3. Reducing IOP: Eye drops of epinephrine, timolol, or clonidine was needed singly or jointly for common patient, carbonic anhydrase inhibitor orally when the IOP is higher than 30mmHg and mannitol of intravenous drip when the IOP is higher than 40mmHg.

4. The antiviral treatment systemically or implanting long-acting agents may be helpful to reduce the frequency of attack, but it has worrying and serious side effects and costs too much. [12]

1.6. The outstanding clinical questions and the main points of the chapter

It was considered in the early years that PSS have a favorable prognosis without glaucomatous damage of optic disk and visual field, however, a number of authors have confirmed that part of the PSS cases suffered from glaucomatous damage similar to that in primary glaucoma patients in recent years. A lot of questions remained vague such as monocular or binocular explode, age of onset, the detailed features of its IOP and KP, the incidence and degree and relating factors of glaucomatous damage, especially the clinical approaches via which the damage occurred and disease complicated with PSS. These brought about to two undesirable consequences: on the one hand, PSS patients were misdiagnosed as primary glaucoma and received incorrect treatment even led to serious adverse consequences due to the lack of knowledge on the clinical characteristics of PSS; on the other hand, most cases of PSS combined with primary glaucoma especially those with primary angle-closed glaucoma were failed to be diagnosed correctly without delay, thus the best opportunity of treatment was lost ; severe damage occurred.

In recent decades, although there were some clinical observations reported by a number of authors on these clinical problems mentioned above, no report of continuous and systematic study was found. A mountain of work in this field had been done in our hospital and some research results were obtained. A brief introduction of our results will be shown in this chapter in combination with the research achievements of other authors.

2. The main results of our clinical research

The main results of our clinical research included 4 fields as follows: the clinical characteristics of PSS; the glaucomatous optic nerve damage in PSS patients; the clinical approach of optic nerve damage in PSS patients; other diseases concomitant with PSS.

2.1. Study on the clinical characteristics of the PSS

The research about clinical characteristics of the PSS included four aspects: clinical observation and analysis of monocular primary open-angle glaucoma(POAG) and binocular PSS; clinical features of elderly PSS patients; characteristics and clinical value of the intraocular pressure and the C-value in PSS patients ; the characteristic of postural intraocular pressure change in PSS patients.

2.1.1. Clinical observation and analysis of monocular primary open-angle glaucoma and binocular PSS

Background: As we knew, most of POAG patients are binocularly involved, while monocular attack is one of typical features of PSS. However, clinically suspected monocular POAG patients are not rare and binocular PSS cases are often reported. So following questions should be put forward based on the facts as follows [3, 11, 14]: Does monocular POAG really exist? What are the differences between monocular and binocularly involved PSS cases? Is there any relationship between the monocular POAG and binocular PSS?

Objects and methods: A long-term, systematic clinical observation and analysis were completed on 121 cases with tentative diagnosis of POAG (22 cases of monocular) and 126 cases of PSS (17 cases of which was binocular). (See figure2)

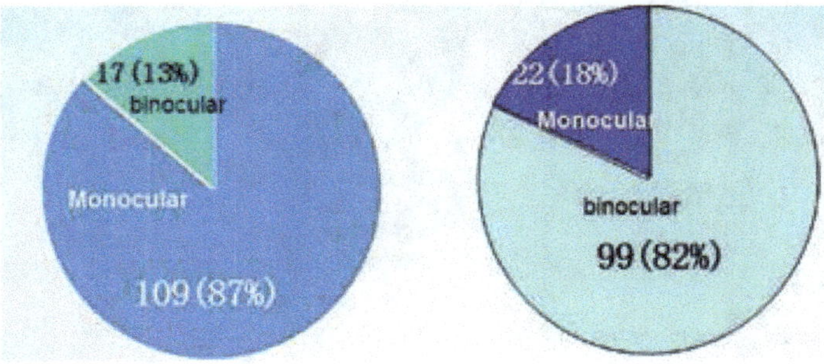

Figure 2. Distribution of monocular and binocular cases in PSS and POAG

Results

1. Glaucomatous visual field damage of monocular/ binocular PSS and binocular POAG

analysis of the clinical data of patients without doubt with the chi-square test showed: (1) The incidence of glaucomatous visual field damage in binocular PSS (15/16) was much higher than that in monocular cases(30/85), (X^2=27.43, P<0.01). (2) The damage in 26 of 30 monocular cases were in early stage, while that in 9 of 15 binocular cases were in middle/ last stage, the difference was significant(X^2=3.53, P<0.01). (3) There is no significant difference in incidence and degree of glaucomatous visual field damage between binocular PSS and binocular POAG.(See Table 2)

2. Visual field damage in binocular PSS

15 of 17 binocular PSS cases were confirmed with glaucomatous visual field damage, that was much more serious than in monocular cases; however, no remarkable difference was found between the course of disease in monocular and binocular cases. (See Figure3)

The result suggests that the course of disease cannot explain the severity of visual field damage in binocular PSS. We speculate that binocular PSS may be more relevant to POAG essentially through the following two ways. First, the insufficiency in adjusting IOP results in combination with POAG in some cases; secondly, the weak resistance of optic nerve to high IOP make it easy for a cumulative effect of high intraocular pressure during attacks of pure PSS to bring about visual field damage.

2. Results of clinical follow-up to monocular POAG

The results of clinical follow-up observation on the 22 cases with clinically suspected monocular POAG are as follows: 15 of the 22 cases were confirmed not to be POAG, 9 of them had been proved to be PSS. Although no definite diagnoses were made in the other 7 cases, but

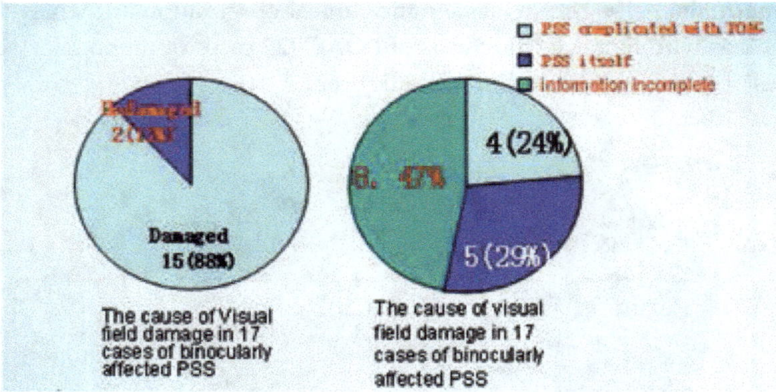

Figure 3. Results of visual field examination and defect in binocular PSS.

clinical manifestations contradictory with POAG were found in most cases, 3 of them were suspected of PSS.(See Figure4)

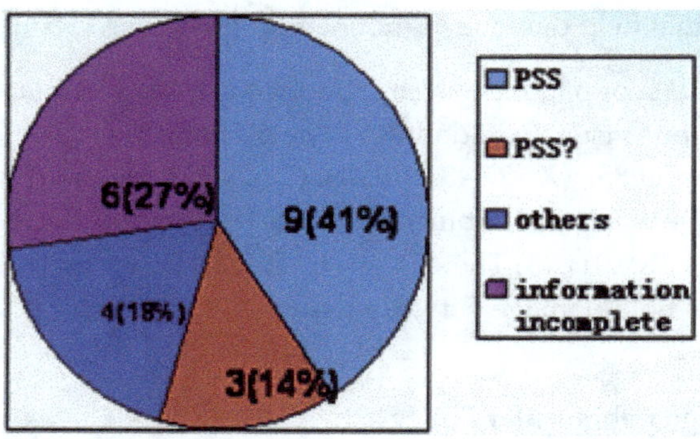

Figure 4. Results of clinical follow-up to monocular POAG.

The result suggests that the diagnosis of monocular POAG should be very careful, in addition to angle closure glaucoma and other secondary glaucoma, PSS which appears late or last transitorily should not be ignored. Close attention to slit lamp examination for KP and its relationship with IOP should be paid for such cases.

All in all, it cannot be stated too strongly: we should be very deliberative when making a diagnosis of monocular POAG or binocular PSS, as half part of suspicious monocular POAG cases were confirmed with PSS after clinical follow-up, and there was a closer connection between binocular PSS and POAG. [15]

2.1.2. Clinical observation of aged PSS cases

Background: Among the cases of PSS, the 50s are rare; the 60s are seldom. What is the feature of the aged PSS cases?

Objects and methods: The clinical data of 14 cases aged above 50 with a definite diagnosis of PSS collected in the past 4 years were summarized and analyzed. Clinical data met all the requirements were obtained in 11cases. The cases aged from 50 to 73 years old, with an average of 61.4 years. One case had a course of the disease beyond 30 years, 4 beyond 10 years and 6 beyond 5 years.

Results: Visual acuity of more than half of the cases was inferior to 0.5, 9 of 11 cases had visual field damage that was of moderate or advanced stage in most cases.

Conclusion: The aged PSS cases had a longer course of the disease and much more frequent and serious visual function damage. [16, 17, 18]

2.1.3. The characteristics and clinical value of the intraocular pressure and the C-value in PSS cases

Background: It is generally acknowledged that IOP of the attacked eye increased and C-value of attack eye decreased in episodes, and both were normal in intermission. Individual author reported that the IOP of the affected eye was lower than that of the fellow one in part of cases, and C-value was higher. It was not confirmed that whether this phenomenon could be considered as the unique characteristic of PSS and what clinical significance should it mean. [3, 19, 20]

Objective and methods: Binocular IOP measurement and tonography were done in 90 cases of PSS; According to the symptom, sign and results of examination for IOP, fundus, visual field, our cases were divided into 3 groups. Group A (typical type): with a normal optic disc, visual field and the diagnostic tests for glaucoma in intermission. Group B (development type): with a damaged optic disc and visual field; except for high intraocular pressure in episodes, binocular IOP and C values were normal. Group C (mixed type): with a damaged optic disc, visual field and abnormal results of binocular IOP, IOP diurnal variation and C value in both episodes and intermission. Another group case of primary glaucoma with a great fluctuation and difference in IOP level between his or her right and left eye was taken as the control group.

Results: IOP of PSS cases in group A and B increased in episodes, and were obviously higher than that of the fellow eye; C-value of them decreased and was lower. In intermission, binocular IOP and C-value turned normal, moreover, IOP of attacked eye was lower than that of the fellow one, and its C-value was higher. It means that binocular IOP and C-value in episodes and intermission were crossed-over.

Crossed-over phenomenon of binocular IOP and C-value had not appeared in the control group (primary glaucoma) as well as Group C (PSS combined with POAG).

Conclusion: Such an inference could be deduced based on our results that Crossed-over phenomenon of IOP and C-value was one characteristic for pure PSS cases, it is conducive to distinguish pure PSS from primary glaucoma and PSS combined with POAG to observe this phenomenon.

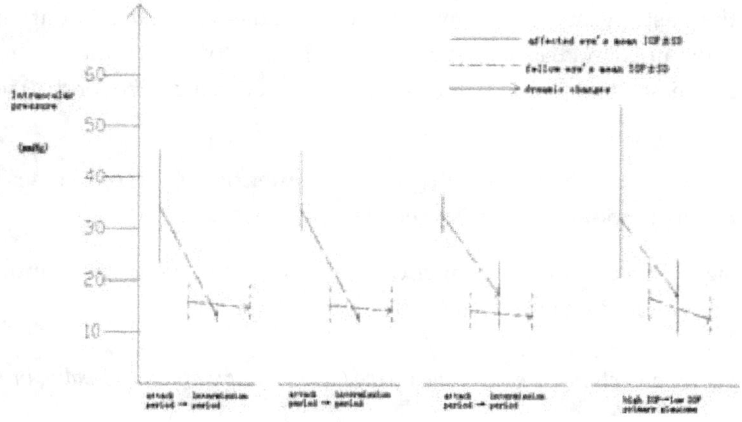

Figure 5. The difference of C-value and its dynamic changes between 3 PSS groups (A, B, C) and primary glaucoma

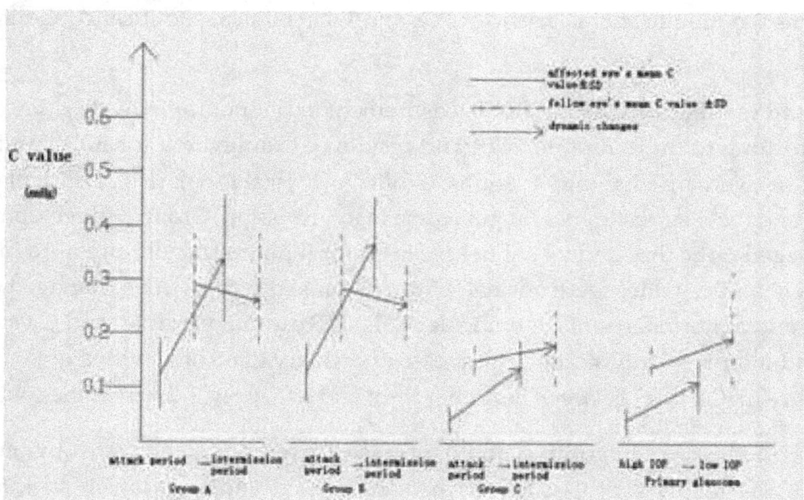

Figure 6. The difference of IOP and its dynamic changes between 3 PSS groups (A, B, C) and primary glaucoma

2.1.4. The characteristics of postural IOP change in PSS cases

Background: It is well known that the recumbent IOP is higher than sedentary one in most of people; however, such an IOP change in PSS cases was not reported so far.

Objective: The cases of PSS with regular IOP change, 42 cases of POAG and 61 cases of PACG with a great wave in IOP level. [21]

Methods: IOP measurement was performed with a handheld applanation tonometer before and after lying for five and thirty minutes, and a tonography was finished 1~3 days before or after postural IOP measurement. (See Figure7)

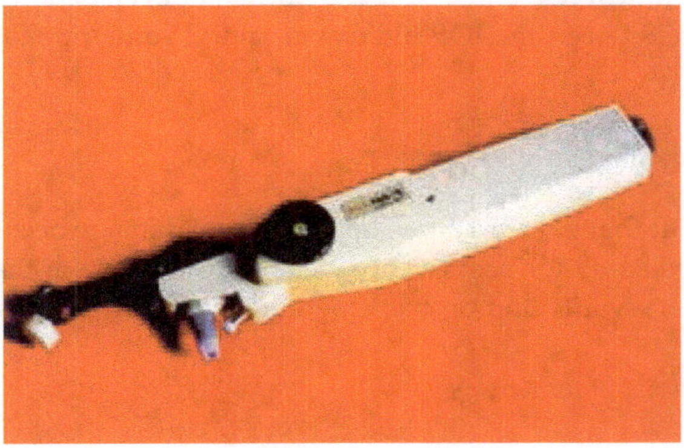

Figure 7. Handheld applanation tonometer.

Results: 1) Recumbent IOP is much higher than sedentary one in cases of all groups, however, their rising degrees after lying were different.2) There was no significant difference in rising degrees after lying in three kinds of glaucoma when IOP was high; when the IOP turned normal, however, the rising degrees in POAG, PACG were much higher than in PSS. 3) When the sedentary IOP is higher than 24mmHg, the number of cases with recumbent IOP elevated more than 5mmHg in three kinds glaucoma wasn't different statistically; When the sedentary IOP is lower than 24mmHg, cases with recumbent IOP elevated more than 5mmHg were rare in PSS group, much less than that in the other two groups. 4) The IOP increment after lying in the attacked eye of PSS cases in episodes was much higher than that of the fellow eye and the both eye in intermission. 5) The IOP increment was related to C value significantly for POAG when IOP was high and normal, for PACG when IOP was normal only; but wasn't related for PSS no matter IOP was high or normal.

Conclusion: Measurement of postural IOP change is beneficial to diagnose suspicious glaucoma cases with a normal or slightly elevated IOP, it may be as valuable as tonography clinically but more convenient, comfort and safer than tonography, complications such as corneal scratches were rarely seen in the measurement of postural IOP change

Discussion: Different pathogenesis of the three kinds of glaucoma brought about the different pattern in correlation between the IOP increment and C value in different conditions. PACG is caused by the closed anterior chamber angle, when the IOP is high, the increased IOP is related to C value significantly as the closed anterior chamber angle loses the ability to reduce IOP, however, the adjustability recovery as the anterior chamber angle open partly when the IOP is low. Degeneration of trabecular meshwork which result in more and more futile eduction function of aqueous humour was the primary mechanism for the increased IOP in POAG, so the IOP increment in POAG cases is related to C value significantly whenever the

IOP is high or low as the adjustability for IOP had been declining eventually. PSS is a secondary glaucoma for which the intermittent increased release of PGs maybe the primary mechanism. Increases PGs may expand the blood vessels and recedes eduction function of trabecular meshwork. On the contrary, the diluent PGs in remission promotes eduction function of aqueous humour and inturn IOP and C value to normal or even better. Therefore, there is no significant correlation between the IOP increment and C value no matter IOP was high or normal. [20, 22, 23]

2.2. The visual field damage in PSS cases

Although reports about that glaucomatous optical neural damage occurred in some cases of PSS were constantly released for past twenty years, we saw little of the systematic research aimed at the incidence, severity and probable relating facts of the damage. [3, 9]

2.2.1. Incidence and severity of the damage

Objective: To study the incidence and severity of the visual field damage in PSS cases.

Methods: Visual field examinations at regular intervals with perimeter of Goldmann or Humphrey 750 type were completed in 145 cases of PSS followed up for 5 to 15 years and 166 cases of POAG observed meanwhile (as the control). [17]

Results: The prevalence of visual field damage in PSS and POAG was 35.43% and 93.42% (P<0.001), 72.11% of the field damage in PSS cases was of early or suspected stage, 78.92% of that in POAG cases was of middle or late stage(P<0.001), 10% of PSS cases suffered a field damage of middle or late stage, 2 became absolute blind and one case had developed into bullous keratitis at last.(See Figure8)

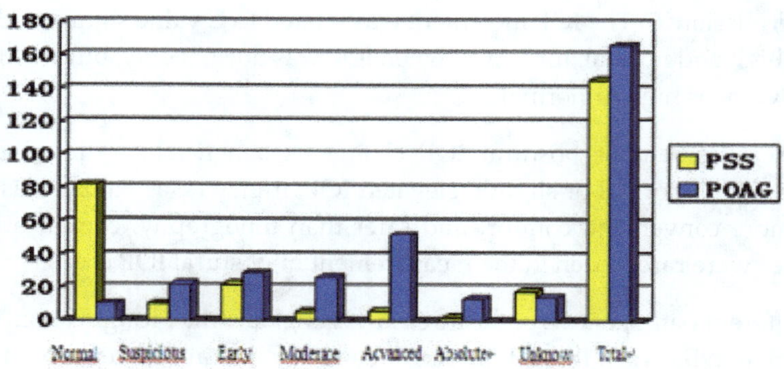

Figure 8. The stage distribution of visual field damage in PSS and POAG.

Conclusions: Even though the visual field damage in cases of PSS was less and slighter than that in cases of POAG, it is necessary to treat PSS efficiently and timely, as recurrent attacks of PSS for long period would result in a sad outcome like POAG.

2.2.2. *The characteristic of the visual field damage in PSS*

Objective: To study the characteristic of the visual field damage in PSS.

Methods: Compare the visual field damage in glaucoma cases with higher and lower IOP (PSS belongs to that with higher IOP). [24]

Results: 1) The visual field damage in cases with lower IOP is less and slighter than that in cases with higher IOP. 2) Paracentral, arcuate and ring scotoma was more seen in cases with normal IOP, while constriction of visual field and nasal field were more common in cases with higher IOP. 3) Most of the visual field damages in cases with higher IOP come from the periphery. (See Figure 9)

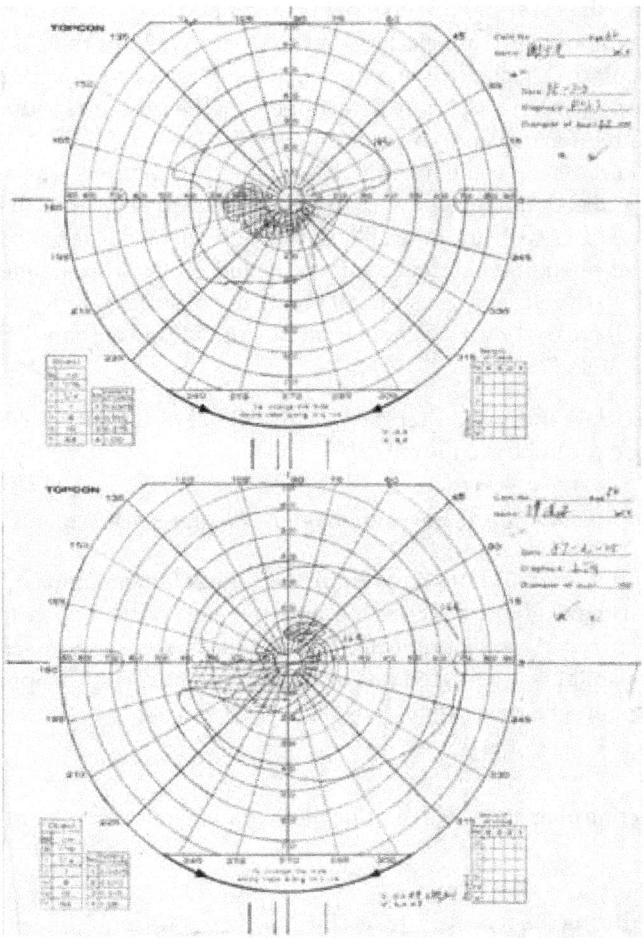

Figure 9. Visual field of a PSS case and a LTG case. The visual field damages in PSS case exist in the periphery area(A), on the contrary, those in glaucoma case with normal IOP exist in the centre area(B).

Conclusions: There are difference in visual field defects between higher IOP patients and lower IOP patients.

2.2.3. *Relating factors of the visual field damage in PSS*

Objective: To study the relating factors of the visual field damage in PSS.

Methods: Analysis the clinical data of 145 PSS cases and 166 POAG cases for recent 15 years.Results about the incidence and severity of visual field damage in the two kinds of glaucoma had been showed above.

Results: 1) Compared with the undamaged group of PSS, the damaged cases were older and with longer course of the disease while there was no remarkable difference in the averaged IOP value during crisis. 2) There was a much higher risk for the visual field damage in binocular cases of PSS. Most of the cases of PSS reported were monocular affected, but later, there were reports about some binocularly affected cases. In our study, 15 of the 35 cases with definite damage were binocularly affected while only one of the 82 cases without damage was affected binocularly. It needs further study to determine whether there is different pathological mechanism for the monocular and binocularly involved cases of PSS. 3) IOP manifestation: although no great difference in the average IOP value during crisis was found between the two groups of PSS, the damage group showed a higher average IOP between crises and included much more cases with an abnormal diurnal and nocturnal variance of IOP or without the IOP crossed-over phenomenon than the undamaged group. These data indicated that the adjustment of IOP between crises was insufficient in those PSS patients with visual field damage. Loss of IOP crossed-over phenomenon meant that other than PSS there were some factors affecting the IOP. [25]

Conclusions: These data indicated that the harmful effect of the raised IOP during crises of PSS on the optic disc could be accumulated.

2.3. The clinical approach of optic nerve damage in Posner Schlossman syndrome

In recent years a number of authors have confirmed that glaucomatous optic nerve damage similar to that in primary glaucoma cases occurred in part of the PSS cases, but the clinical approach of the occurrence was not reported. Clinical data of cases with PSS during a period of 25 years in our hospital was collected and analyzed, and four clinical approaches via which the damage occurred in PSS cases were deduced.

Propose

To investigate the clinical approaches of optic nerve damage in PSS patients.

Methods

208 cases with PSS during the recent 25 years collected in our hospital(male 124 cases, female84 cases), from 9 to 71 years old, with an average of 39.56±12.80. Diagnosis standard for PSS was basically accorded to clinical features described by Posner and Schlossman, except for the cases who suffered binocularly or had damage were contained in. [23, 26]

Research project of first diagnosis at the first attendance in our hospital

History, eyesight, intraocular pressure of episode and intermission, depth of anterior chamber, gonioscope or UBM, intraocular pressure during 24 hours in intermission without eyedrops more than five days, panretinal scope or OCT, FFA in episode of part cases, and so on.

Analytical methods

1. Analysis for damage

Standard: repeatable glaucomatous visual field damage and corresponding fundus performance

2. Stage division standard of glaucomatous visual field damage(see Table2)

Without defect	static visual field: no more than 2 clusters of spots with sensitivity reduces more than 5dB, no spot with sensitivity reduces more than 5dB; dynamic visual field: no nasal step and temporal quadrantanopsia more than 10 degrees, no significantly constriction of visual field (except for refractive interstitial lesions and retinopathy)
Early stage	paracentral scotoma, nasal step, temporal quadrantanopsia, arcuate scotoma not linked with physiological blind spot
Moderate stage	arcuate scotoma linked with physiological blind spot, nasal hemianopsia,ring scotoma, constriction of visual field more than 30 degrees,
Advanced stage	tubular visual field
Absolute stage	no light perception

Table 2. Staging standard of glaucomatous visual field defect

3. Classification method

According to the results of comprehensive and dynamical analysis of the clinical data of each cases and classification method as shown in table 3, each case was discriminated for the clinical approach of optic nerve damage. [20,21,22,24,27,28]

	A		B		C		D	
	Early stage	**Later stage**	**Early stage**	**later stage**	**Early stage**	**later stage**	**Early stage**	**later stage**
Age of onset	middle-aged and aged people		middle-aged and aged people		most middle-aged and aged people		middle-aged and aged people	
Family history of glaucoma	usually not		usually not		sometimes have		most have	
Monocular/ binoculus	monocular		monocular		moncocular KP, binocular high IOP or eyes alternate		monocular KP,binocular high IOP	
Typical PSS course	positive	positive	positive	negative	Intermittent attack with binocular high IOP		positive	negative

		A		B		C		D	
		Early stage	Later stage	Early stage	later stage	Early stage	later stage	Early stage	later stage
IOP	Episodes: Sick eye	rise	rise	rise	rise	higher	higher	rise	rise
	Episodes: another eye	normal	normal	normal	normal	high	high	high*/normal	high*/normal
	Intermission: Sick eye	normal	normal	normal	rise	high	high	high*/normal	high*/normal
	Intermission: another eye	normal	normal	normal	normal	high	high	high*/normal	high*/normal
	Cross phenomenon of IOP	positive		positive	negative	negative	negative	positive */ negative	positive */ negative
	IOP of 24 hours in period of intermittent	normal	normal	normal	abnormal	abnormal	abnormal	abnormal */ normal	abnormal */ normal
Anterior chamber depth		normal	normal	normal	normal	normal	normal	A little shallow	Very shallow
Anterior chamber angle		medium width	medium width	medium width	medium width	medium width	medium width	narrow II-III	narrow III-IV

Table 3. Classification method of the clinical approach for optic nerve damage in PSS

Results

1. Incidence and stage distribution of glaucomatous optic nerve damage

190 cases of 208 patients with PSS had a set of complete material. There were 71 cases (34.1%) with optic nerve damage, in which 12 cases (16.9%) regarded as suspicious damage, 59 cases(83.1%) regarded as definite damage.

Stage distribution of glaucomatous optic nerve damage was shown in Table 4:

Early stage	Moderate stage	Advanced stage	Absolute stage	total
35	11	11	2	59
59.32%	18.64%	18.64%	3.39%	100%

Table 4. Stage of glaucomatous optic nerve damage in 59 cases regarded as clear damage

2. The clinical approach of optic nerve damage

Four clinical approaches via which the damage occurred in PSS were deduced, they were represented as Type A, B, C and D.

Type A Cumulative effect of repeated episode of high intraocular pressure of pure PSS leads to visual field damage: 27 cases

Type B Recurrent attacks of PSS which results in secondary trabecular meshwork damage causes secondary open-angle glaucoma: 6 cases

Type C PSS combined with primary open-angle glaucoma: 19 cases

Type D PSS combined with primary closed-angle glaucoma: 7 cases

Composition of the clinical approach in 59 cases regarded as definite glaucomatous optic nerve damage was showed in Figure10

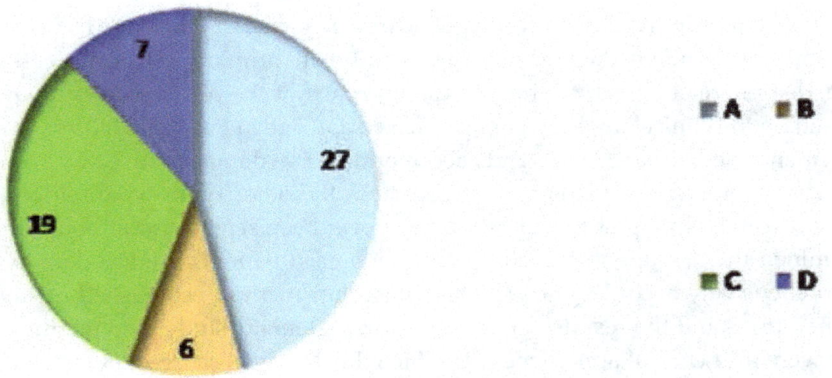

Figure 10. The distribution of clinical approach of optic nerve damage in PSS.

Distribution of stage of visual field damage in different optic nerve damage approacheswas showed in Table 5.

	Early stage	moderate stage	advanced stage	absolute stage	total
Type A	17	7	1	2	27
Type B	2	2	2	0	6
Type C	5	7	7	0	19
Type D	2	3	2	0	7

Table 5. Visual field damage in different type of PSS patients

There is no significant difference in the stage distribution of visual field damage in different type of PSS patients. (X^2=6.904, P>0.05).Make the early and moderate stage as one group, advanced and absolute stage as another group, Statistical result shows that there is significant difference in the stage distribution of visual field damage in different type of PSS patients. The incidence of early stage of glaucomatous visual field damage in Type A (63%) was higher. While 7 of 19 Type C cases were in advanced stage.

Conclusion: Most cases in type A suffered an early stage damage, and most in other types suffered a moderate or advanced stage damage, but there were 2 cases in type A who had gone to absolute stage.

Discussion

1. The clinical approach of optic nerve damage in Posner-Schlossman syndrome.

In the past PSS was considered to be a self-limited disease and has a favorable prognosis, however, in recent years a number of authors have confirmed that part of the PSS cases suffered glaucomatous optic nerve damage similar to those in primary glaucoma cases, but the incidence, degree, related factors and clinical approach of the occurrence is unknown. This part focused on the clinical approach of optic nerve damage in Posner-Schlossman syndrome after aforementioned researches. Reports about optic nerve damage caused by PSS combined with primary open-angle glaucoma were common; the other types were seldom reported. Systematic research aiming at this question has never been seen so far at home and abroad. We determined the damage approach by analyzing each patient's clinical data dynamically and comprehensively according to the discrimination method established on the basis of relating literatures and the results of our long-term systematic study, and got the conclusion that there were four clinical approaches via which the damage occurred. Beyond all question, further research, supplement and correct is necessary in this field, but the method and result of our study may be a wind vane for the further researches.

2. Clinical features and treatment principle for cases with damage from different clinical approach

(1) Type A Cumulative effect of repeated episodes of high intraocular pressure of pure PSS leads to damage

Clinical features

Except for visual field damage, type A cases complied with the basic characteristics of typical PSS: monocular attacked; intermittently onset of high intraocular pressure with hoar and suet-shaped KP ; normal intraocular pressure(including 24 hours intraocular pressure) of the fellow eye in episode and the both eyes in intermission ; Crossed-over phenomenon and postural changes of IOP; normal anterior chamber depth; wide anterior chamber angle; visual field change of vascular shadow usually appears in episode and recover in intermission at the initial in most cases, and true visual field damage is of mild and early stage usually, but loss of light perception can be seen in a few cases; the attack lasts a long time frequently in middle-aged and aged people for long course, also with higher IOP; heterochromia iridis occurred in later stage in some cases. (See Figure11) [20, 22, 29]

Treatment principle

Enough attention should be paid to treatment for each attack, in which the most important is controlling intraocular pressure timely and effectively. Surgery is necessary for the cases with excessive frequent attacks, heavy damage or obvious progress of his damage.

The surgery method and the time: glaucoma valve or EX-press glaucoma filtration device implantation may be suit for cases with excessive frequent attack, high IOP but light inflammation (intermission or episodes); trabeculectomy could be selected for cases with low attack frequency, high IOP as well as severe inflammation (intermission only).

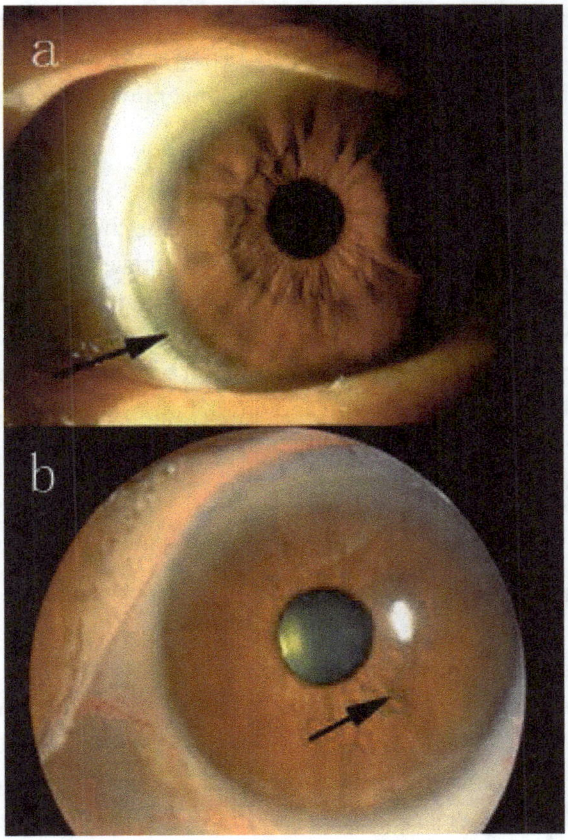

Figure 11. The iridis of a PSS patient.(A)is that of the normal eye,(B) is that of the affected eye.

Typical cases 1) A patient visited our hospital and was diagnosed as glaucomatocyclitis crisis of left eye in other hospital six years ago. In the initial stage, she attacked once or twice per year with duration of 3~7 days for each attack and ceased spontaneously, then the frequency of attack increased and the duration extended. This attack happened one month before this visits to our hospital and stop one week ago without use of any drug. Examination at first visit: Vision 1.0(OU), IOP19.7mmHg(R), 12mmHg (L), anterior chambers of both eyes were not shallow, iris color was symmetrical, KP (-).Fundus examination: C/D0.3(R) 0.6(L), there wasn't other abnormalities. She was diagnosed as secondary glaucoma of left eye. On September 13 (10 days after withdrawal), the 24 hours IOP of both eyes were measured: right eye: 14-18mmHg, left eye 12-14mmHg, Corneal thickness: right eye: 584μm, left eye: 575μm. She was diagnosed as "glaucomatocyclitis crisis in left eye." Another onset lasted for more than 10 days, IOP of the left eye was 43mmHg, there was 2hoar and suet--like KP and faded iris pigment in left eye. There were total seven attacks in one year, with the duration from 1 week to 20 days, during one of which the KP appeared 9day after the occurrence. 24 hours IOP during this episode: right

Eye: 14-19mmHg, left Eye: 23-29mmHg; iris depigmentation of her left eye exacerbated, no abnormal was found with fundus angiography. The recent onset occurred in September this year, the medication of hormone and pranopulin continued for 3 months, with another minor attack during thatthis period.

She made another visit to our hospital one year later. It was found that the iris of her left eye appeared a typical "rain dozen sand samples", meanwhile, there were two off-white round medium-sized lipid-like KP and she was diagnosed as "left eye glaucomatocyclitic crisis with heterochromatic iris." Since then, the attack occurred more frequently, with frequency of 1 to 2 times per month, the visual field damage exacerbated. She was hospitalized in our department, and the surgery of glaucoma valve implantation was performed. Postoperative intraocular pressure: 19mmHg for her right eye and 6mmHg for her left eye:, visual acuity1.0 left eye (with pin hole) for her both eye, and the syndrome did not attack postoperation. (Clinical data please see Figure 12)

Typical Case 2)

A patient was hospitalized in our hospital for the reason of "intermittent pain of left eye for 25years, decrease of vision for 20 years, blind for 1 year". The patient had a history of intermittent episodes of pain and blurred vision with his left eye for 25 years, which occurred 1 to 2 times per month with the duration of 3 to 5 days, and than self-cured. In many hospitals he was diagnosed as "glaucomatocyclitic crisis" and treated with medication irregularly The occurrence becomes more frequently in the recent 10 years, and the duration longer, and the vision recessions gradually. In the intermittent period, he was hospitalized for systematic examination. The visual acuity was 1.0 for his right eye and no light perception for his left eye. All the results of IOP, tonography, 24 hours IOP measurement and other tests during the intermittent period were normal for his both eyes. The result of the medical examination at this hospitalization showed as following: his right eye had a corrected visual acuity of 1.0, IOP 14mmHg, C/D 0.4, wide anterior chamber angle; his left eye had no light perception, intraocular pressure 56mmHg, C / D1.0, width of N1 ~ N3 for the anterior chamber angle with some small limited adhesions; corneal edema, a dozen of round lipid-like KP.

Without any treatment, the IOP of his fell to 14mmHg within one week. All results of examinations including 24 hours IOP measurement, drinking water experiment, dark room prone test for his right eye were normal. Laboratory results of systemic body check were normal.

His left eye still had attacks of PSS after he left hospital and each attack was self-limited. The IOP and 24-hour IOP during the intermittent period were measured to be normal, and his left eye had an IOP lower than that of his right eye, a typical IOP cross phenomenon appeared every time. Three years later, the fundus and visual field of his right eye kept normal. (Clinical data see Figure 13)

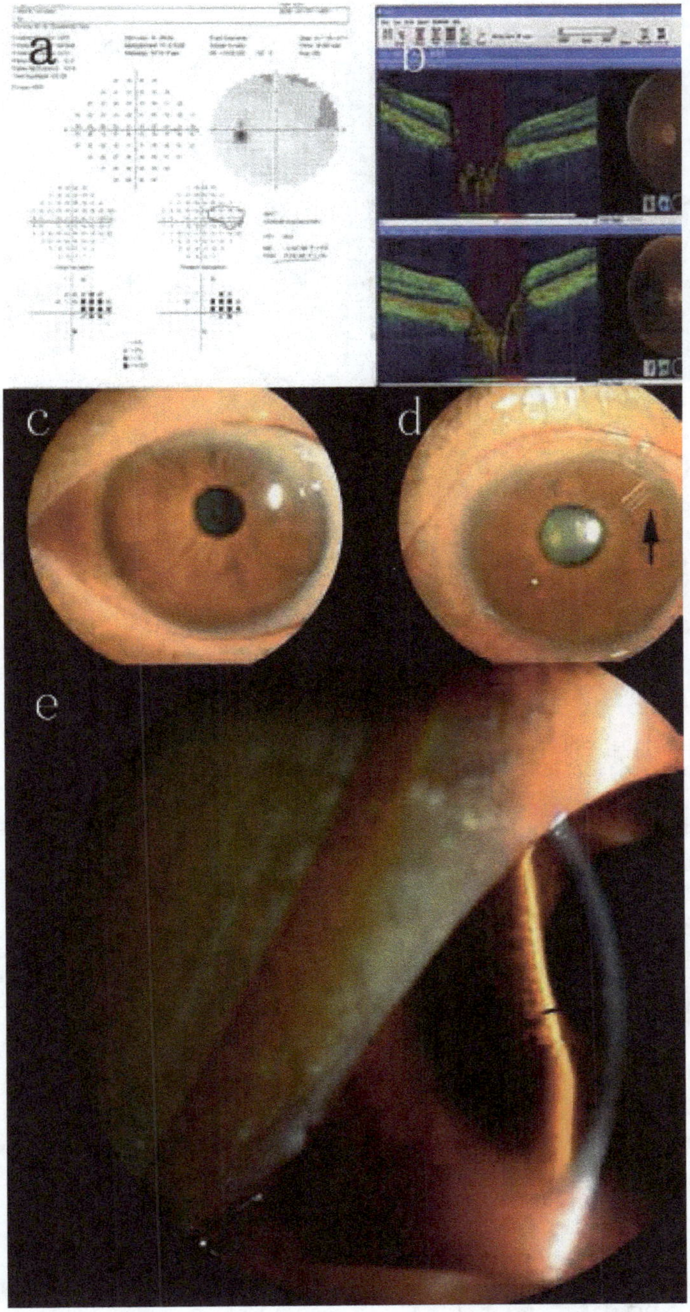

Figure 12. Clinical data of a cases suffered from PSS with glaucomatous optic nerve damage combined with heterochromia iris (Clinical number 488368).Visual field (A) and Optical Coherence Tomography (B) indicate glaucoma damages;Anterio segment of normal right eye(C) and left eye(D),arrow shows heterochmia iris and KP in the attacked eye(E).

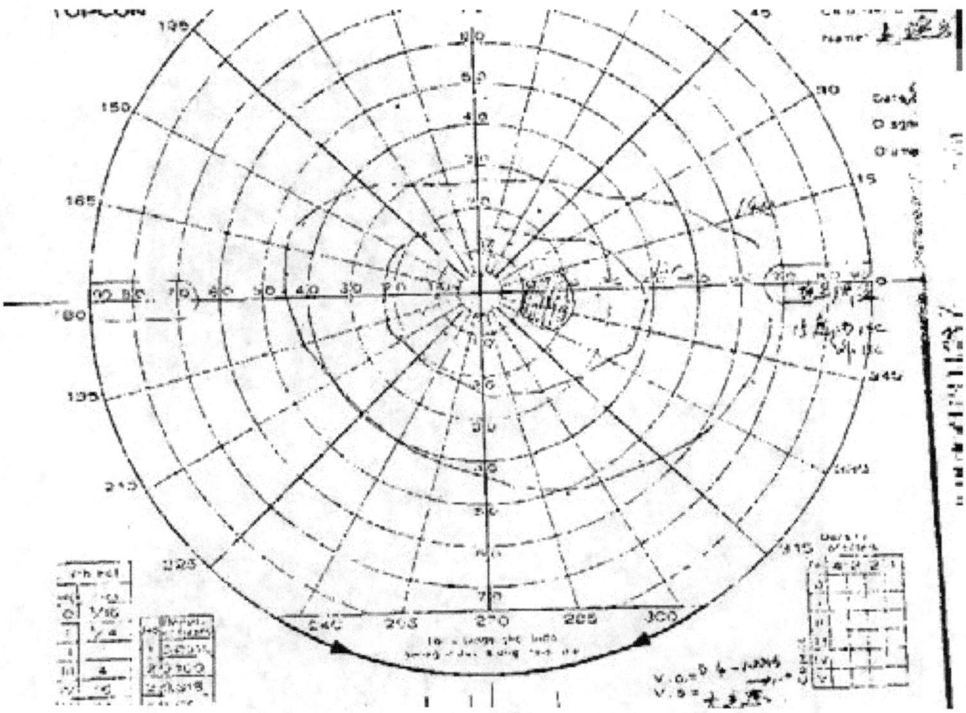

Figure 13. Visual field of the right eye of patient (Clinical number 241163).PSS results in blind of his left eye, but the visual field of his right eye without PSS is normal.

(2) Type B secondary open-angle glaucoma from secondary damage to trabecular meshwork by recurrent attacks of PSS

Clinical features

Type B cases complied with the basic characteristics (above mentioned) of typical PSS in early stage. These characteristics lost eventually as the damage to trabecular meshwork gradually accelerated, the attack takes place more frequently and lasts a longer and longer time with a higher and higher IOP, and serious visual field damage developed at last.[30, 31] However, the fundus, visual field, IOP in intermittent and episode of the fellow eye maintained normal. Patients of this type usually had a long course of the disease with an older age.

Treatment principle

It is necessary to reduce IOP with drugs according to extent and characteristics of elevated IOP and diminish inflammation with hormone of weak effect on elevating IOP for short time, for example, lotemax. PGA is useful and myotic is prohibitive. Surgery or other treatment (SLT,

trabeculectomy, glaucoma valve or EX-press implantation) should be taken into account according to the IOP level controlled by drugs in intermittent and the situation of visual field damage.

Typical case

A patient was diagnosed as "left eye PSS" with the complain of vision decline associated with distending pain of his left eye in other hospitals five years ago. The medical records of other hospitals showed: IOP and other relating examinations of the right eye in episode and these in intermittent period of his both eyes was normal at the initial stage. The visual acuity decreased gradually, IOP fluctuated from 32 to 48 mmHg in recent years. He was hospitalized in our hospital three times, the results of clinical observation showed: IOP including 24 hours IOP in intermittent period, the fundus and visual field of his right eye appeared normal; while IOP of his left eye was high frequently and higher when PSS attacked, 24 hours IOP in intermittent period appeared abnormal including the highest IOP and IOP variation. The left eye was diagnosed as secondary open-angle glaucoma from secondary damage to trabecular meshwork by recurrent attacks of PSS, and then a trabecuectomy was performed on his left eye. Postoperative IOP of his left eye was from 12 to 10mmHg in intermittent period, 20 to 31 mmHg in episodes, while his right eye kept normal in all ways. (Clinical data see Figure 14)

(3) Type C PSS combined with primary open-angle glaucoma

Clinical features

Monocular/ binocular paroxysmal increased IOP with mild cyclitis; wide anterior chamber angle; binocular abnormal IOP and visual field damage; high average IOP; great fluctuation of IOP level; absence of IOP cross phenomenon; PSS attacks at the same eye in most cases; at the two eyes alternately or at the same time in a few cases; visual field damage was serious, and more serious in the eye often attacked by PSS.[27, 32]

Treatment principle

Enough attention should be given to the treatment for cases of this type, whose incidence reached up to 31% as reported. Drug treatment is similar to that of POAG, but in episode of PSS, corticosteroid is useful transitorily, while PGA and myotic is prohibitive. Indication of surgery is similar to that of POAG, but classical trabeculectomy should be performed in intermission, and the effect and safety of non-penetrating trabeculectomy, implantation of Ahmed glaucoma valve or EX-PRESS Glaucoma Filtration Device has not been confirmed. Laser trabeculoplasty(ALT), Selective laser trabeculoplasty (SLT) or Pneumatic trabeculoplasty (PNT) should be adopted in intermission, however, there has no related report. [11, 33, 34, 35]

Typical cases

A patient reported of discomfort and blurred vision of her left eye for more than 1 year, the patient was diagnosed as POAG in other hospital 10 days ago. Clinical date of that time showed: KP (-), IOP16.3/42.7(R/L), and she was treated with Travoprost Eye Drops to her left eye and brimonidine and brinzolamide to the both eye. 1 week after treatment, her IOP turned to 36/17(R/L), the treatment had been changed to travoprost, brimonidine and brinzolamide for the both eye. The results of examination in our hospital showed as follows: visual acuity R1.0 (-1.25DS),L0.05(-3.75DS), IOP17(OU); absence of conjunctiva hyperemia; cup/disc ratios 0.8 OD and0.9OS,and inferior RNFLD(by OCT:) in the both eye; severe glaucomatous visual

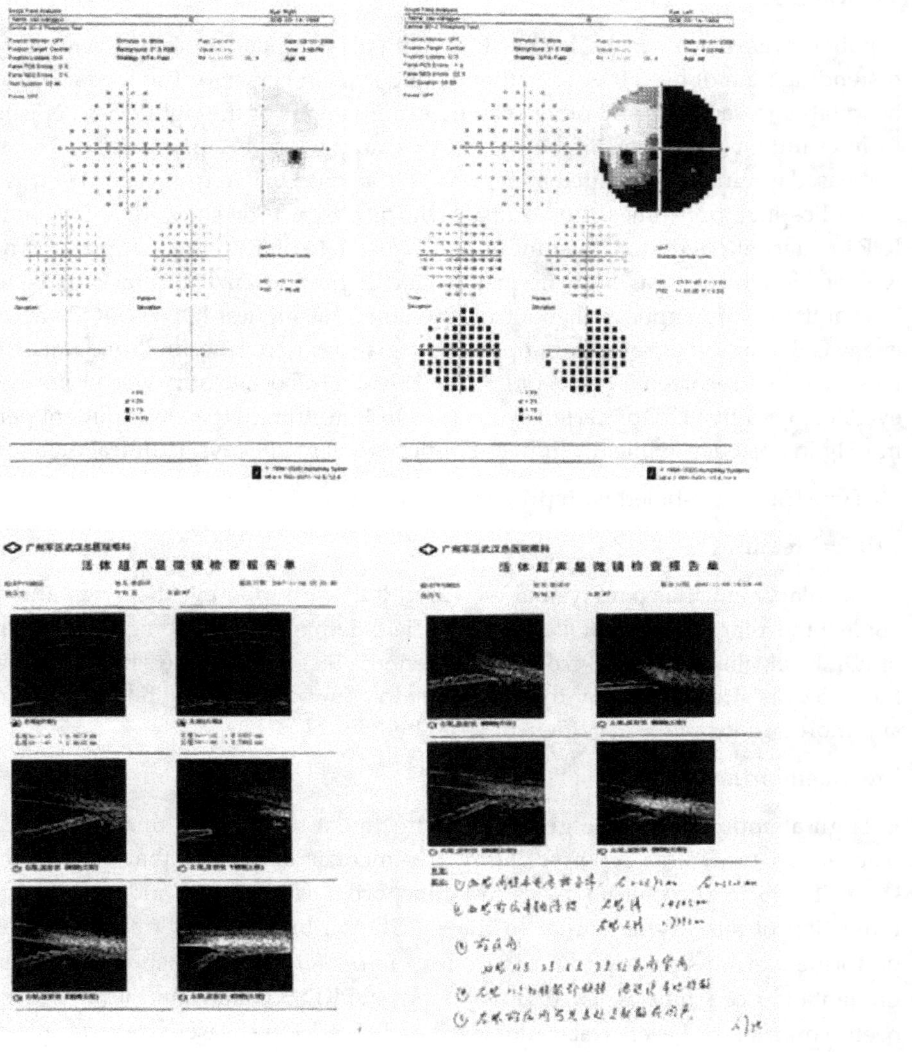

Figure 14. Clinical data of a patient suffered from PSS with glaucomatous optic nerve damange due to secondary open angle glaucoma (Clinical number 813064).Normal visual field in right eye(A) and advanced visual field defect in left eye (B);UBM shows the normol right eye and the affected left eye post-operation(C).

field damage in both eye, extended latent time and descended amplitude on VEP; CCT:540/520 (R/L),corneal endothelium cells 1730/2747(R/L); center anterior chamber depth ≥3.0mm and open anterior chamber angle in every direction for the both eye by UBM. She was diagnosed as binocular POAG, and treated successively with travatan, alphagan and brinzolamide to binoculus, but her IOP was not controlled well. Thus, a trabeculectomy was performed the left eye. Two weeksafter the operation, the filtration bubble turned fibrosed, and IOP increased. By 3 times of pin-delamination with 5-fluorouracil and eyeball massage, IOP was controlled on 12 to 14 mmHg. Her right eye was treated with travatan, carteolol hydrochloride and brimonidine, IOP wascontrolled from 12 to 14 mmHg. She was discharged from hospital. Four months later, the right eye appeared 5 small rounds and mutton-fat like KP, IOP increased to 19mmHg. A week later, KP played down, IOP descended to 12 mmHg. A month later; KP appeared again, IOP increased to 37, after treatment in hospital for a week, the IOP decreased to 12 mmHg. She was diagnosed as POAG combined with PSS. Two months later PSS of her right attacked again, IOP increased to 44 mmHg; visual field damage has progressed remarkably. FFA showed optic atrophy without any other abnormal. She was hospitalized again, and a implantation of Ahmed valve to her right eye was done on the next day. During the operation, the valve appeared out of control; we dealt it well with removable restraint line processing; the IOP and anterior chamber stability was controlled. 2 month after the operation, the IOP increased to 22 mmHg because of the draining disc was packaged. By pin-delamination and eyeball massage, IOP was controlled near to 20mmHg. Carteolol hydrochloride was added and the IOP was controlled well in intermittent, but PSS attacked frequently and the IOP was out of control during episode. She was hospitalized once more and the right eye was treated with no-penetrating glaucoma surgery. One month after surgery, the IOP was controlled well, binocular IOP was 10mmHg. 2 month after surgery, PSS attackwas seen in her right eye again, IOP increased to 20 mmHg. This attack faded a week later and IOP of her both maintained 14mmHg below until now. (Clinical data please see Figure 15)

(4) Type D PSS combined with primary closed-angle glaucoma

Research status

Except for our data, there had been only two individual reports about PSS combined with PCAG in China and none in abroad. Cases of PSS combined with PCAG at home are much more than those in abroad due to the higher incidence of PCAG as well as PSS at home. In 2004 we reported 6 cases and completed a systematic clinical analysis. It was often reminded by many ophthalmologists that cases of PSS had be mistaken as PACG, but enough attention has not been paid to this type of PSS. [18, 28, 36, 37, 38]

Clinical features

There is a typical history of PSS attack with binocular shallow anterior chamber and narrow or closed anterior chamber angle. PSS hardly attacked synchronously with PACG, the anterior chamber angle is open in episodes of PSS. Type D cases complied with the basic characteristics of typical PSS in early stage: binocular IOP is normal in intermission; with cross phenomenon of IOP; however, when PACG became more advanced, although the IOP of the PSS attacked eye was much higher than that of the unattacked eye in the episode of PSS, binocular IOP turned higher than normal even in intermission of PSS without obvious cross phenomenon. Most cases were diagnosed as PACG previously, PSS appeared after the treatment for PACG had been completed and the anterior chamber angle been opened, a few cases were typical PSS with narrow anterior chamber angle when they were young; PACG appeared as anterior chamber angle became narrower and narrower with age. Most of the cases of this type were elder with a longer course of PSS and a more advanced visual field damage.

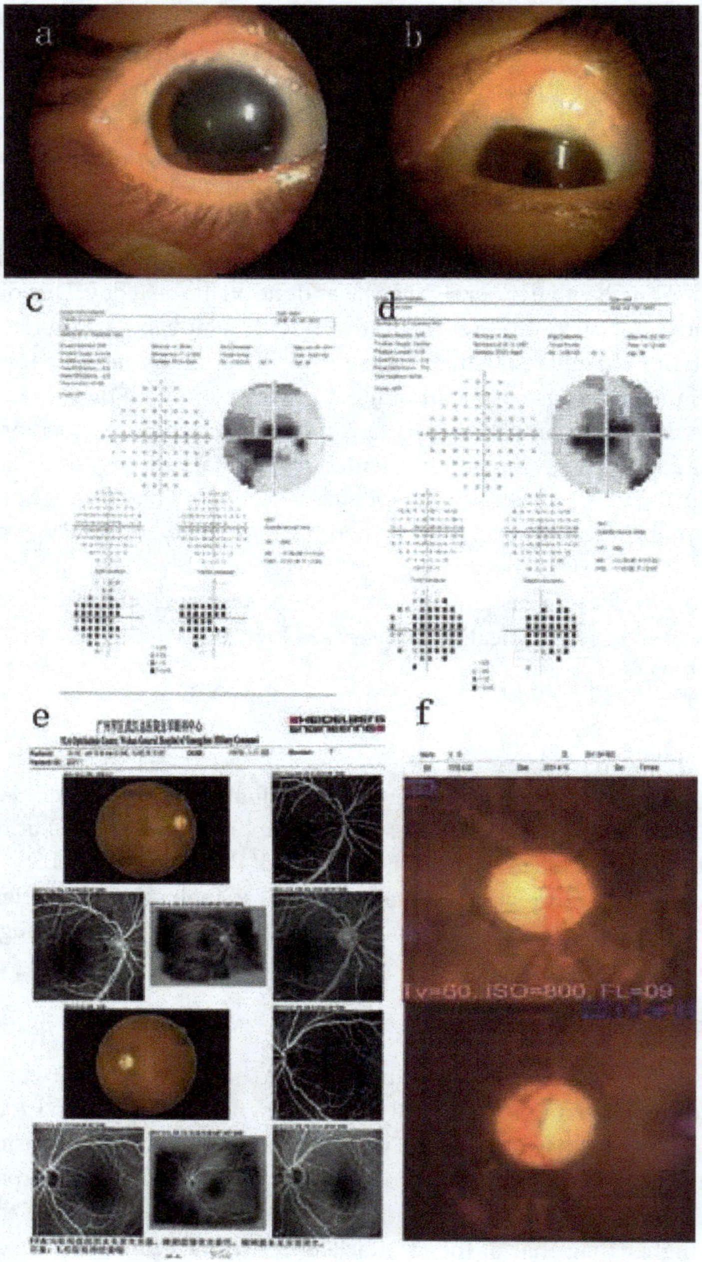

Figure 15. Clinical data of patient suffered from PSS(right eye) with glaucomatous optic nerve damange combined with POAG(both eye),the right eye is treated with Ahmed value implantation surgery(A),the left eye is treated with normal trabeculectomy(B), visual field of right eye(C) and left eye(D)show typical glaucoma damages,the fundus angiography indicates no vasular disorder except of optic atrophy(E) and the optic cups of right eye and lefr eye are non-symmetrical.

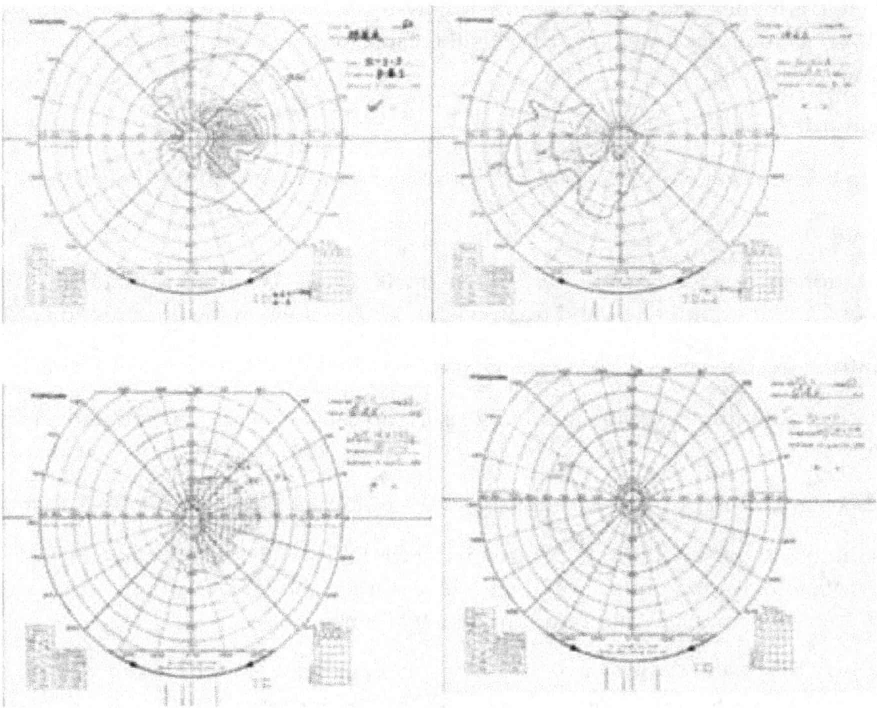

Figure 16. Visual field of patient (Clinical number 232036)with binocular PSS combined with POAG. After drug treatment,the damage of binocular visual field between 1991(A) and 1998(B) has no significant advance.

Diagnosis standard

The first is that the anterior chamber angle is open when PSS is diagnosed at episode, either in the intermission of PACG or after PACG was treated with Laser/surgery/drug; the second is that the cases complied with the basic characteristics of typical PSS described by Posner-Schlossman. In our study, 2 cases was diagnosed as PSS at a younger age with binocular narrow anterior chamber angle (first was narrow II, narrow III-IV four years later), 5 cases was diagnosed as PSS after treatment of PACG (similar to the two cases reported at home).[28, 39]

Diagnostic summary

To find out PACG complicated with PSS as soon as possible, it is necessary to carry out a set of comprehensive and careful examinations relating to PACG in the intermission of PSS for PSS patients with factors as follows: the old-aged, with a serious visual field damage, longer course of the disease, with a shallow anterior chamber or an narrow anterior chamber angle, and binocularly attacked.

When IOP appeared as repeated, intermittent and sudden elevation in a patient with PACG whose anterior chamber angle had been opened and the IOP been controlled well for a period after treatment by means of laser and/or surgery and/or drugs, it is very important to pay sufficient attention to the depth of the binocular anterior chamber and anterior chamber angle when the IOP is higher, and to make clinical follow-up observations for KP and its relationship with IOP, so as to ascertain whether PSS is the cause of elevating IOP, so that unnecessary surgery can be avoided.

Treatment principles

According to condition of PACG, laser and/or surgery and/or drugs may become options.

Laser treatment:

1. Indications of that for cases of PSS combined with PACG is similar to that PACG patients, except for that examination and treatment should be done in the intermission of PSS;
2. Curative effect on cases with typical cross phenomenon of IOP should be better;
3. The iris surrounding excision mouth by laser must be thoroughly penetrated and the hole should be big enough;
4. Corticosteroids and drugs for reducing IOP should be sufficient after laser operation;
5. It is import to pay attention to the treatment for PSS which continue to attack after laser therapy, and to the monitor of IOP and its dynamic change. Additional drug treatment even trabeculectomy should be adopted timely when necessary;[27]

It is necessary to prevent the attack of PACG in either episodes or intermission of PSS for these untreated PACG cases with the appropriate use of miosis drug.

Typical cases 1)

A patient was diagnosed as "PSS" in our hospital because of pain and discomfort of his right eye, then he was diagnosed as "acute angle-closure glaucoma " in other hospital because of severe sore of his both eyes and switched to our hospital after remission seven years later.

Examination revealed mutton-fat like KP in the right eye. His right eye was diagnosed as PSS combined with PACG with analysis by synthesis combining history and test results of IOP, fundus, visual field and anterior chamber angle. The right eye was treated with "glaucoma drainage surgery" and the left eye with "YAG laser iridectomy ".

IOP of his both appeared stable for six months after operation, then the right eye was attacked by PSS once again. This attack of PSS appeared as typical KP, open angle and slightly increased IOP. (Clinical data please see Figure 17)

Typical cases 2)

A patient came to our clinic because of “repeated intermittent attacks of eye pain and impaired vision for her left eye and right eye as well for more than 14 years”. She was treated with YAG laser iridotomy in other hospital for PACG binocularly twice each. Her left eye had been still attacked intermittently ever since. Clinical date from her medical record showed that KP and IOP rising appeared nearly simultaneously on each episode and the IOP turned persistently higher than normal even if in intermission since 2 years ago and the drugs could not control the IOP well. Examination at this time showed: Vision R 1.0, L 0.4; IOP R 14 mmHg and L 46

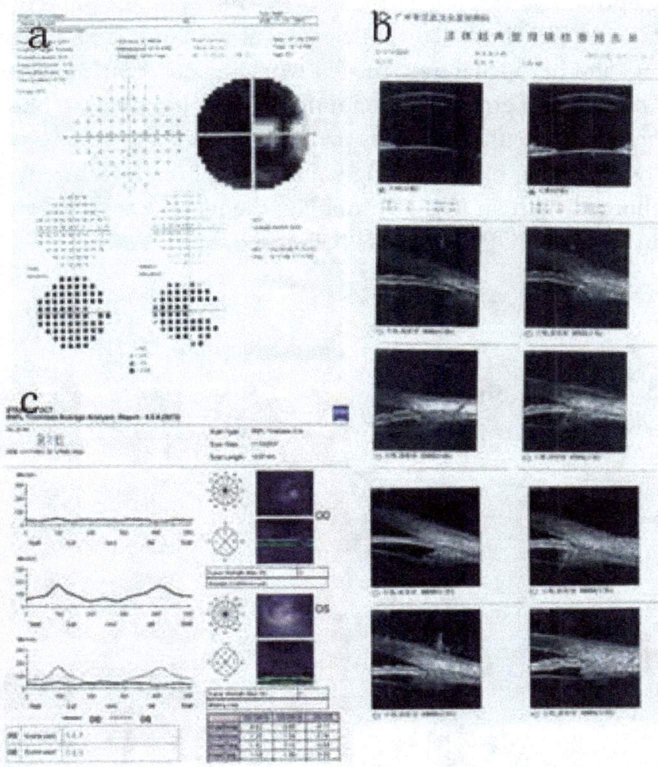

Figure 17. Typical clinical data of patient (Clinical number :406013)with diagnosis of right PSS combined with binocular PACG and treatment with classical trabeculectomy.The visual field show advanced glaucoma damange (A),OCT(C) also shows retinal nerve fiber layer defect.UBM indicate binocular closed angle(B).

mmHg; two mutton-fat like KP in the left eye ; shallow anterior chamber and angle multiple adhesions in both eyes; several trace of laser therapy on iris of her both eye, the only peetrated hole on the right eye be covered with fibrous membrane, and that on the left eye be too small; cup/disc ratios R 0.4and L 0.8.A diagnosis of "binocular PACG complicated with PSS in left eye" was established. A complementary laser therapy was given to her right eye just at that moment; after this laser therapy, her right had been kept well until now with only the help of 2% Carteolol Hydrochloride eye drops twice a day. Three weeks later, when this attack of PSS faded away, she was hospitalized in our hospital, and a trabeculectomy was performed on her left eye, and she was discharged 10 days after a IOP of 14mmHg. Six weeks after the surgery, an attack of PSS occurred with a IOP of 32mmHg and lasted a week; such attack occurred once or twice a year after that with a maximal IOP of 25mmHg. The IOP in intermission had maintained near 15mmHg during the first 4 years, but the result of 24h IOP measurement showed 13~20mmHg in the right eye and 15~24mmHg in the left eye. Iris heterochromia appeared in the left eye. Such a therapeutic schedule was established and kept 3 years since then: 2% Carteolol Hydrochloride Eye Drops twice a day to the both eye in intermission of PSS; 2% Carteolol twice a day plus brimonidine 3 times a day with shortly use of Lotemax for the left eye during episode of PSS. IOP of the both eye maintained15mmHg or below, and the visual field maintained stable in the 3 years. Several attacks of PSS had been recorded with a IOP up to 40mmHg, and her visual field turned worsen, and "rain dozen sand-like" appearance in the iris of her left eye got more pronounced in the last 2 years. She was hospitalized once more, and another trabeculectomy was performedon the left eye near the first one, at the end of which the two filtering blebs (an original and a just manufactured) were merged into one. She was discharged with an IOP of 12mmHg; the left eye was no longer attacked after this trabeculectomy, and the IOP kept stable.(Clinical data see Figure 18)

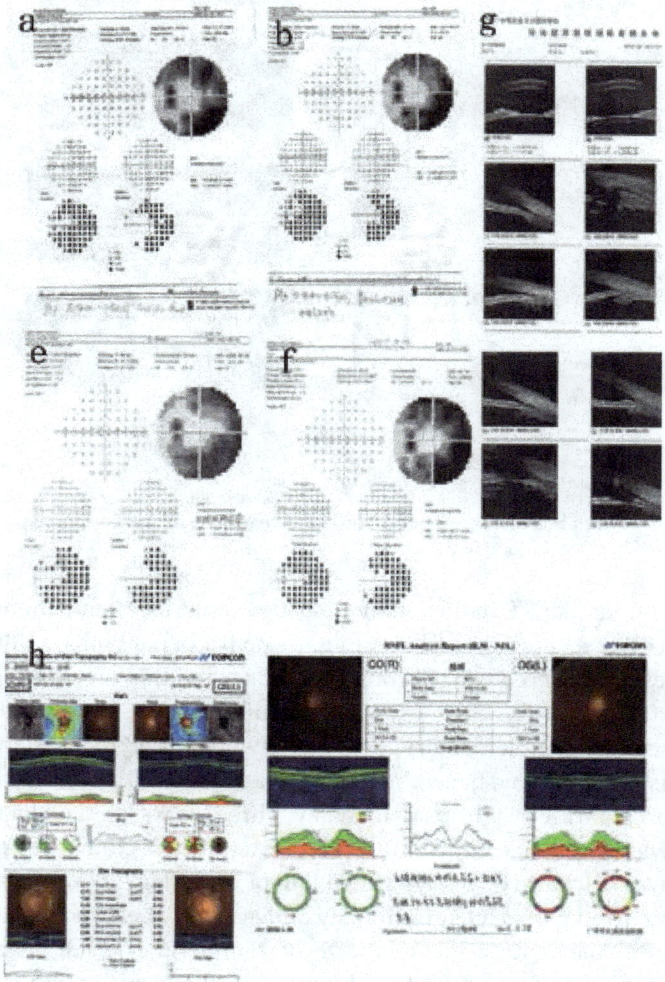

Figure 18. Typical clinical data of patient (Clinical number :341555)with diagnosis of left PSS combined with binocular closed-angle glaucoma. The visual fields of right eye(A) and left eye(B) become worse 4years later(C) and (D),UBM indicate binocular aqueous humour outflow after the 1 st trabeculectomy(E) and the OCT results show serious retinal nerve fiber layer defect in left eye(F).

3. Differential diagnosis and main points in diagnosis and treatment of complications of PSS

On the one hand, PSS is often misdiagnosed as other diseases, other diseases are often misdiagnosed as PSS; on the other hand, PSS can also be merged with or cause other diseases. Although the differential diagnosis of these conditions is complex, but we should be able to complete the work well through a careful clinical observation and analyzation rely on the basic characteristics of PSS described by Posner and Schlossman and new discoveries introduced above.,,.

3.1. The differential diagnosis of PSS and other diseases.

3.1.1. Analysis the situation of misdiagnosis

There were a total of 37 articles about misdiagnosis of PSS among the domestic documents about PSS since 1990. Here are the results of our analysis of these documents.

1. Other diseases misdiagnosed as PSS

There were 5 cases in which Fuchs syndrome was misdiagnosed as PSS, in 5 cases viral keratitis misdiagnosed as PSS and in 4 cases acute retinal necrosis misdiagnosed as PSS.

2. PSS misdiagnosed as other diseases

There were 76 cases of PSS misdiagnosed as acute angle-closure glaucoma, 42 misdiagnosed as iridocyclitis, 42 cases misdiagnosed as primary open-angle glaucoma, 22 cases misdiagnosed as uveitis, 4 cases misdiagnosed as conjunctivitis, 4 cases misdiagnosed as Fuch's syndrome, 1 case misdiagnosed as high intraocular pressure and1 case misdiagnosed as keratitis.

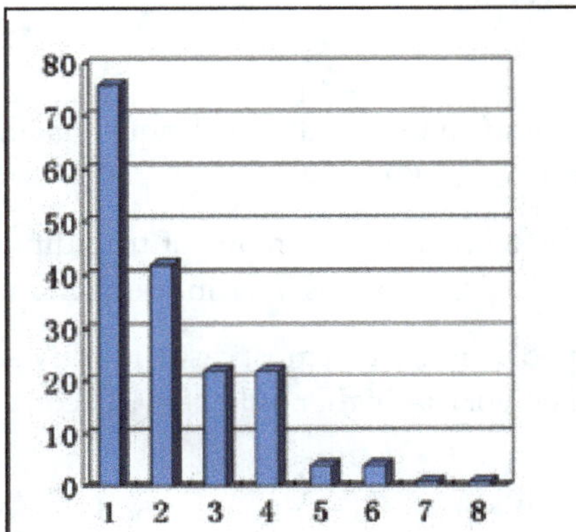

1. misdiagnosed as acute angle-closure glaucoma
2. misdiagnosed as iridocyclitis
3. misdiagnosed as POAG
4. misdiagnosed as uveitis
5. misdiagnosed as conjunctivitis
6. misdiagnosed as Fuch 's syndrome
7. misdiagnosed as high intraocular pressure
8. misdiagnosed as keratitis

Figure 19. Number of cases of PSS misdiagnosed as other diseases

3. About the harms of misdiagnosis for the patients.PSS patients were misdiagnosed as primary glaucoma and inappropriate treated, even the surgery that should not be done had been performed. Primary glaucoma merged with PSS were missed diagnosis, result in the lost the optimal timing of treatment. Such diseases as Fuch's syndrome, acute retinal necrosis and viral keratitis were misdiagnosed as PSS, lead to the delay of treatment.

	PSS	POAG	PCAG
age at first onset	usually under the age of 50 years	middle-aged or older	
KP	Yes, accompany with elevated IOP	No	pigmented KP sometimes after a outburst
Anterior chamber angle			or closed
Affected eye	most	most binocular	binocular, usually
Visual field damage	Little and light, more began in the peripheral, usually	usually binocular and centrally located	more binocular, often irregular
IOP	In episodes the is normal, in intermission both eyes are normal	invariably	Invariably or paroxysmal
IOP cross	Yes	No	No in chronic cases, Yes in acute cases sometimes after an outburst
postrualar IOP change	Not related to C value no matter IOP is high or low	Related to C value no matter IOP is high or low	Related to C value only when IOP is high

Table 6. The key points about differential diagnosis between PSS and POAG or PACG

3.1.2. The differential diagnosis of several kinds of common diseases

1. The differential diagnosis of PSS and other glaucomaThe differential diagnosis between PSS and POAG or PACG can be carried out in reference to table 7. [23 24, 27, 28, 40]

2. The differential diagnosis of PSS and other uveitis

The characteristics of common uveitis

Iridocyclitis: Ciliary hyperemia, eyesight drops significantly, smaller KP, aqueous humor of turbidity, fast and heavy adhesion of iris, higher or lower IOP.

Choroiditis: significantly dropped vision, with or without KP, vitreous of turbidity, no iris adhesion usually, lower IOP, corresponding pathological changes in retinal and choroiditis.

All uveitis: ciliary hyperemia, significantly dropped vision, KP in most cases, muddy aqueous humor, vitreous of turbidity, fast and heavy adhesion of iris, higher or lower IOP, corresponding pathological changes in retinal and choroiditis.

Intermediate uveitis: a kind of uveitis limited in the pars plana of ciliary body, peripheral retina and vitreous base, without any clinical symptoms in some cases or with muscae volitantes, blurred vision and temporary myopia in most cases, normal or mild declined vision in most cases but significant vision loss in case with cystoid macular edema and other complications or sudden severe vision loss in case with acute vitreous hemorrhage, retinal detachment,, mild to moderate anterior segment inflammation in most cases but severe ciliary hyperemia, a large number of KP, obvious aqueous flare and a lot of inflammatory cells in the anterior chamber in a few cases at first onset with severe anterior segment reaction occasionally, change in the vitreous and the pars plana of ciliary body (the most common and important performance of the disease) such as vitreous inflammatory cells, snow ball turbidity due to cell agglutination, snowbank like lesion stretches from the pars plana and vitreous base into vitreous cavity, vitreous degeneration, hemorrhage and hyperplastic vitreous retinopathy at late stage, a variety of retinopathy, such as macular edema, diffuse retinal edema, retinal vasculitis and perivascular inflammation, exudation, hemorrhage, retinal neovascularization, hyperplastic retinopathy, retinal detachment, usually normal IOP in early time but a persistent high IOP once elevated, sporadic KP with no association with IOP.

3. The differential diagnosis of PSS and keratitis

Keratitis

Sign Obvious hyperaemia, matrix and endothelial change, KP with different forms mainly distributed in lesion site of the cornealand seldom inhealthy area.

Characteristics The eye with angle-closure glaucoma induced by keratitis have the basic characteristics of angle-closure glaucoma; A monocular open-angle glaucoma would occurred in the affected eye if keratitis spread to the trabecular meshwork with an intraocular pressure changes over the cornea edema.

Course of disease:They are not self-limited and repeated outbreaks tend to occur.

3.2. Main points in diagnosis and treatment of complications of PSS

Other kinds of glaucoma which PSS concurred with or lead to were not introduced before. PSS can also concur with or cause iris heterochromia, ischemic optic neuropathy, complicated cataract and other diseases, such as retinal detachment. Main points in diagnosis and treatment of these complications were briefly introduced as follows:

3.2.1. PSS combined with iris heterochromia

Typical cases

Case 1) A patient consulted at our hospital because his left eye suffered from intermittent recurrent pain and blurred vision for more than one year. Intraday examinations showed: best corrected visual acuity is 1.0/ 0.6(R/L), IOP: 16.7/ 13.7(R/L) mmHg, FFA in both eyes are normal, optic cup in his left eye is expand. He was suspected of glaucoma. Intermittent recurrent pain and blurred vision kept to attack his left eye for more than half a year after then. These attacks usually ceased a few days late, with or without the help of 0.5% timolol eye drop and other drugs. During this period, the highest IOP record of his left eye was 35mmHg with a normal record of his right eye. The patient returned to our hospital one year later after stopping use of any drugs for two weeks. Ophthalmologic examination at this time showed: visual acuity1.2

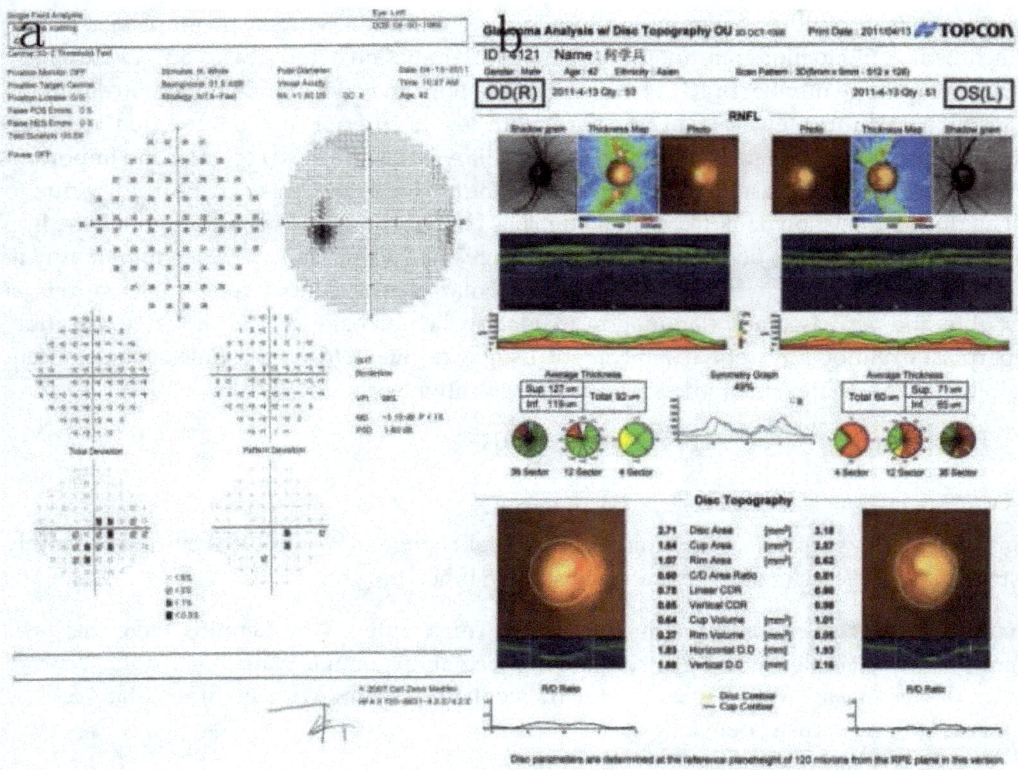

Figure 20. Typical clinical data of patient (ID :11041302)with diagnosis of left PSS combined with iris heterochromia. The visual fields of left eye show nasal defect (A) ,binocular OCTresults indicate ocular cups expand (B)and (C) obvious retinal nerve fiber layer defect (C).

both eyes, IOP 17/15(R/L)mmHg, a lot of small lipid-like KP in the inferior of the left cornea, "rain dozen sand-like" appearance in the iris of his left eye, C/D rate 0.6/0.7(R/L),CCT 553/560(R/L). Results of his visual field and OCT showed in Figure below. UBM showed wide-angle in the both eyes. Fundus fluorescein angiography and contrast sensitivity revealed no special finds. 24 hours IOP measurements (2 weeks after KP disappeared): 13~16/ 12~15(R/L)mmHg. Diagnosis of "PSS complicated with iris heterochromia" for his left eye was confirmed than. He was asked to treat every onset of the disease in time with drugs dropping IOP as well as anti-inflammatory medicine. (Clinical data see Figure 20)

Case 2) A patient was admitted to our hospital because her right eye suffered from repeated episodes of pain with blurred vision for more than nine years, and her vision decreased 3 months, with a primary diagnosis of "secondary glaucoma" for her right eye. A lot of intermittent recurrent pain and blurred vision had attacked her right eye from nine years ago, 2 or 3 times a year. Each attack lasted about one week, than resolved spontaneously. Three months ago her sense of vision went to recession. She felt that her right eye was attacked again recent days, so she can to our hospital. Ophthalmologic examination in this time showed: visual

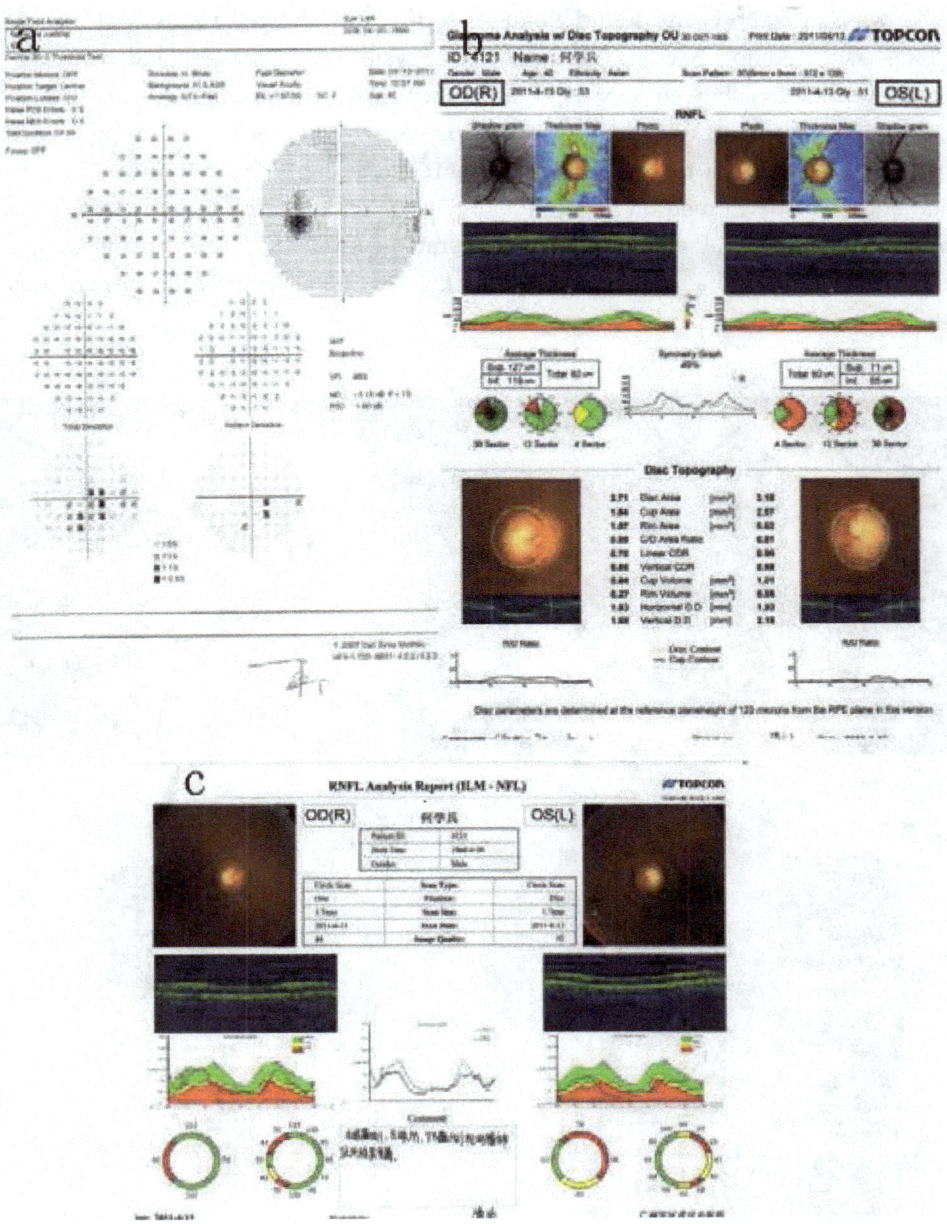

Figure 21. Typical clinical data of patient (ID :11041302)with diagnosis of left PSS combined with iris heterochromia. The visual fields of left eye show nasal defect(A),binocular OCT results indicate ocular cups expand(B) and (C) obvious retinal nerve fiber layer defect (C).

acuity: 0.15/ 1.0(R/L), IOP: 43/12(R/L) mmHg, mist edema in her cornea of her right eye with a lot of fat-like KP, pale and "rain scatting beach-like" appearance in her left iris with a round pupil about 3mm in diameter, her optic disk appeared pale in color with a C/D 0.9, her anterior chamber was not shallow, ultrasound biomicroscopy (UBM) showed a wide angle in both eye. Her left eye showed no KP with a C/D less 0.3. Her systemic examination and routine inspection and examination showed no special finds. Treatment with drugs dropping IOP such as carteolol and brimonidine and mannitol as well as steroids loteprednol kept about a week, KP significantly reduced but the intraocular pressure is still high. Operation of Ahmed valve implantation was performed on her right eye two weeks later. She was discharged a week postoperative with an IOP of 9mmHg in the operated eye. Her IOP was controlled well with fewer attacks of PSS and a stable visual field in the recent 3 years after the surgery. (Clinical data see Figure 21)

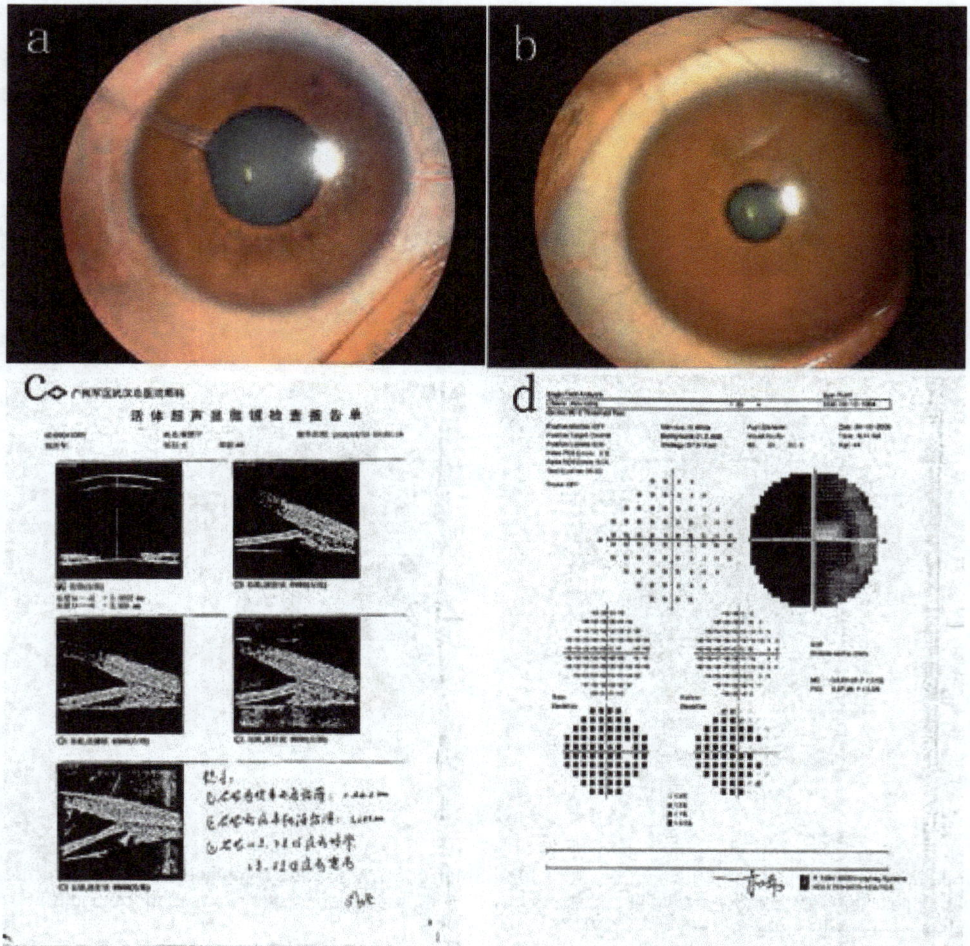

Figure 22. Typical clinical data of patient (Clinical number :437614)with diagnosis of right PSS combined with iris disorder. The right eye is after Ahmed implantation and arrow indicate iris heterochromia(A),the left eye is normal(B).UBM indicate a wild angle in right eye (C),but the visual field show serious damanges in right eye(D).

Discussion

1. Clinical performance of PSS complicated with iris heterochromia

Four cases of PSS complicated with iris heterochromia were reported [40]. They were two males and two females aged 35 to 45 years. In addition to typical PSS performance, the iris showed "rain scatting sand-like" appearance in all of the 4 patients. All of them are monocular repeatedly attacked at the same eye. Each attack kept 3 to 7 days with a significantly increased IOP up to30.00 ~ 60.00mnHg and a few of fat-like KP, than relieve itself or extinct with the help of medication. Intraocular pressure (including 24 hours intraocular pressure) in intermittent period appeared normal after discontinuation of all medication with a typical crossed-over phenomenon.

2. Key-points in the differential diagnosis between PSS complicated with iris heterochromatic and FHI (Fuchs heterochromic iridicyclitis).The two diseases are different clinically in the following five aspects: the attacked eye and sex of patients, manifestation of intraocular pressure, character of KP, appearance of the Lens and glaucomatous damage of optic nerve and visual field.

(1) The attacked eye and sex of patients

Most of PSS cases had monocular presentation, a few of cases were binocular, but usually one eye was affected at a time, in extremely rare cases was binocularly attacked simultaneously. Male patients were more common than female in PSS. FH is generally believed that no gender more predisposed than the other more than 90% of the cases were monocularly affected.

(2) Manifestation of intraocular pressure

The IOP in patients of PSS with iris heterochromatic appeared as an intermittent and abruptly rising when the attack comes with the appearance of typical KP in pure PSS patients. IOP elevation in patients of PSS with iris heterochromatic usually lasted 3 ~ 10days, and then turned to subside spontaneously with the disappearance of the KP after this period, it is also sensitive to drugs dropping IOP and anti-inflammatory medicine. On the contrary, IOP of patient with FH appeared normal in the initial stage for a long time, after that, elevated in part of the cases gradually; however, once the intraocular pressure elevated, it often appeared persistently higher, although there maybe some fluctuations. The elevated IOP and KP in patient with FH had no characteristic of intermittent, were difficult to be controlled and poorly responded to corticosteroids therapy. The IOP in patients with PSS complicated with iris heterochromia kept the characteristic of crossed-over, that is, the IOP of the attacked eye was higher than that of contra lateral eye during the episode but lower(3 ~ 5mmHg) than the other eye between attacks. IOP in patients with Fuchs syndrome had no such characteristic, once elevated; it is always higher if untreated.

(3) Keratic Precipitates

The KP in patient with PSS complicated with iris heterochromia appeared only in a short period during the attack in most cases. This KP is of following characteristics: small round suet-like, medium sized, isolated, with no pigment in initial stage, mainly located in the lower part of the cornea, usually disappeared naturally within a few days after or before IOP reduction. On the contrary, KP in patients with Fuchs syndrome has different characteristics as following: persistence for very long time even always in most cases, white transparent small dot or star-like coexisting with pigmented KP, diffuse distribution in the cornea, sometimes connected each other with fibrous filaments, poor response to corticosteroids therapy. (Clinical data see Figure 22)

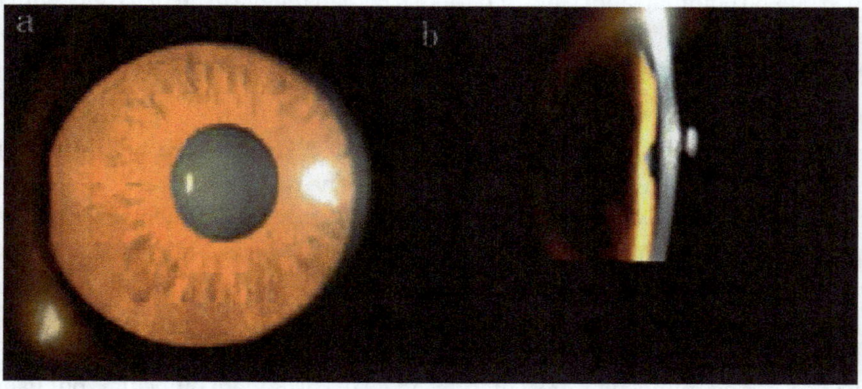

Figure 23. Heterochromatic iris and KP in FHI. There is a typical iris such as "rain dozen sand-like"(A) arrow shows a lot of star-like KPs(B).

(4) Lens situation

Fuchs syndrome complicated with cataract is common at later stage; however the complicated cataract is uncommon in the PSS cases with iris heterochromia.

(5) Glaucomatous retinal and visual damage

Glaucomatous damage in PSS cases appeared later and to a lesser extent, however that of FH cases occur earlier and quicker.

3.2.2. PSS combined with ischemic optic neuropathy

Typical cases

A patient came to our hospital because her vision of the left eye sudden dropped 2 months ago. She was examined 2 months ago: visual acuity: 1.0/ 0.5(R/L) IOP: 17.3/ 15(R/L) mmHg. The optic disc of her left eye was pale, visual field showed an inferior fan like defect. Fundus fluorescein angiography(FFA) of her left eye showed ischemic optic neuropathy. The anterior segment, fundus, vision, and FFA of her right eye were normal. She was diagnosed as "left eye ischemic optic neuropathy". She was admitted to our hospital, and examinations showed: visual acuity: 1.0/ 0.15(R/L). IOP: 17.3/ 50.62(R/L), anterior chamber of both eyes were not shallow, Right eye showed no abnormality. Left cornea had mild edema and there was a medium size fat-like KP below the pupil. The boundary of optic papillae in left eye was clear, the color was off white, and the C / D was about 0.3,the angle of left eye was N1 ~ N2. Systemic examination such as X-ray, electrocardiogram and routine laboratory tests were normal. Visual field of right eye was normal and that of the left eye showed a centripetal narrow with an inferior fan like defect. She was diagnosed as "Left eye PSS, complicated with ischemic optic neuropathy", and treated with drugs for reducing IOP and nutrition curing to optic nerve for about a weak. She was discharged with IOP 12mmHg disappeared KP, vision 0.2 of her left eye. (Clinical data see Figure 23)

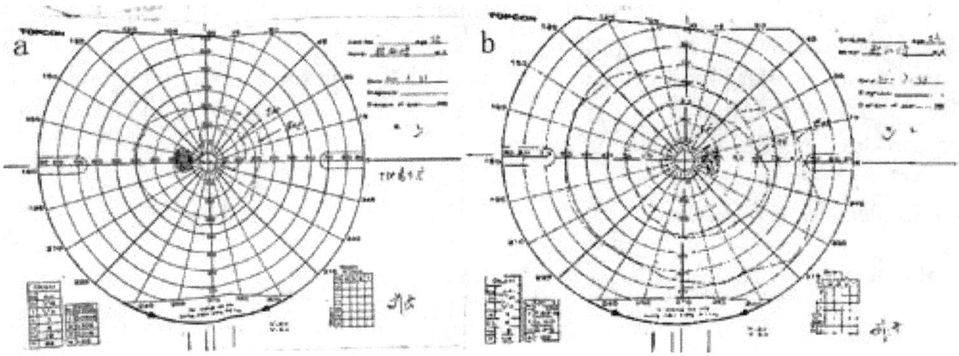

Figure 24. visual field of patient (Clinical number :294450) The case suffered from left eye PSS combined with ischemic optic neuropathy. inferior visual field defect and serious contraction of left(A),and that of the normal right eye(B).

Discussion

In 2003 1 case of PSS complicated with non-arteritic anterior ischemic optic neuropathy (AION) was reported. The vision of the case improved significantly after the attack of PSS had been controlled, but the vision and optic neuropathy damaged continually. The authors emphasized that the IOP of PSS patients complicated with AION should be promptly controlled as it is one of the risk factors [41]. It is useful to use drugs with dual role of reducing IOP and improving retinal blood supply in intermittent period. Our case appeared a sudden vision loss and significant discomfort two months ago. The result of examinations in other hospital such as visual field defect of arcuate below and FFA supported the diagnosis of left eye ischemic optic neuropathy. Results of examinations, reaction to treatment and course of the disease during her hospitalization in our hospital In July 2000 conformed with diagnostic criteria of PSS. The structure of the optic nerve, damage of blood vessels and blood state are related to ischemic optic neuropathy, the severely sudden rising of IOP during attack of PSS maybe the inducing factors. So it is necessary to reduce the IOP during each attack of PSS as soon and effective as possible for the cases of PSS combined with ischemic optic neuropathy or with the risk factors for that.

3.2.3. PSS combined with rhegmatogenous retinal detachment

Typical cases

A patient was hospitalized in our hospital for the reason that there was shadow before his right eye with a diagnose of rhegmatogenous retinal detachment. The IOP of his right eye elevated to 29 mmHg 3 days after hospitalization and a fat-like KP appeared in his right eye, than he was diagnosed as rhegmatogenous retinal detachment combined with PSS. Retinal detachment surgery (Condensation+cerclage+scleral pressure technique) were done after reducing IOP with the treatment of drugs. Postoperative recovery was good. PSS recurred 4 months later and recovered 5 days late.

Discussion

The pathogenesis of PSS combined with rhegmatogenous retinal detachment is unknown. Increased concentration of PG (especially PGE) resulted from retinal S-antigen entered into the vitreous cavity after blood-eye barrier breakdown during the formation of retinal breaks may leads to the inflammation of the uvea, and the higher concentration of PGs and inflammatory products results in the IOP elevation.

3.2.4. PSS combined with cataract

Typical cases

A patient complained of recurrent pain and decreased vision of her right eye for four years. Results of examinations intraday showed: visual acuity:0.08/ 0.4(R/L); corrected visual acuityR: 0.3(-0.75DS/1.50DC*111),L: 0.9(-1.25DS/-0.50DC*83) ;IOP: 12/ 14(R/L) mmHg; a few of time worn pigmented KP on the central and lower part of her clear corneal; round pupil about3mm in diameter; normal iris, opacification of posterior capsule of lens; C/D of optic papillaeo.4.Her left eye appeared normal. She was hospitalized with the diagnosis of PSS and was treated with carteolol, brimonidine, mannitol for reducing IOP, tobradex for anti-inflammation and methycobal to maintain optic nerve. She was discharged once the attack of PSS faded away every time. The PSS attacked her1 to 2 month a time, her vision of right eye declined gradually without other discomfort. (Clinical data see Figure 24)

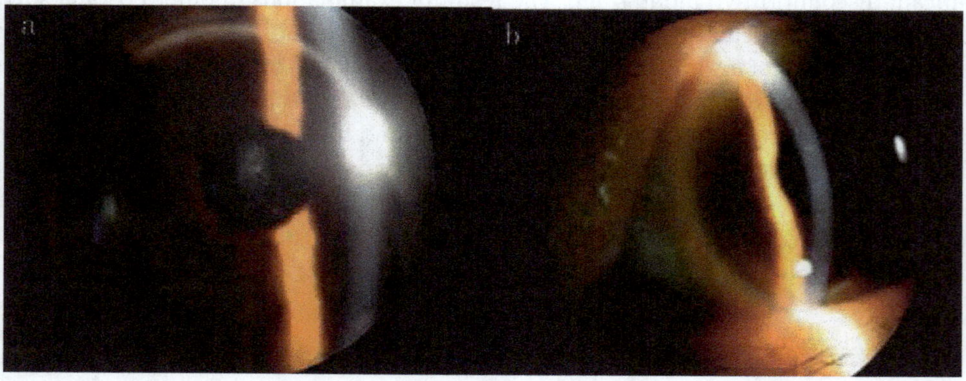

Figure 25. Anterior segment slit-lamp photography of patient (Clinical number 394998) with the diagnosis of PSS combined with cataract.Arrows show an opacities area at posterior capsule (A) and few typical fat-shaped KPs(B).

Discussion

The possible pathogenesis: repeated onset of IOP elevation and anterior segment inflammation cause disorders of nutrition and metabolism of the lens.

Surgical opportunity: Cataract surgery should be done after the inflammation has been subsidized for more than 3 months. The rest of the indication is the same to the conventional cataract. Considering the PSS is an inflammation of the nature of the disease and the literature PSS patients of corneal endothelial cell density is low, PSS patients combined cataract surgery methods should also do more thinking. Femtosecond laser cataract surgery with accurate positioning, and the advantage of less influence on corneal endothelial, compared with the phaco, whether merger of cataract in patients with PSS has advantages, is worth our discussion.[42]

Prospect

With the deepening of the research on PSS, the pathogenic factors, pathogenesis, clinical characteristics, especially the clinical pathway via which the glaucoma optic nerve damage occurred in PSS cases will become clearer. For example, if hormone treatment was used excessively in PSS cases, would glueoeortieoid-induced glaucoma take place? If a poor blood supply to the optic disc of a patient with PSS or a weak structure of the papilla of optic nerve or a lower intracranial pressure, in such cases, would a normal-tension glaucoma appear? All these problems need to be continuously explored through our joint efforts.

Author details

He-Zheng Zhou*, Wen-Shan Jiang, Han-Guang Jie, Chang Feng, Wen-Qiang Zhang, Qian Ye, Jian-Guo Wu, Yan-Ping Song and Qin Ding

*Address all correspondence to: zhoueye@qq.com

Department of Ophthalmology, Wuhan General Hospital of Guangzhou Command, China

References

[1] Posener A, Schlossman A. Syndrome of unilateral attacks of glaucoma with cyclic-symptoms. Arch opthalmol.1948,39:5-28

[2] Theodore FH. Observation on glaucomatocycliticcrisis(Posner Schloddman Syndrome).Br J Ophthalmol.1952,36:207-213

[3] Dao-Ping Lu, Ran-Ran Xi. [Clinical analyzation of 177 cases with Posner Schloddman Syndrome]. Chin J Ophthalmology. 1982,18:34-37

[4] Paivonsalo HT, Tuminen J, Vaahtoranta LH, et al. Incidence and prevalence of differentuneitis,entilies in Filand. Acta Ophthalmology Scand.1997, 75:76~81.

[5] Kanjiro M. The relationship between elevation of intraocular pressure and prostaglandin in cases with glaucomatocyclitic crisis. clinical ophthalmology. 1975,29:689-692

[6] Yamamoto S, Pavan-Langston D, Tada R, et al. Possible role of herpes simplex virusin the origin of Posner-Schlossman syndrome. Am J Ophthalmol.1995, 119: 796-798

[7] Yang SY, Chen MJ, Chen KH, et al. Cytomegalovirus and herpes simplex virus ascauses of bilateral anterior uveitis in an immunocompetent patient. J Chin Med Assoc. 2011,74:48-50

[8] Blich-Michel E, Dussaix E, Cerqueti P, et al. Possible role of cytomegalovirus infection in the etiology of the Posner-Schlossman syndrome. IntOphthalmol. 1987,11:95-96

[9] Chee SP, Jap A. Presumed Fuchs heterochromiciridocyclitis and Posner-Schlossmansyndrome: comparison of cytomegalovirus-positive and negative eyes. Am2008,146:883-889

[10] CY Choi, MS Kim, JM Kim, SH Park, KH Park, C Hong. Association between Helicobacter pylori infection and Posner–Schlossman syndrome. Eye. 2010, [11] Zhi-Hui Li, Xun-ChuanJi, Shu-Chu Chen, et al. [The Long-term follow-up of PosnerSchloddman Syndrome]. Chin J Ophthalmology. 1982,18:306-308

[11] Nan-Xiang Peng. [Clinical analyzation of 52 cases with Posner Schloddman Syndrome].Contemporary Medicine.2008, 5:141-141

[12] Wen-Xue Hu. [Clinical observation of early stage of Posner-Schlossman syndrome].Int J Ophthalmology. 2011; 11: 1980-1982

[13] Puri P, Verma D. Bilateral glaucomatocyclitic crisis in a patient with Holmes Adiesyndrome. J Postgrad Med.1998,44:76-77

[14] Yu-Hong Wang, Xing-Huai Sun. [Clinical analysization of the the operative effect inpatients with glaucomatocyclitic crisis]. Chinese Journal of Practical Ophthalmology. 2005, 10:23-30

[15] Wen-Bing Zhou, Shou-Xiong Peng. [glaucomatocyclitic crisis and Primary Open-angle Glaucoma]. Chinese Ophthalmic Res.1994,12:34-36

[16] He-Zheng Zhou, Yuan-Hong Du. [The related factors about Posner-Schlossman syndrome damage of visual field].Chinese Journal of Practical Ophthalmology. 2002,10:768~769

[17] Hua-Xin Chen, He-Zheng Zhou, Bai-Chuan Wang et al.[The Clinical Observation of14 cases elderly Posner-Schlossmansyndrome]. Military medical journal of South-China. 2007; 21: 43-45

[18] Raitta C, Vannas A. Glaucomatocyclitic crisis. Arch Ophthalmology. 1977, 95:608-612

[19] He-Zheng Zhou, Yi-Jia Yang. [Characteristics and clinical value of the intraocular-pressure and the C-value in Posner Schloddman Syndrome]. Chinese Journal ofPractical Ophthalmology.1992, 10:143-145

[20] Ying-Bo Shui, Hou-Ren Wei. [Influence of Postural Change on Intraocular Pressureof Normal Eyes]. Chinese Ophthalmic Res. 1987; 3 : 182-185

[21] He-Zheng Zhou. [Tonography and postural change of intraocular pressure in patients with glaucoma]. Chinese Journal of Practical Ophthalmology.1991,9:598-602

[22] He-Zheng Zhou, Wen-Shan Jiang. [Differential diagnosis of Posner-Schlossman syndrome]. Military medical journal of South China.2012,2:32-35

[23] He-Zheng Zhou, Yuan-Hong Du, Yan-Ping Song, Guang-Jie Wang, Jian-Guo Wu. [Visual field damage of glaucomatocyclitic crisis and its relating factors]. Fourth MilMed Univ.2001,22:1674-1677

[24] Yi-Lin Tang. [Clinical analysis of damage of visual field with Posner Schlossmanps-syndrome]. International Journal of Ophthalmology. 2010,10:1204-1205

[25] Jap A, Sivakumar M, Chee SP. Is Posner-Schlossman syndrome benign? Ophthalmology.2001,108:913-991

[26] He-Zheng Zhou, Bai-Chuan Wang, Xiong Zhou. [Unilateral Primary Open-Angle-Glaucomaand BilateralPosner-Schlossman syndrome]. Chin J Misdiagn. 2001,1:334-336

[27] He-Zheng Zhou, Wen-Qiang Zhang, Bai-ChuanWang. [Glaucomatocyclitic crisiswith primary close-Angle glaucoma]. International Journal of Ophthalmology,2004,4(5): 844-847

[28] Darchuk V, Sampaolesi J, Mato L, Nicoli C, SampaolesiR.Optic nerve head behavior-in Posner-Schlossman syndrome. IntOphthalmol,2001;23:373-379

[29] Rong-Xin Wu. [Operative effect in 1 Case with Posner-Schlossman syndrome].Ocular trauma professional eye disease magazine. 2002,24:328

[30] Lei Sheng, Yu-Pu Li, Gui-LanLan. [1 Case of Posner-Schlossmansyndrome].Chinese-Journal of Practical Ophthalmology.2008,26:572

[31] Bo Zhao, Da-Yong Bai, Hui Zhao.et al. [Posner-Schlossman syndrome and primaryopen-angle glaucoma]. Chin J Pract Ophthalmology. 2004,22:142-143

[32] Xiu-Feng Ke, Dan-Ning Z, Li Yuan. [Observation the clinical operation curative effectof Posner-Schlossman syndrome]. Chinese Journal of Practical Ophthalmology. 2007,6:642-643

[33] Dinakaran S, Kayarkar V. Trabeculectomy in the management of Posner-Schlossman-syndrome. Ophthalmic SurgLasers.2002,33:321-322

[34] Stavrou P, Murray PI. Does trabeculectomy influence the course of uveitis? OculImmunolInflamm. 1999,7:103-108

[35] Xiao-Ping Zhang, Ji-Zhong Chen, Ru-Yong Song,[Analyze the Diagnostic of Posner-Schlossman syndrome]. Journal of clinical ophthalmology.2002,10:137-139

[36] Jin-Fu Ying, Ling-Ling Wu, [Posner-Schlossman syndrome complicated with Primary Closed-Angle Glaucoma]. Chinese Journal of Practical Ophthalmology. 1993.11:491-492

[37] Chang-lin Zhao, Han-Ping Xie. [A case report of primary angle closure glaucoma accompanied by glaucomatocyclitic crisis]. Acta Academiae Medicinae Militaris Tertiae. 2004.10.25; 26: 1798

[38] Li-Hong Guan. [2 cases of Posner-Schlossman syndrome complicated with Primary Closed-Angle Glaucoma]. Modern Medicine & Health. 2008, 24: 152

[39] Wen-Shan Jiang, He-ZhengZhou,Yun-Hui Chen, Ling Hong [Differential diagnosisof the Posner-Schlossman syndrome with heterochromic iris and the Fuchs syndrome—clinial report about three cases]. International Journal of Ophthalmology, 2009; 9 (9): 1762-1763

[40] Irak I, Katz BJ, Zabriskie NA, Zimmerman PL.Posner-Schlossman syndrome andnonarteritic anterior ischemic optic neuropathy. J Neuroophthalmol. 2003,23: 264-267

[41] Schultz T, Conrad – Hengerer I, Hengerer FH, et al. Intraocular pressure variation during femtosecond laser – assisted cataract surgery using a fluid–filled interface. J Cataract Refract Surg 2013; 39 (1): 22–27

10

Regional Immune, Hormonal and Mediatory Mechanisms Responsible for Function of "Immune Privilege of an Eye" at Senile and Complicated Cataracts

Artashes A. Zilfyan and Arto V. Zilfyan

1. Introduction

Nowadays, in current biology and medicine the subject of wide discussion present paracrine and autocrine immune, endocrine and mediatory mechanisms functioning of which in all the integrative systems of the organism are realized due to principles of interregulation and interdependence. It is not excluded that similar mechanisms are also engaged in eye tunics, moreover that the hematoophthalmic barrier is characterized by a more stable selective permeability (as compared to other histohematic barriers) towards a wide range of endogenous active biological compounds of immune, hormonal and mediatory origin.

In this concern, to our mind, studies aimed at elucidation of autonomous mechanisms engaged in sustaining the immune and endocrine homeostasis in the eye tunics are rather promising.

Hence, during the last 40 years the subject of special investigation became scientific research works relevant to the aspects of pathogenesis "active immunological tolerance" originating in eye tunics as a response to baring of antigenic determinants in eye tunics and tissues at a wide range of ophthalmological diseases. The entire symptom complex of *in situ* occurring immunological reactions is defined in modern ophthalmology as "anterior chamber associated immune deviation" (ACAID).

At the same time, regional mechanisms responsible for ACAID function are studied rather insufficiently.

In the mentioned aspect, cells identified in certain eye tunics should become the subject of specific discussion; besides their "main functions' these cells are provided with the immune, hormonal and mediatory activity as well. The matter is *in situ* synthesis of transforming growth factor-$_{\beta\text{-}2}$, cortisol, fibronectin, availability of receptors to prolactin and prostaglandins E_2.

This chapter will bring to the attention of readers the analysis of scientific evidence and our own research findings obtained during the last 10 years in respect of possible regional immune, hormonal and mediatory mechanisms engaged in formation and abolition of ACAID function.

To avoid artificially expanded volume of this chapter, we considered to be expedient to supplement the narrative description of own research results with Tables and Schemes, excluding all the methodic approaches to selection of patient cohorts, methods of investigation, which were comprehensively presented within our previous studies (Zilfyan A., 2009; 2012; 2013).

We should only mention those groups of patients under study in the aqueous humor of which we determined the spectrum of the above-mentioned endogenously active substances of the immune, hormonal and mediatory nature.

The first (control) group included patients with senile non-complicated cataract, the second group involved patients with cataracts occurring on the background of primary open-angle glaucoma and the third group embraced patients with cataracts on the background of glaucoma and pseudoexfoliative syndrome, the fourth group made patients with cataracts on the background of "arterial hypertension", the fifth group – cataracts on the background of diabetes mellitus and the sixth group was composed of patients with cataract on the background of previous eye injury.

To our mind, it was rather reasonable that we did not include in the current chapter issues dealing with the role of intracorporeal resident gram-negative and gram-positive microorganisms, as well as viruses, *Chlamidiae, Toxoplasmas*, etc. Despite the bulk of evidence-frequently of contradictory character – mechanisms of "bacterial translocation" of the above-mentioned microorganisms in the aspect of their passage through the hematoophthalmic barrier and/or penetration of their secretion and decomposition products into the eye tunics are almost none-investigated.

Similar approach was used by us regarding the role of pro-and anti-inflammatory immunocytokines, because of a known controversy of available scientific data on their role in mechanisms responsible for formation of reactions responsible for ACAID function. The controversial character of scientific publications to a known extent is connected with dose-dependent and pleiotropic potencies of immunocytokines even towards the same "immunocompetent" cells localized in the eye tunics.

2. Immune shifts in mechanisms of formation and abolition of the active immunological tolerance responsible for ACAID function

The term "immune privilege of an eye" implies the entire complex of regional immune cell-mediated and humoral reactions aimed at prevention of inflammatory and dystrophic processes development in tunics and fluid sections (slices) of an eye under conditions of a wide range of ophthalmologic maladies.

At the same time, this term first of all reflects the state of "local immune homeostasis" under conditions of normal functioning of an eye. The complete cascade of local protective/adaptive mechanisms is aimed to form immunological processes, which in total are defined as anterior chamber associated immune deviation (ACAID). To our mind based on available scientific publications, the general scheme of immunopathological process can be presented as the following chronologically occurring stages:

1. As a result of interaction of different pathogenetic factors there occurs "baring" (uncovering) of antigenic determinants (Orge Y., Gungor S., 1984; D'Orazio T., Niederkorn J., 1998; Sonoda A. et al., 2000; Camelo S. et al., 2005).
2. As a response to acquiring of antigenic properties by tissues of an eye in the region of damage (injury) there occurs no activation of the antibody formation process, as reactions of active immunological tolerance there prevail to dominate (Murray P. et al., 1990; Lightman S., Towler H., 1992; Fu T. et al., 2004; Kitaichi N. et al., 2005).
3. No formation of immune complexes occurs as under conditions of pathology there is engaged the regional mechanism preventing activation of the compliment (Streilein J., Stein-Streilein J., 2000).
4. Mechanisms of immune suppression (inhibition of antibody formation) are conditioned by targeted (directed) activation of T-suppressory and killer (killing) subpopulation (Wilbanks C., Streilein J., 1990; Muhaya M. et al., 1999).
5. Directed activation of T-killer lymphocytes occurs due to production of TGF_{β} (Streilein J. et al., 1992; Abrahamian A. et al., 1995; Fleenor D. et al., 2006).
6. The high level of CD_8 is mainly conditioned by the fact that in the region of eye tissues damage there occurs activation of the main histocompatibility class I complex, which functions as the initial factor ensuring triggering of receptor mechanisms underlying activation and proliferation of T-killer lymphocyte populations (Nishi O. et al., 1982; Martin W. et al., 1995; Bakunowicz L. et al., 1997; Muhaya M. et al., 1999).

It should be emphasized that certain pathogenetic mechanisms/links underlying induction and course of ACAID in case of non-complicated and complicated cataracts are currently the subject of a wide discussion (Orge Y., Gungor S., 1984; Uenoyama K. et al., 1989; Streilein J. et al., 1992; Zhou Z. et al., 1996; Cinatl et al., 2000; Robinson M. et al., 2000; Kawakami M. et al., 2005).

As a rule, the main reason of ACAID induction is 1-or 2-stage surgical intervention, as a result of which there occurs "baring" (uncovering) of antigenic determinants of lens tissues. As a result, in the "immunocompetent" tunics of an eye there occurs the synthesis of specific autoantibodies targeted to tissues of lens; by this latter are caused local processes of autoimmune aggression are caused being conditioned by the damaging action of both autoantibodies and locally formed immune complexes.

The activation of reactions of local humoral immunity is accompanied by significant increase of IgG levels in aqueous humor (in anterior and posterior chambers of eyes), due to which the aqueous humor is a rather informative media for studies on mechanisms of both formation and abolition of ACAID. At the same time, all the above-mentioned links underlying abolition of ACAID in case of cataracts are studied rather insufficiently.

It should be emphasized that regional immune mechanisms responsible for *in situ* formation of the active immunological tolerance, which ensures the ACAID function, is most comprehensively studied at senile non-complicated cataracts. At the same time, only single, sometimes even contradictory evidence is available on the course of the regional immune reactions engaged at complicated cataracts.

In our previous investigation (Zilfyan A., 2009) we studied the shifts of CD_4, CD_8 and IgG in the aqueous humor of patients with complicated cataracts: at cataracts on the background of primary open-angle glaucoma, pseudoexpfoliative glaucoma, diabetes mellitus, arterial hypertension, prior eye trauma.

The results of enzyme immunoassays for CD_4 and CD_8 in aqueous humor of patients are presented as Table 1.

Study groups (n=40)	Indices studied					
	CD_4			CD_8		
	M	*m*	*p*	*M*	*m*	*p*
I	10.7	± 2.1		53.9	±5.3	
II	28.4	±3.6	<0.0005	22.05	±5.4	<0.0005
III	30.2	±2.9	<0.0005	18.15	±2.3	<0.0005
IV	14.2	±2.4	*<0.25*	48.8	±4.2	<0.25
V	11.0	±2.5	"/>0.4	50.21	±2.54	<0.4
VI	17.5	±2.0	<0.025	33.7	±4.99	<0.005

Notes: *M* – mean; *m* – standard error of mean; *p* – confidence interval (indices of complicated cataracts as related to senile cataracts).

Table 1. The content of CD_4 (*unit/ml*) and CD_8 (*unit/ml*) in aqueous humor of patients with senile and complicated cataracts.

As obvious from the Table, at complicated cataracts (study groups II and III) already in pre-surgery period in the aqueous humor there was a marked decrease of CD_8 on the background of CD_4 increase in the aqueous humor of the same cohort of patients.

It is rather remarkable that upon the 2-factor statistical analysis strong reverse correlation dependence was revealed between the studied indices (correlation index made-0.893 and-0.940, appropriately). Apparently, at complicated cataracts in study groups II and III the antigenic determinants in post-barrier eye tunics were bared already in pre-surgery period;

relatively high levels of IgG revealed in the aqueous humor of the specified cohort of patients signified to this latter (Table 2).

Study groups (n=40)	IgG content		
	M	*m*	*p*
I	9.025	±0.73	
II	16.82	±2.20	<0.005
III	25.05	±2.25	<0.0005
IV	8.75	±1.71	"/>0.40
V	10.1	±0.74	<0.25
VI	14.57	±2.05	<0.025

Notes: *M* – mean; *m* – standard error of mean; *p* – confidence interval (indices of complicated cataracts as related to senile cataracts).

Table 2. IgG content (*IU/ml*) in the aqueous humor of patients with senile and complicated cataracts.

It appears, that in this precise case the intercellular mechanisms, which are conditioned by the cooperative activity of B-helper subpopulations and B-lymphocytic populations in the immune competent eye tunics and, first of all, of the ciliary body, are engaged in eye tunics; these latter eventually bring to the synthesis of anti-tissue autoantibodies. The performed 2-factor correlation analysis also signifies in favour of this circumstance: strong direct correlation dependence was revealed between CD_4 and IgG high levels in the aqueous humor of patients of the II and III study groups (correlation index made-0.891 and-0.935, appropriately). It should be mentioned that similar picture of immunological shifts was also observed in study group VI, i.e. at cataracts occurring on the background of trauma. Therefore, it is not excluded that prior trauma can be considered as a provoking factor bringing forth impairment of the immune homeostasis. In the aqueous humor of patients from all other study groups of complicated cataracts (groups IV and V) we registered CD_8, CD_4 and IgG indices similar to those registered in the aqueous humor of patients with senile cataracts.

The results of performed immunological analysis for IgG determination in aqueous humor of patients with senile and complicated cataracts are conformed by available data of scientific publications. In particular, N. Stambuk et al. (1994) established that IgG level in aqueous humor of patients with complicated cataracts was significantly higher than in patients with senile cataracts.

Thus performed, the comparative analysis in all study groups, though with due circumspection, signifies that at senile cataracts and, in all probability, at cataracts occurring on the background of diabetes mellitus and arterial hypertension during the pre-surgery period the regional immune homeostasis is not disturbed, i.e. only those mechanisms are engaged, which ensure the function of ACAID at norm.

At the same time, based on the studies performed by the above-mentioned authors (Lightman S., Towler H., 1992; Sonoda A. et al., 2000; Fu T. et al., 2004; Camelo S. et al., 2005; Kitaichi N. et al., 2005) it is difficult to consider if there is adequacy of inflammatory process, which occurs in eye post-barrier tunics as a response to surgery-related trauma, to what extent the local protective mechanisms work characterizing the immune deviation as related to "bared" autoantigens of the specified tunics. To our mind, it is possible to judge about the character and intensity of the inflammatory process in eye post-barrier tissues only under conditions of the lens transplantation into heterogenous sites of the organism. This problem was successfully solved by Japanese researchers already in 1989 (Uenoyama K. et al., 1989). The authors performed experiments aimed to study tissue specific shifts upon lens transplantation into the eye and intraperitoneally. Due to the complex approach with the use of cytological, immune-histochemical and electron microscopy methods the authors revealed that the degree of inflammatory reaction, the intensity of lymphomacrophagial infiltration were considerably more expressed at the site of lens transplantation, i.e.-in the peritoneum.

At the same time, even in patient with senile non-complicated cataract the surgery-related trauma might provoke disturbance of ACAID function, because as a response to baring of eye tunics antigenic determinants there occurrs the regional autoimmune process. The post-surgery period in those patients and the performed corrective therapy in the prevailing majority of cases proceed without complications; this latter allows us considering that the traumatic injury occurring in the course of surgery intervention is fraught with development of *in situ* immunopathological disorders, which are of exceptionally temporary, transient character.

3. Cortisol-and prolactin-dependent mechanisms responsible for formation and abolition of the ACAID function

In current scientific publications there is only scarce evidence according to which in certain eye tunics the cells of epithelial genesis and fibroblastic line – apart from their main function – also possess the hormone-producing property to synthesize cortisol (Chong A., Aw S., 1986). Due to experimental studies (Southern A. et al., 1979), the presence of receptors to glucocorticoids in cells of ciliary body and the cornea was established, whereas translocation of glucocorticoids from the surface towards the cell nuclei occurred during a rather short period of time. It is reasonable to mention another circumstance of no less importance. The authors failed to reveal similar mechanism of reception and translocation, which is characteristic for glucocorticoids, as related to a wide range of hormones: testosterone, estradiol, progesterone, T_3 and T_4. It was established that biological effects of cortisol are realized within the sclera, cornea, ciliary body and, mostly important, in the lens capsule (Kasavina B. et al., 1977). According to S. Rauz and associates (2001; 2003), cortisol is secreted in the ciliary body of both actually healthy contingent and in patients with the primary open-angle glaucoma.

Currently, the opinion dominates that the fundamental function of cortisol in eye tunics is sustaining the optimal level of intraocular pressure. Furthermore, this function has a dual realization: through regulation of the regional immune homeostasis and potentiating the adrenergic effect towards the system of vascularization in specific eye tunics (Jacob E. et al., 1996; Rauz S. et al., 2001).

Nowadays, the role of prolactin appears more disputable. At cataracts and uveitides the presence of prolactin was revealed in the anterior chamber of the eye (Pleyer U. et al., 1991). Efforts were done to interpret biological effects of prolactin within the specific eye structures functioning. In particular, S. Duenas and co-workers (2004) allow for the possibility of intraocular synthesis of prolactin within the blood vessels of retina. At retinopathies, the mentioned authors revealed a high level of prolactin in the anterior chamber of the eye. It is important to emphasize that authors did not reveal any correlation dependence between prolactin levels in the anterior chamber of the eye and in blood serum. Despite the fact that of prolactin revealment in tunics and liquid media of the eye, the role of this hormone in the integrative activity of the eye remains unstudied.

To our mind, the role of in situ produced hormones, cortisol and prolactin, in eye tissues is more versatile and is far beyond the functions ensuring processes of ion exchange and intraocular pressure regulation.

We propose a hypothesis according to which cortisol and prolactin play an important role in establishment of ACAID function through modulation of immunological processes in the aspects of both activation and/or inhibition of specific T-and B-populations and also targeted synthesis of cytokines with adaptogenic spectrum of action.

The mentioned supposition is confirmed by literary data, according to which in the mammalian organism cortisol and prolactin possess immunomodulatory functions. In particular, it is established that prolactin and cortisol at physiological concentrations maintain the stability of the immune homeostasis. However, at high concentrations cortisol acts as a factor that selectively inhibits the activity of T-killer and T-helper cytotoxic lymphocytes (Pazirandeh A. et al., 2002; Lindeman D., Racke K., 2003; Visser J. et al., 2003), while prolactin activates a number of cytokines (IL-I, VI, TNF, as well as γ-IFN in central and periphery organs of immunogenesis (Matera L., 1986; Yarilin A., Belyakov I., 1996). Furthermore, prolactin – in a dose dependent mode – activates B-lympocytic population (Berczi I. et al., 1981; McMurrey R. et al., 1991; Lahat N. et al., 1993).

As shown by the results of our earlier performed immune enzyme assays (Zilfyan A., 2009; 2012; 2013) (Table 3) in the aqueous humor of patients with complicated cataracts (cataract occurring on the background of primary open-angle and pseudoexfoliative glaucoma and cataract occurring on the background of preceding trauma) the level of cortisol significantly increased as compared to control.

The highest indices were recorded by us in aqueous humor of the III group patients: at cataracts occurring on the background of pseudoexfoliative glaucoma.

Until present it was considered to be established that the main function of cortisol in the eye tunics was to regulate the intraocular pressure (Jacob E. et al., 1996; Rauz S. et al., 2001). At the same time, due to results obtained, a supposition might be done: the revealed high concen-

Study groups (n=40)	Cortisol content					
	aqueous humor			blood serum		
	M	*m*	*p*	*M*	*m*	*p*
I	12.90	± 0.64		56.90	±4.15	
II	23.38	±1.46	<0.0005	64.84	±7.28	<0.25
III	30.4	±1.56	<0.0005	50.70	±6.91	<0.25
IV	14.10	±0.61	*<0.1*	115.60	±16.88	<0.005
V	9.70	±2.69	<0.25	70.50	±10.41	<0.25
VI	14.05	±0.69	<0.25	68.60	±8.13	<0.25

Notes: *M* – mean; *m* – standard error of mean; *p* – confidence interval (indices of complicated cataracts as related to senile cataracts).

Table 3. The content of cortisol (*pg/ml*) in blood serum and aqueous humor of patients with senile and *complicated cataracts.*

trations of cortisol in the aqueous humor of patients from study groups II, VI and, especially, from group III might produce alterative (damaging) action towards immunocompetent cells of the anterior chamber of the eye, because the cytotoxic effect of cortisol immunocompetent cells of organs of immunogenesis and blood is considered to be established long ago (Bell P., Munck A., 1973; Carr D., Blalock J. et al., 1989). Moreover, we considered it reasonable to the interpret data obtained on shifts of cortisol content in aqueous humor of patients with cataracts taking into account rather informative evidence on dose-dependent impact of cortisol towards the functional state of lymphocytic populations (Pazirandeh A. et al., 2002). The authors studied the direct hormonal influence of endogenous levels of glucocorticoids to thymocytes and peripheral T-lymphocytic subpopulations in transgenic mice with the altered sensitivity to glucocorticoids. According to mentioned researchers, 2-fold increase of sensitivity to glucocorticoids in the organism of transgenic mice was accompanied with the profound alterative changes in thymocytes followed by a marked increase in number of all T-lymphocytic subpopulations in the cortical layer of thymus.

To our mind, it is not ruled out that in mechanisms of ACAID formation and functioning precisely similar cortisol-dependent mechanism of reactions balanced functioning – simultaneously ensuring processes of proliferation and apoptosis of T-lymphocytic subpopulations in tunics and anterior chamber of an eye – is engaged.

At the same time, we cannot exclude that cortisol high concentrations recorded by us in the aqueous humor of patients from study groups II, III and VI might be the provoking factor in the aspect of an abrupt enhancement of apoptosis processes in the immunocompetent cells of eye tunics and the cells of inflammatory reaction in the anterior chamber of the eye.

As seen in studies performed by our group a conclusion might be drawn that in organisms of mammals cortisol plays an important role in processes promoting ACAID functioning (Zilfyan A., 2009; Zilfyan A.A., Zilfyan A.V., 2013).

Moreover, at complicated cataracts (groups II, III and IV), especially at cataracts occurring on the background of the open-angle and pseudoexfoliative glaucoma, we should assign to cortisol an important role in mechanisms infringing the normal course of immunological reactions in tunics and the anterior chamber of an eye ensuring ACAID – in the aspect of abolishing the processes promoting *in situ* active and immunological tolerance.

Significant shifts were also observed on the part of prolactin determined in the aqueous humor of patients with complicated cataracts. In particular, in the aqueous humor of patients with complicated cataracts (study groups II, III and VI) relatively high level of prolactin was recorded. In the remaining patients with complicated cataracts (study groups IV, V) indices of prolactin were similar to those determined in aqueous humor of patients with senile cataracts (Table 4).

Study groups (n=40)	Prolactin content					
	aqueous humor			blood serum		
	M	*m*	*p*	*M*	*m*	*p*
I	0.34	±0.045		7.0	±3.6	
II	1.10	±0.08	<0.0005	9.5	±1.6	<0.10
III	2.23	±0.22	<0.0005	9.1	±2.2	<0.25
IV	0.300	±0.046	*<0.40*	7.50	±0.57	<0.25
V	0.49	±0.09	<0.10	6.40	±1.45	<0.40
VI	14.05	±0.07	*p*<0.0005	10.90	±3.66	<0.25

Notes: *M* – mean; *m* – standard error of mean; *p* – confidence interval (indices of complicated cataracts as related to senile cataracts).

Table 4. The content of prolactin (*ng/ml*) in aqueous humor and blood serum of patients with senile and complicated cataracts.

In the available literature the evidence on the role of prolactin in mechanisms of ACAID formation is lacking.

At the same time it is known that the organism of mammals prolactin possesses a profound stimulant action towards the specific subpopulations of lymphocytes and the cells of monocyte and lymphocyte line – in the aspect of synthesizing a number of immunocytokines: tumor necrosis factor alpha,-beta ($TNF_{\alpha,\beta}$), interleukins-IL-I, IL-II, IL-VI and γ-interferon. It is known that at senile and complicated cataracts relatively high levels of some pro-and anti-inflammatory cytokines (TNF, IL-I, IL-II, IL-IV, IL-VI, IL-X) are determined in the aqueous humor (Stambuk N. et al., 1994; Slepova O.S. et al., 1998; Patel J. et al., 2006; Sawada H., et al., 2010).

In consideration of the existing immune endocrine interrelations of prolactin and proinflammatory cytokines we can suppose that relatively high prolactin concentrations revealed by us in the aqueous humor of study groups II and III patients might be the cause of the enhanced synthesis of proinflammatory cytokines by immonocompetent cells of some eye tunics and cells of lymphocyte-monocyte line localized in the aqueous humor. This is one of the probable prolactin-dependent mechanisms underlying infringement of ACAID function at complicated cataracts.

Under conditions of pathology, i.e. at complicated cataracts, in the anterior chamber of the eye there might be also engaged another prolactin-dependent mechanism bringing to ACAID abolition. It is not excluded that prolactin acts as a co-factor participating in activation of *in situ* reaction of humoral immunity through the selective effect to B-cellular populations of eye tunics and the inflammatory exudates of the anterior chamber of the eye. Apparently, under conditions of increased prolactin content in the aqueous humor with precedent baring of antigenic determinants of eye tunics, prolactin in its turn stimulates the antigen-dependent function of B-lymphocyte populations. In favour of the proposed supposition also signify rather informative literary data depicting a direct dose-dependent stimulant effect of prolactin to the B-lymphocyte populations (Berczi I. et al., 1981; McMurray R. et al., 1991; Lahat N. et al., 1993).

On the base of our own findings and comparing them with the available scientific data on the role of prolactin in the immunological processes and its revealment in the anterior chamber of the eyes the following conclusion might be drawn. Prolactin-dependent mechanisms, which, on the one hand, stimulate the local synthesis of proinflammatory cytokines and, on the other hand, activate processes of *in situ* B-lymphocyte populations proliferation and thus worsen the course of an earlier developed autoimmune process in post-barrier tunics and the anterior chamber of the eye, are also engaged in mechanisms of ACAID abolition at complicated cataracts.

4. Fibronectin and prostaglandins E_2-dependent mechanisms responsible for abolition of reactions promoting the ACAID function

In our previous studies (Zilfyan A., 2009; 2012) data were presented on the important role of fibronectin and PgE_2 produced in the eye tunics regarding the mechanisms of disorders in the drainage function of the trabecular meshwork and the increase of intraocular pressure at complicated cataracts: cataracts occurring on the background of primary open-angle and pseudoexfoliative glaucoma.

At the same time, till present, the role of fibronectin and prostaglandins E_2 (PgE_2) at senile non-complicated cataract and complicated cataracts never became the subject of a special investigation.

Only scarce evidence is available that fibronectin is produced by keratocytes of the cornea, ciliary body and cells of the trabecular meshwork of the eye (Tripathi B., et al., 2004; Hindman

H. et al., 2010; Wordinger R.J. et al., 2007). The enhanced synthesis of fibronectin in the mentioned eye tunics might bring to activation of fibroplastic processes finally terminating in fibrosis of the eye tunics, including the lens. However, the role of fibronectin in processes of ACAID function formation and abolition is not studied. At the same time it is considered to be established that fibronectin might enhance phagocytosis; on the surface of macrophages there are receptors to fibronectin (Kuznik B. et al., 1989). Therefore, it is not excluded that fibronectin at a number of eye diseases might play a leading role in activation of macrophages of the eye tunics and the anterior chamber of the eye: both in the aspect of phagocytosis and synthesis of pro-inflammatory cytokines: interleukin-I (IL-I) and tumor necrosis factors alpha and beta (TNF-$_{\alpha,\beta}$) (Slepova O. et al., 1998; Sawada H. et al., 2010).

As demonstrated by our results of the performed immune enzyme assays, in patients of the study group II, i.e. at cataracts occurring on the background of primary open-angle and pseudoexfoliative glaucoma, relatively high indices of fibronectin were revealed in the aqueous humor (Table 5).

Study groups (n=40)	**Fibronectin content**		
	M	*m*	*p*
I	11.26	± 0.099	
II	20.71	±2.37	<0.005
III	33.83	±5.97	<0.005
IV	13.43	±2.57	*<0.25*
V	12.76	±1.14	*<0.25*
VI	12.04	±1.12	<0.40

Notes: *M* – mean; *m* – standard error of mean; *p* – confidence interval (indices of complicated cataracts as related to senile cataracts).

Table 5. The content of fibronectin (*ng/ml*) in the aqueous humor of patients with senile and complicated cataracts.

The highest indices of the cytokine were recorded by us in the aqueous humor of patients with cataract occurring on the background of pseudoexfoliative glaucoma (as compared to indices of the control group).

In all other study groups of patients with complicated cataracts low indices of fibronectin were determined in the aqueous humor; these indices were similar to those recorded in the aqueous humor of patients with senile cataracts.

Let us consider the role of fibronectin in processes of ACAID function formation and abolition. It is considered to be established that macrophages of eye tunics and aqueous humor play a role of in processes of pro-and anti-inflammatory cytokines synthesis; the balanced synthesis of mentioned cytokines ensures the normal course of reactions supporting ACAID.

Study groups (n=40)	Prostaglandins E_2 content		
	M	*m*	*p*
I	43.05	± 4.13	
II	66.11	±7.40	<0.01
III	76.64	±7.78	<0.005
IV	48.03	±3.02	*<0.25*
V	49.60	±6.37	*<0.25*
VI	58.96	±2.81	<0.25

Notes: *M* – mean; *m* – standard error of mean; *p* – confidence interval (indices of complicated cataracts as related to senile cataracts).

Table 6. Shifts in content of PgE_2 (*pg/ml*) in the aqueous humor of patients with senile and complicated cataracts.

As already mentioned by us earlier, at a number of diseases, including the complicated cataracts, this balance is broken and macrophages begin to produce immunocytokines – primarily of the proinflammatory – character: TNF_2 and IL I. Therefore, a role of no less importance should be assigned to macrophages in processes of abolishing reactions responsible for ACAID function.

At the same time, it is considered to be established that fibronectin has an ability to activate the cytokine function of macrophages. Hence, it is not excluded that at complicated cataracts fibronectin-dependent mechanisms are engaged in mechanisms of ACAID functions infringement; specified mechanisms are realized at the level of the regional monocyte-macrophageal system.

In our further research the shifts in PgE_2content in the aqueous humor of patients with senile and complicated cataracts were studied. There is only rather scarce literature on synthesis of prostaglandins in eye tunics. The local synthesis of prostaglandins was revealed only in epithelial cells of the lens capsule and was proved by experiments of O. Nishi and co-workers (1982), who performed model *in vitro* tests; in case of cataract surgery the isolated lens was placed in the incubation medium. Alongside with incubation time increase the content of prostaglandins in the incubation medium markedly increased. At the same time, in some eye tunics – the ciliary body, retina, sclera and trabecular meshwork of the anterior chamber angle receptors to PgE_2 were identified (Toris C. et al., 2008). The role of PgE_2 in maintaining the drainage function is widely discussed (Podos S. et al., 1972).

However, the role of PgE_2 in mechanisms of ACAID formation and infringement is almost not investigated. As shown by results of our own studies, the level of PgE_2 in aqueous humor of patients from study groups II, III and VI markedly increased as compared to the level of PgE_2 in the aqueous humor of the control group patients (Table 6).

The highest values were observed in aqueous humor of patients with cataract on the background of pseudoexfoliative glaucoma. In all other groups of complicated cataracts low indices were recorded in the aqueous humor; these indices were similar to those determined in aqueous humor of the control group patients. The high level of PgE_2 at complicated cataracts (study groups II, III, VI) might be considered as a factor bringing to disorder of the eye trabecular meshwork drainage function; moreover that on its cells receptors to PgE_2 were revealed. Despite the presence of receptors to PgE_2 in different eye tunics, epithelial cells of the lens capsule are the only possible source of PgE_2 local synthesis. Therefore, it is not ruled out that in complicated cataracts the lens cells are engaged in an enhanced synthesis of E_2 group prostaglandins, which might influence the course and duration of reactions promoting abolition of the ACAID function.

Our supposition is also grounded by data of scientific publications dealing with the functional activity of PgE_2 towards the numerous integrative systems of the organism, including the immune system. In particular, it is considered to be established long ago, that PgE_2 inhibit the synthesis of cytotoxic lymphocytes: T-suppressor and T-killer lymphocyte subpopulations. Hence, it is not excluded, that the high level of PgE_2 in the aqueous humor of patients with complicated cataracts (study groups II, III and VI) might be considered as a factor producing immunosuppressive action to cytotoxic lymphocytes localized in eye tunics and the aqueous humor; the latter is fraught with abolishing the reactions responsible for *in situ* abolition of ACAID function.

This is the precise reason for formation of "favourable" conditions for *in situ* intensification of autoimmune reactions in the post-surgery period under conditions of infringed integrity of the lens capsule and baring of its antigenic determinants; moreover, at complicated cataracts the immune stimulant mechanisms aimed at activation of T-cytotoxic lymphocytes is infringed already at the pre-surgery stage.

The investigation of E.L. Nelson (1976) also signified to the important role of prostaglandins in induction of local inflammatory processes. According to author, different traumatic injuries of the eye are followed with the enhanced synthesis of E_2 and $F_{2\alpha}$ in the iris and other eye tissues, as a result of which the content of mentioned prostaglandins in the aqueous humor is significantly increased. The enhancement of mentioned processes is accompanied with vasodilatation, increased permeability of micro-vessels, and increased protein content in the aqueous humor.

Apart from this, the mentioned author proposed a supposition, according to which at traumatic injuries of the eye leucocytes of inflammatory exudates in the aqueous humor might serve as a source of prostaglandins synthesis.

Furthermore, as considered by the authors, the cascade of molecular and cellular processes at induction of inflammatory process in eye tunics is eventually terminated by the reaction that, to a considerable degree, is conditioned by prostaglandins. On the other hand, the high level of PgE_2 in the aqueous humor, to a known extent, reflects *in situ* formation of protective-adaptive mechanisms – in the aspect of correlation of synthesis processes of specific pro-inflammatory cytokines produced in the post-barrier tunics of the eye as well.

It is a common knowledge that prostaglandins of E and F group inhibit the synthesis of IL I in macrophages and leucocytes. Apparently, the similar mechanism is engaged in post-barrier eye tunics both at norm and in case of some eye diseases. The following fact signifies in favour of the latter circumstance: at endotoxin-induced experimental uveitis in rabbit despite the expressed inflammatory reaction in post-barrier eye tunics the level of IL-I in the aqueous humor did not increase (Kulkarni P.S., 1991). It is not excluded that PgE_2 serve as a factor preventing the increase of IL-I and IL-II production in immunocompetent cells.

5. The role of transforming growth factor in pathogenesis of cataracts and glaucomas

Nowadays rather informative evidence is available on the role of $TGF_{\beta\text{-}2}$ in the mechanisms of immunological tolerance activation at senile and complicated cataracts. High regional immunological tolerance in eye tunics is ensured through the enhanced $TGF_{\beta\text{-}2}$ synthesis by the cells of eye tunics: ciliary body, cornea, and retina (Stefan C. et al., 2008; Dawes L. et al., 2009; Hindman H. et al., 2010; Pattabiraman P., Rao P., 2010).

It is established that the active immunological tolerance at senile non-complicated cataracts is targeted at activation of T-helper and T-suppressor subpopulations in immune competent cells of the eye; these latter play an important role in prevention of autoimmune reactions aimed to produce antibodies against the lens tissues (Streilein J. et al., 1992; Wilbanks G. et al., 1992).

In the most relief mode the entire cascade of immunological shifts is presented in the aqueous humor of patients with senile and complicated cataracts, as a result of which currently the aqueous humor is considered as a rather informative bio-object characterizing the course of immunological reactions responsible for anterior chamber associated immune deviation (ACAID) formation.

In the specified aspect there are rather informative scientific publications, according to which at senile non-complicated cataracts during the post-surgery period is engaged the similar $TGF_{\beta\text{-}2}$-dependent mechanism that underlies the suppresson of local humoral immunity reactions through *in situ* activation of cytotoxic lymphocytes (Fleenor D. et al., 2006; Streilein J. et al., 1992).

At the same time our own investigation (Zilfyan A., 2009) allowed establishing that unlike senile non-complicated cataracts occurring on the background of glaucoma and pseudoexfoliative syndrome already in the pre-surgery period in eye tunics there originated immunopathological disorders manifested as activation of reactions responsible for antibody formation (high level of CD_4 and IgG in the aqueous humor – on the background of a marked decrease in CD_8 level).

Data obtained signify in favour of the fact, according to which $TGF_{\beta\text{-}2}$-dependent mechanism engaged in ACAID formation is actually not the single one at complicated cataracts (Zilfyan A.A., Zilfyan A.V., 2013).

Thus, our studies revealed that at complicated cataracts in the aqueous humor there is a marked increase of cortisol, prolactin and PgE_2 (Zilfyan A., 2009; 2012). Moreover, high concentrations of mentioned hormones and PgE_2 are conditioned by their "non-arrival" from the periphery (as a result of increase in hematoophthalmic barrier permeability), or most likely, as a result of the enhanced synthesis in the eye tunics.

According to the proposed concept, relatively high concentrations of the above-mentioned biologically active compounds might act as endogenous factors activating *in situ* reactions of humoral immunity, because their selective influence towards the immune competent cells T-helpers and B-cellular populations is considered to be established (Goodwin J., Ceuppens J., 1983; McMurray R. et al., 1991; Lahat N. et al., 1993;).

Thus, in cases of complicated cataracts we revealed earlier unknown mediatory mechanisms engaged in launching the humoral immunity reactions, which apart the surgery-related trauma produce rather unfavourable impacts to the course of the regional pathological process.

In the light of data thus obtained, the role of $TGF_{\beta-2}$ in glaucomatous pathogenesis should be considered from the alternative standpoint. In particular, $TGF_{\beta-2}$ produced in the cornea and the ciliary body stimulates *in situ* synthesis of insulin-like growth factor-1 (IGF-1) and fibronectin, i.e. precisely those cytokines the excessive concentrations of which are considered as *provoking* factors hindering the normal outflow of the aqueous humor; this latter is fraught with the increase of aqueous humor in glaucoma.

Our previous studies also signify to the existence / presence of the similar $TGF_{\beta-2}$-dependent mechanism (Zilfyan A., 2013); it was demonstrated that at complicated cataracts on the background of glaucoma and pseudoexfoliative syndrome high concentrations of fibronectin and IGF-1 are determined in the aqueous humor (compared to those recorded in the aqueous humor of patients with senile non-complicated cataract).

Hence, the role of $TGF_{\beta-2}$ in pathogenesis of cataracts and glaucomas is far from being unambiguous. In particular, on the one hand, in senile non-complicated cataract $TGF_{\beta-2}$ modulates in the eye tunics processes of active immune tolerance aimed at prevention of autoimmune aggression against the antigenic determinants of the lens; on the other hand,-the same cytokine produced a rather unfavourable impact to the course and duration of glaucomas through its direct and/or indirect impact to the processes of fibronectin and IGF-1 enhanced synthesis in the trabecular meshwork of the eye. The excessive accumulation of both cytokines brings to impaired function of the eye anterior chamber trabecular meshwork, thus eventually accompanied by the increase of intraocular pressure.

On the basis of studies performed, within the entire context of available published data, from the qualitatively new positions we should consider the established, earlier unknown, $TGF_{\beta-2}$-independent hormonal mediatory mechanisms underlying the abolition of reactions responsible for ACAID formation and the increase of intraocular pressure at complicated cataracts.

6. Conclusion

Currently existing term "immune privilege of an eye" is mostly associated with evolutionary secured mechanisms, which ensure the regional immune homeostasis in eye tunics and in the eye liquid media both at norm and pathology. In particular, at cataracts in some eye tunics there are engaged mechanisms promoting the "active immunological tolerance" that is selectively targeted against the "bared" (revealed) antigenic determinants of the lens tissues. In modern ophthalmology the symptom complex of immune reactions occurring in eye tunics is defined as "anterior chamber associated immune deviation – ACAID".

Hence, it is considered to be proved that at senile non-complicated cataracts in the post-surgery period there are *in situ* activated immune processes, which manifest as activation of cytotoxic lymphocytes (T-suppressors and T-killers) due to which the "active immunological tolerance" is formed averting the processes of autoimmune aggression against the bared antigenic tissues of the lens.

Based on the evidence of available modern literature and our own research findings new earlier unknown hormonal mediatory mechanisms appear to the proscenium of the stage; those mechanisms at complicated cataracts are responsible for abolition of reactions promoting the ACAID function.

Thereupon, from qualitatively new positions should be considered the role of cortisol, prolactin fibronectin, $TGF_{\beta\text{-}2}$ and PgE_2, which are produced in specific eye tunics, in mechanisms of *in situ* realization of the immune reactions responsible for ACAID formation and abolition. It should be emphasized that all the above-mentioned biologically active substances in case of complicated cataracts (cataracts on the background of anterior open-angle glaucoma and pseudoexfoliative glaucoma) act as "provoking" factors, which take an active part in both impairment of the eye trabecular meshwork drainage function and the increase of intraocular pressure.

At the same time, in complicated cataracts the specified factors might take an active part in abolishing the reactions providing the "active immunological tolerance" through *in situ* activity of cytotoxic lymphocytes and activation of autoimmune processes targeted against the antigenic determinants of the eye tissues and tunics.

Based on the analysis of the available literature and the presented own studies we consider it purposeful to present to the attention of the readers the main regional immune and hormonal-mediatory mechanisms responsible for ACAID formation and abolition in senile and complicated cataracts also depicting them in detail as summary Schemes 1 and 2.

Immune and hormonal-mediatory factors engaged in ACAID formation at non-complicated cataracts are presented as Scheme 1.

During the surgery intervention for phacoemulsification of cataract (PhEC) there occurs baring of antigenic determinants of the lens tissues (BADLT). According to available evidence of scientific publications, 3 mechanisms are engaged in ACAID formation.

The first mechanism is associated with the activation of $TGF_{\beta\text{-}2}$ synthesis in the eye cornea, ciliary body and retina as a result of which there occurs stimulation of cytotoxic lymphocytes (T-ct).

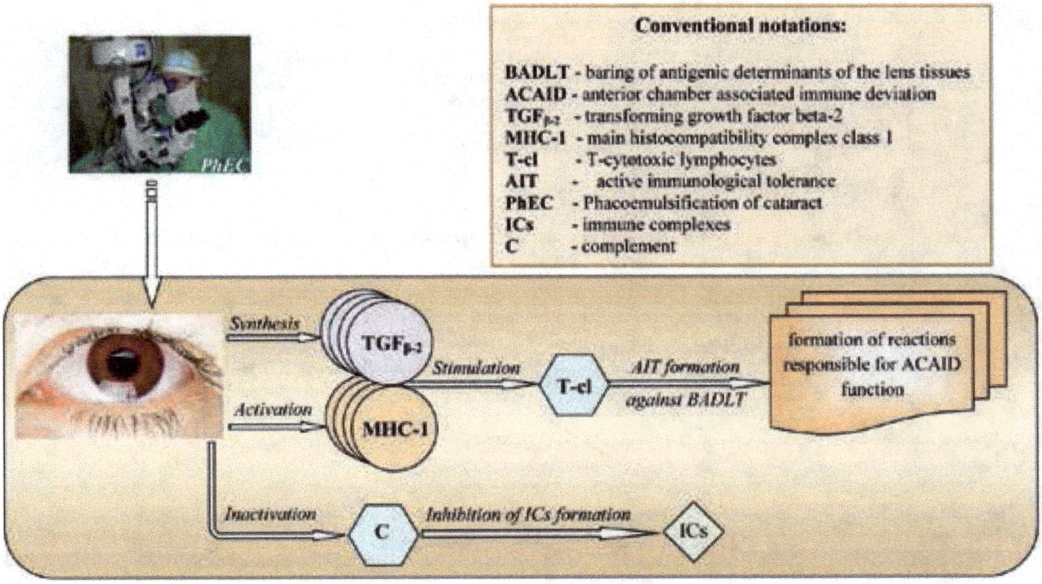

Scheme 1. Regional immune andmediatory mechanisms responsible for ACAID function.

As a result of the targeted stimulation of T-suppressor and T-killer subpopulations there occurs an active immunological tolerance (AIT) against the bared antigenic determinants of lens tissues, in particular through inhibition of activity in T-helper subpopulation of lymphocytes.

The second mechanism is associated with *in situ* activation of the main histocompatibility complex class 1 (MHC-1) with the subsequent activation of T-killer subpopulations.

The third mechanism is associated with *in situ* inactivation of the complement (C); therefore, the formation of immune complexes (IC) does not occur.

As a result, one of the possible mechanisms of autoaggression is excluded through deposition of the immune complexes on the lens tissues followed by their subsequent impairment.

According to the bulk of scientific data, similar mechanism is engaged in the post-surgery period at senile non-complicated cataracts.

From the result of our investigations we do not exclude that ACAID function is also engaged in cataracts occurring on the background of diabetes mellitus and arterial hypertension, because in both cases the recovery process was without complications, even without the aseptic autoimmune iridocyclitis.

Thus performed, our studies allowed establishing that at specific types of complicated cataracts (cataract on the background of primary open-angle and pseudoexfoliative glaucoma) regional immune mechanisms responsible for ACAID function were impaired (Scheme 2).

Thus, in both cases after the performed phacoemulsification of cataract (PhEC) and baring of antigenic determinants of the lens tissues (BADLT) the aqueous humor levels of cortisol (Cor)

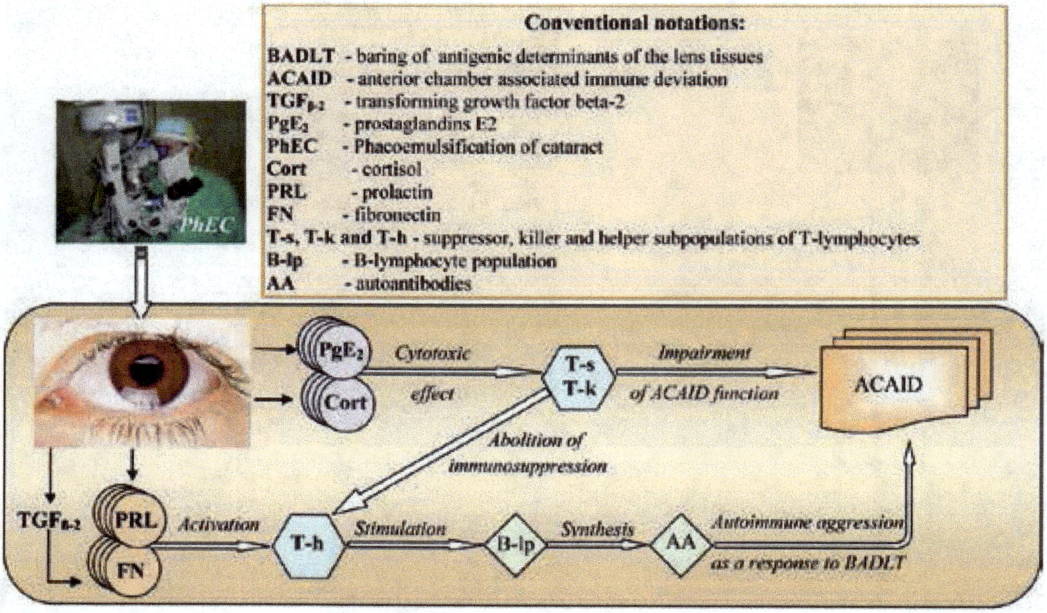

Scheme 2. Regional immune and hormonal mediatory mechanisms responsible for abolishing the ACAID function at complicated cataracts.

and PgE_2 increased. Both factors had unidirectional cytotoxic action towards the specific lymphocytic subpopulations – T-suppressors and T-killers (T-s, T-k). Hence, there occurred the abolition of the immunosuppressive action of those latter to the T-helper subpopulation of lymphocytes (T-h). Against this background we recorded high concentrations of prolactin (PRL) and fibronectin (FN) in the aqueous humor. The FN high level was conditioned by the stimulant influence of transforming growth factor beta-2 ($TGF_{\beta\text{-}2}$) towards the eye cornea cells and the trabecular meshwork. Both factors, prolactin (PRL) and fibronectin (FN), activate T-helper subpopulation of lymphocytes (T-h). As a result of surgery-related impairment of the lens tissues on the background of cytotoxic lymphocytes-abolished suppression there occurs stimulation of T-helper subpopulation that is fraught with formation of autoantibodies (AA) against the impaired tissues of lens followed with their autoimmunoaggrression towards both impaired and "structurally" preserved tissues of lens.

As a rule, such a complication as aseptic autoimmune iridocyclitis developed in the specified contingent of patients during the post-surgery period.

Undoubtedly, the presented Schemes 1 and 2 are not ultimate; moreover, they are not comprehensive. These Schemes should be supplemented (enriched) with new evidence on the role of earlier unknown biologically active substances of immune, hormonal, mediatory genesis, which are produced in eye tunics, in formation of in situ reactions responsible for formation and abolition of the ACAID function.

Author details

Artashes A. Zilfyan[1] and Arto V. Zilfyan[2*]

*Address all correspondence to: namj@ysmu.am

1 Scientific-Research Center, Yerevan State Medical University, Yerevan, Armenia

2 "Shengavit" Medical Center, Yerevan, Armenia

References

[1] Abrahamian A., Xi M., Donnelly J., Rockey J. Effect of interferon-gamma on the expression of transforming growth factor-beta by human corneal fibroblasts: role in corneal immunoseclusion. J. Interferon Cytokine Res. 1995; 15(4): 323-330.

[2] Bakunowicz L., Lazarczyk A., Moniuszko T. et al. Levels of selected cytokines in aqueous humor of patients with cataract extraction. Klin. Oczna. 1997; 99(4): 235-237.

[3] Bell P., Munck A. Steroid-binding properties and stabilization of cytoplasmic glucocorticoid receptors from rat thymus cells. Biochem. J. 1973; 136(1): 97-107.

[4] Berczi I., Nagy E., Kovacs K., Horvath E. Regulation of humoral immunity in rats by pituitary hormones. Acta Endocrinol. Copenhagen. 1981: 98: 506-513.

[5] Camelo S., Kezic J., McMenamin P. Anterior chamber-associated immune deviation: a review of the anatomical evidence for the afferent arm of this unusual experimental model of ocular immune responses. Clin. Exper. Ophthalmol. 2005; 33(4): 426-432.

[6] Carr D., Blalock J. A molecular basis for intersystem communication between the immune and neuroendocrine systems. Int. Rev. Immunol. 1989; 4(3): 213-228.

[7] Chong A., Aw S. Postmortem endocrine levels in the vitreous humor. Ann. Acad. Med. Singapore. 1986; 15 (4): 606-609.

[8] Cinatl J., Blaheta R., Bittoova M., Scholz M., Margraf S., Vogel J., Cinatl J., Deorr H. Decreased neutrophil adhesion to human cytomegalovirus-infected retinal pigment epithelial cells is mediated by virus-induced up-regulation of Fas ligand independent of neutrophil apoptosis. J. Immunol. 2000; 165(8): 4405-4413.

[9] D'Orazio T., Niederkorn J. The nature of antigen in the eye has a profound effect on the cytoki milieu and resultant immune response. Eur. J. Immunnol. 1998; 28(5): 1544-1553.

[10] Dawes L.J., Sleeman M.A., Anderson I.K., Reddan J.R., Wormstone I.M. TGFbeta/Smad4-dependent and-independent regulation of human lens epithelial cells. Invest. Ophthalmol. Vis. Sci. 2009 Nov; 50(11): 5318-5327. Epub 2009 Jun 10.

[11] Duenas Z., Rivera J., Quiroz-Mercado H., Aranda J., Macotela Y., Montes de Oca P., Lopez-Barrera F., Nava G., Guerrero J., Suarez A., De Regil M., Martinez de la Escalera G., Clapp C. Prolactin in eyes of patients with retinopathy of prematurity: implications for vascular regression. Invest. Ophthalmol. Vis. Sci. 2004; 45(7): 2049-2055.

[12] Fleenor D., Shepard A., Hellberg P., Jacobson N., Pang I., Clark A. TGFbeta2-induced changes in human trabecular meshwork: implications for intraocular pressure. Invest. Ophthalmol. Vis. Sci. 2006: 47(1): 226-234.

[13] Fu T., Yang P., Huang X., Zhou H., Li F., Huang Q. Preventive effect of anterior chamber associated immune deviation on endotoxin-induced uveitis. Zhonghua Yi Xue Za Zhi. 2004; 84(18): 1562-1566.

[14] Goodwin J.S., Ceuppens J. Regulation of the immune response by prostaglandins. J. Clin. Immunol. 1983; 3(4): 295-315.

[15] Hindman H.B., Swanton J.N., Phipps R.P., Sime P.J., Huxlin K.R. Differences in the TGF-{beta}1-induced profibrotic response of anterior and posterior corneal keratocytes in vitro. Invest. Ophthalmol. Vis. Sci. 2010 Apr; 51(4): 1935-1942. Epub 2009 Nov 11.

[16] Jacob E., FitzSimon J., Brubaker R. Combined corticosteroid and catecholamine stimulation of aqueous humor flow. Ophthalmology. 1996; 103: 1303-1308.

[17] Kasavina B., Ukhina T., Churakova T. Distribution of labeled cortisol in the tissues and media of the eye. Bull. Exp. Biol. Med. 1977; 83: 401-402.

[18] Kawakami M., Nakata J., Ohguro N., Yoshihara S., Inoue T., Tatekawa T., Ikegame K., Oka Y., Kawase I., Ogawa H. A case of immune recovery vitritis induced by donor leukocyte infusion for the treatment of cytomegalovirus retinitis. Eur. J. Haematol. 2005; 75(4): 352-354.

[19] Kitaichi N., Namba K., Taylor A. Inducible immune regulation following autoimmune disease in the immune-privileged eye. J. Leukoc. Biol. 2005; 77(4): 496-502.

[20] Kulkarni P.S. The role of endogenous eicosanoids in rabbit-intraocular inflammation. J. Ocul. Pharmacol. 1991; 7(3): 227-241.

[21] Kuznik B., Vasiliev N., Zybikov N. [Immunogenesis, homeostasis and non-specific resistance of the organism][published in Russian]. Moscow. Medicina ("Medicine" Publishers). 1989. 320p.

[22] Lahat N., Shitler R., Zlotnik A.Y., Merin G. Early IL-2/sIL-2R surge following surgery leads to temporary immune refractoriness. Clinical and Experim. Immun. 1993 June; 92(3): 482-486.

[23] Lightman S., Towler H. Immunopathology and altered immunity in posterior uveitis in man: a review. Curr. Eye Res. 1992; 11(Suppl.): 11-15.

[24] Lindemann D., Racke K. Glucocorticoid inhibition of interleukin-4 (IL-4) and interleukin-13 (IL-13) induced up-regulation of arginase in rat airway fibroblasts. Naunyn Schmiedebergs Arch. Pharmacol. 2003; 368(6): 546-550.

[25] Martin W., Egan R., Stevens J., Woodward J.G. Lens-specific expression of a major histocompatibility complex class I molecule disrupts normal lens development and induces cataracts in transgenic mice. Invest. Ophthalmol. Vis. Sci. 1995; 36(6): 1144-1154.

[26] Matera L. Endocrine, paracrine and autocrine actions of prolactin on immune cells. Life Sci. 1986; 59(8): 593-614.

[27] McMurray R., Keisler D., Kanuckel K., Izui S., Walker S.E. Prolactin influences autoimmune disease activity in the female B/W mouse. J. Immunol. 1991; 147: 3780-3787.

[28] Muhaya M., Calder V., Towler H. et al. Characterization of phenotype and cytokine profiles of T-cell lines derived from vitreous humor in ocular inflammation in man. Clin. Exp. Immunol. 1999; 116(3): 410-414.

[29] Murray P., Hoekzema R., Luyendijk L., Konings S., Kijlstra A. Analysis of aqueous humor immunoglobulin G in uveitis by enzyme-linked immunosorbent assay, isoelectric focusing, and immunoblotting. Invest. Ophthalmol. Vis. Sci. 1990: 31(10): 2129-2135.

[30] Nelson E.L. Prostaglandins and inflammation in the eye. Review. Mod. Probl Ophthalmol. 1976; 16: 125-130.

[31] Nishi O., Nishi K., Imanishi M. Synthesis of interleukin-1 and prostaglandin E2 by lens epithelial cells of human cataracts. Br. J. Ophthalmol. 1982; 76: 338-341.

[32] Orge Y., Gungor S. Immunological etiopathogenesis of senile and complicated cataract. Microbiol Bul. 1984; 18(3): 145-153.

[33] Patel J.I., Hykin P.G., Cree I.A. Diabetic cataract removal: postoperative progression of maculopathy – growth factor and clinical analysis. Br. J. Ophthalmol. 2006; Jun; 90(6) 697-701. Epub 2006 Mar 15

[34] Pattabiraman P.P., Rao P.V. Mechanistic basis of Rho GTPase-induced extracellular matrix synthesis in trabecular meshwork cells. Am. J. Phys. Cell Phys. 2010 Mar; 298(3): 749-763. Epub 2009 Nov 25.

[35] Pazirandeh A., Xue Y., Prestegaard T., Jondal M., Okret S. Effects of altered glucocorticoid sensitivity in the T cell lineage on thymocyte and T cell homeostasis. FASEB J. 2002; 16(7): 727-729.

[36] Pleyer U., Gupta D., Weidle E., Lisch W., Zierhut M., Thiel H. Elevated prolactin levels in human aqueous humor of patients with anterior uveitis. Graefes. Arch. Clin.

Exp. Ophthalmol. 1991; 229(5): 447-451.

[37] Pleyer U., Yang J., Knapp S., Schacke H., Schemes N., Orlic N., Otasevic L., De Ruijter M., Ritter T., Keipert S. Effects of a selective glucocorticoid receptor agonist on experimental keratoplasty. Graefes. Arch. Clin. Exp. Ophthalmol. 2005; 243(5): 450-455.

[38] Podos S.M., Jaffe B.M., Becker B. Prostaglandinsand glaucoma. Br. Med. J. 1972 Oct 28; 4(5834): 232.

[39] Rauz S., Cheung C., Wood P., Coca-Prados M., Walker E., Murray P., Stewart P. Inhibition of 11β-hydroxysteroid dehydrogenase type 1 lowers intraocular pressure in patients with ocular hypertension. QJM. 2003; 96(7): 481-490.

[40] Rauz S., Walker E., Shackleton C., Hewison M., Murray P., Stewart P. Expression and putative role of 11 beta-hydroxysteroid dehydrogenase isozymes within the human eye. Invest. Ophthalmol. Vis. Sci. 2001; 42(9): 2037-2042.

[41] Robinson M., Reed G., Csaky K., Polis M., Whitcup S. Immune-recovery uveitis in patients with cytomegalovirus retinitis taking highly active antiretroviral therapy. Am. J. Ophthalmol. 2000: 130(1): 103-106.

[42] Sawada H., Fukuchi T., Tanaka T. Abe H. Tumor necrosis factor-alpha concentrations in the aqueous humor of patients with glaucoma. Invest. Ophthalmol. Vis. Sci. 2010 Feb; 51(2): 903-906.

[43] Slepova O.S., Gerasimenko V.A. Makarov V.P., Kushnir V.N., Zakharov G.Iu., Bykovskaia G.N., Vartanian I.R., Sadrislamova L.F. [Comparative study of the role of cytokines in different forms of eye diseases. 1. Tumor necrosis factor-alpha][Article in Russian]. Vestn. Ophthalmol. 1998 May-Jun; 114(3): 28-32.

[44] Sonoda A., Sonoda Y., Muramatu R., Streilein J., Usui M. ACAID induced by allogeneic corneal tissue promotes subsequent survival of orthotopic corneal grafts. Invest. Ophthalmol. Vis. Sci. 2000; 41(3): 790-798.

[45] Southren A., Gordon G., Yeh H., Dunn M., Weinstein B. Nuclear translocation of the cytoplasmic glucocorticoid receptor in the iris-ciliary body of the rabbit. Invest. Ophthalmol. Vis. Sci. 1979; 18(5): 517-521.

[46] Stambuk N., Curkovic T., Trbojevic-Cepe M., Dujmov I. Interleukin-4, IgG and oligoclonal IgG in aqueous humor of cataract patients. Graefes Arch. Clin. Exp. Ophthalmol. 1994; 232(2): 103-106.

[47] Stefan C., Dragomir L., Dumitrică D.M., Ursaciuc C., Dobre M., Surcel M. [TGF-beta-2 involvements in open angle glaucoma][published in Romanian]. Oftalmologia. 2008; 52: 110-112.

[48] Streilein J., Stein-Streilein J. Does innate immune privilege exist? J. Leukoc. Biol. 2000; 67(4): 479-487.

[49] Streilein J., Wilbanks G., Taylor A., Cousins S. Eye-derived cytokines and the immu-

nosuppressive intraocular microenvironment: a review. Curr. Eye Res. 1992: 11(Suppl.): 41-47.

[50] Toris C.B., Gabelt B.T., Kaufman P.L. Update on the mechanism of action of topical prostaglandins for intraocular pressure reduction. Surv. Ophthalmol. 2008; 53: 107-120.

[51] Tripathi B.J., Tripathi R.C., Chen J., Gotsis S., Li J. Trabecular cell expression of fibronectin and MMP-3 is modulated by aqueous humor growth factors. Exp. Eye Res. 2004; 78: 653-660.

[52] Uenoyama K., Kanagawa R., Tamura M., Matoba M., Enomoto Y., Ohmi S. Experimental intraocular lens implantation in the rabbit eye and in the mouse peritoneal space. Part IV: Cell adhesion, fibroblast-like cell, and lymphocytic cluster observed on the implanted lens surface. J. Cataract. Refract. Surg. 1989; 15(5): 559-566.

[53] Visser J. Sparing interleukin-10 receptor expression by glucocorticoids is a prerequisite for the synergistic immunosuppressive effects of interleukin-10 and glucocorticoids. Transplantation 2003; 76(10): 1534-1535.

[54] Wilbanks G., Mammolenti M., Streilein J. Studies on the induction of anterior chamber-associated immune deviation (ACAID). III. Induction of ACAID depends upon intraocular transforming growth factor-beta. Eur. J. Immunol. 1992; 22(1): 165-173.

[55] Wilbanks G., Streilein J. Characterization of suppressor cells in anterior chamber-associated immune deviation (ACAID) induced by soluble antigen. Evidence of two functionally and phenotypically distinct T-suppressor cell populations. Immunol. 1990; 71(3): 383-389.

[56] Wordinger R.J., Fleenor D.L., Hellberg P.E., Pang I.H., Tovar T.O., Zode G.S., Fuller J.A., Clark A.F. Effects of TGF-beta2, BMP-4, and gremlin in the trabecular meshwork: implications for glaucoma. Invest. Ophthalmol. Vis. Sci. 2007 Mar; 48(3): 1191-1200.

[57] Yarilin A., Belyakov I. [Thymus as an organ of endocrine system][Article in Russian]. Immunologiya. 1996. P. 4-10.

[58] Zhou Z., He S., Liang Y. An experimental study of pathomorphology in the iris and ciliary body after intraocular lens implantation. Zhonghua Yan Ke Za Zhi. 1996; 32(6): 421-423.

[59] Zilfyan A.A. Modern Aspects of Glaucoma Pathogenesis Local Factors for Development of Primary Open-Angle Glaucoma Associated with Impairment of Secretory Functions of the Eye Membranes. Chapter 5 in: "Glaucoma – Basic and Clinical Aspects". Edited by Shimon Rumelt. INTECH. Croatia. 2013. P. 75-102.

[60] Zilfyan A.A. Shifts in content of fibronectin, insulin-like growth factor-1 and E_2 prostaglandins in aqueous humor in case of senile and complicated cataracts. The New Armenian Medical Journal. 2012; 6(3): 34-41.

[61] Zilfyan A.A. The role of cortisol, prolactin, CD_4 and CD_8 in induction of anterior chamber associated immune deviation (ACAID) in case of cataracts. The New Armenian Medical Journal. 2009; 3(1): 59-67.

[62] Zilfyan A.A., Zilfyan A.V. Hormonal-Mediatory Mechanisms in the Process of Anterior Chamber Associated Immune Deviation. The New Armenian Medical Journal. 2013; 7(3): 85-88.

Permissions

All chapters in this book were first published by InTech Open; hereby published with permission under the Creative Commons Attribution License or equivalent. Every chapter published in this book has been scrutinized by our experts. Their significance has been extensively debated. The topics covered herein carry significant findings which will fuel the growth of the discipline. They may even be implemented as practical applications or may be referred to as a beginning point for another development.

The contributors of this book come from diverse backgrounds, making this book a truly international effort. This book will bring forth new frontiers with its revolutionizing research information and detailed analysis of the nascent developments around the world.

We would like to thank all the contributing authors for lending their expertise to make the book truly unique. They have played a crucial role in the development of this book. Without their invaluable contributions this book wouldn't have been possible. They have made vital efforts to compile up to date information on the varied aspects of this subject to make this book a valuable addition to the collection of many professionals and students.

This book was conceptualized with the vision of imparting up-to-date information and advanced data in this field. To ensure the same, a matchless editorial board was set up. Every individual on the board went through rigorous rounds of assessment to prove their worth. After which they invested a large part of their time researching and compiling the most relevant data for our readers.

The editorial board has been involved in producing this book since its inception. They have spent rigorous hours researching and exploring the diverse topics which have resulted in the successful publishing of this book. They have passed on their knowledge of decades through this book. To expedite this challenging task, the publisher supported the team at every step. A small team of assistant editors was also appointed to further simplify the editing procedure and attain best results for the readers.

Apart from the editorial board, the designing team has also invested a significant amount of their time in understanding the subject and creating the most relevant covers. They scrutinized every image to scout for the most suitable representation of the subject and create an appropriate cover for the book.

The publishing team has been an ardent support to the editorial, designing and production team. Their endless efforts to recruit the best for this project, has resulted in the accomplishment of this book. They are a veteran in the field of academics and their pool of knowledge is as vast as their experience in printing. Their expertise and guidance has proved useful at every step. Their uncompromising quality standards have made this book an exceptional effort. Their encouragement from time to time has been an inspiration for everyone.

The publisher and the editorial board hope that this book will prove to be a valuable piece of knowledge for researchers, students, practitioners and scholars across the globe.

List of Contributors

Umit Yolcu
Siirt Military Hospital, Ophthalmology, Siirt, Turkey

Omer Faruk Sahin
Etimesgut Military Hospital, Ophthalmology, Ankara, Turkey

Fatih C. Gundogan
GATA Medical School, Ophthalmology, Ankara, Turkey

Felicia Ferreri, Rosa Minniti, Alessandra Polimeni, Lucia Zavettieri, Giuseppina Ferreri and Pasquale Aragona
Institute of Ophthalmology, University of Messina, Italy

Paolo Ferreri
Institute of Ophthalmology, University of Bari, Italy

Vikas Tah
Stoke Mandeville Hospital, UK
Moorfields Eye Hospital London, UK

Kamran Saha, Jason Ho and Stephen Tuft
Moorfields Eye Hospital London, UK

James Myerscough
Colchester University Hospital NHS Foundation Trust, UK

Muhammad Ahad
Stoke Mandeville Hospital, UK

Pranev Sharma
Chelsea and Westminister Hospital, UK

Farihah Tariq
Raigmore Hospital Inverness, UK

Patricio A. Pacheco
Moorfields Eye Hospital, London, UK West Hertfordshire Hospitals, NHS trust, UK

Elliot M. Kirstein
Harper's Point Eye Associates, Cincinnati, Ohio, USA

Ipek Midi
Marmara University Pendik Research and Training Hospital, Department of Neurology, Istanbul, Turkey

Jenni Deveau and Aaron R. Seitz
Department of Psychology, University of California - Riverside, Riverside, CA, USA

Gary Lovcik
Anaheim Hills Optometric Center, Anaheim, CA, USA

Italo Giuffré
Department of Ophthalmology - Medical School - Catholic University of Roma, Italy

He-Zheng Zhou, Wen-Shan Jiang, Han-Guang Jie, Chang Feng, Wen-Qiang Zhang, Qian Ye, Jian-Guo Wu, Yan-Ping Song and Qin Ding
Department of Ophthalmology, Wuhan General Hospital of Guangzhou Command, China

Artashes A. Zilfyan
Scientific-Research Center, Yerevan State Medical University, Yerevan, Armenia

Arto V. Zilfyan
"Shengavit" Medical Center, Yerevan, Armenia

Index

www.ingramcontent.com/pod-product-compliance
Lightning Source LLC
LaVergne TN
LVHW080618210926
848485LV00003B/178